101 MSK Imaging

Volume 1

Series Editor

Rajesh Botchu
Department of Musculoskeletal Radiology
Royal Orthopaedic Hospital
Birmingham, UK

This series provides a quick bird's-eye of key cases in each area relating to musculoskeletal radiology. Images with key findings, differential and take-home points will be of interest to most radiologists, trainees, orthopaedic surgeons, trainees, and allied professionals. This is an easy way to review important and interesting cases of each anatomical area like the Knee, the Shoulder, the Ankle, the Elbow, the Hand, the Spine, and the Hip, but also cases on Ultrasound, and Tumours.

Sonal Saran • Amit Kharat • Rajesh Botchu

101 Knee Imaging Case Series

Springer

Sonal Saran
Department of Diagnostic
and Interventional Radiology
AIIMS Rishikesh
Rishikesh, Uttarakhand, India

Amit Kharat
DeepTek Inc.
Pune, Maharashtra, India

Rajesh Botchu
Department of Musculoskeletal
Radiology
Royal Orthopaedic Hospital
Birmingham, UK

ISSN 3091-2970 ISSN 3091-2989 (electronic)
101 MSK Imaging
ISBN 978-3-032-21566-6 ISBN 978-3-032-21567-3 (eBook)
https://doi.org/10.1007/978-3-032-21567-3

This Springer imprint is published by the registered company Springer Nature Switzerland AG
The registered company address is: Gewerbestrasse 11, 6330 Cham, Switzerland

Preface

The knee, a masterpiece of biomechanical engineering, is also one of the most frequently imaged and clinically challenging joints in musculoskeletal practice. Its intricate interplay of ligaments, menisci, cartilage, and synovial structures presents a continuous learning curve for radiologists and clinicians alike. Interpretation of knee imaging requires not only a firm grasp of anatomy and pathology but also an understanding of the clinical context and a keen eye for subtle, often overlooked findings.

This book, *101 Knee Imaging Case Series*, was born from our collective passion for musculoskeletal radiology and a shared commitment to education. As practising musculoskeletal radiologists, we have firsthand experience with the gaps that can exist between theoretical knowledge and practical, day-to-day case interpretation. Our goal is to bridge that gap by presenting a curated collection of real-world cases that mirror the spectrum of pathology encountered in a busy clinical practice.

The book is intentionally structured to simulate a progressive learning pathway. We have divided the 101 cases into three distinct sections: Easy, Intermediate, and Difficult. The "Easy" cases reinforce fundamental knowledge and classic presentations, building a solid foundation. The "Intermediate" section introduces greater complexity and mimics the nuanced decision-making required in daily reporting. Finally, the "Difficult" cases are designed to challenge even the experienced eye, focusing on rare entities, complex post-operative changes, and diagnostic pitfalls.

Each case is presented in a consistent, reader-friendly format, showcasing key images with a short clinical history on one page. Explanation with annotated images and a concise discussion that highlights the essential teaching points is presented on the following pages for each case. We have ensured that the content is equally valuable for radiology residents and fellows seeking to solidify their musculoskeletal knowledge, as well as for practising consultants—both radiologists and orthopaedic surgeons—who wish to refine their diagnostic acumen and stay up-to-date with challenging scenarios.

We extend our deepest gratitude to our colleagues, mentors, and families for their unwavering support throughout this endeavour. We also thank our patients, whose cases form the very foundation of this educational journey.

It is our sincere hope that this case-based approach will not only enhance your diagnostic confidence but also rekindle the intellectual curiosity that makes musculoskeletal radiology such a rewarding field.

Sonal Saran
Rishikesh, Uttarakhand, India

Amit Kharat
Pune, Maharashtra, India

Rajesh Botchu
Birmingham, UK

Contents

Easy Cases

Most Difficult Cases

Easy Cases

Contents

Case 1

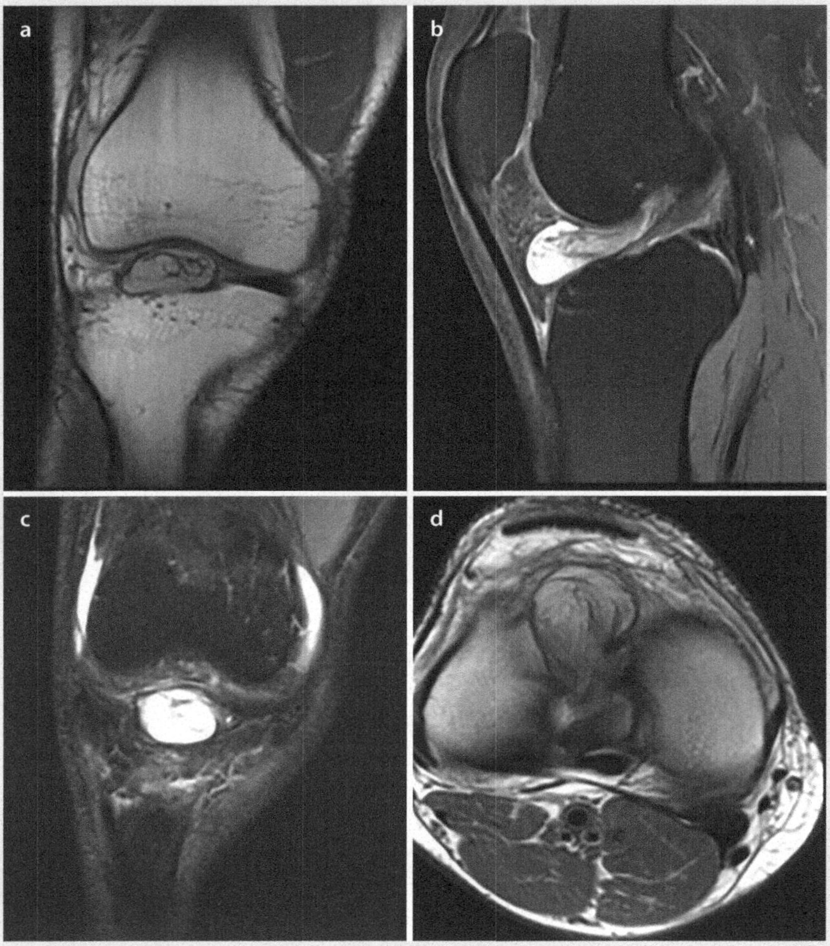

■ A 44-year-old male with a history of knee pain

S. Saran et al., *101 Knee Imaging Case Series*, 101 MSK Imaging 1,
https://doi.org/10.1007/978-3-032-21567-3_1

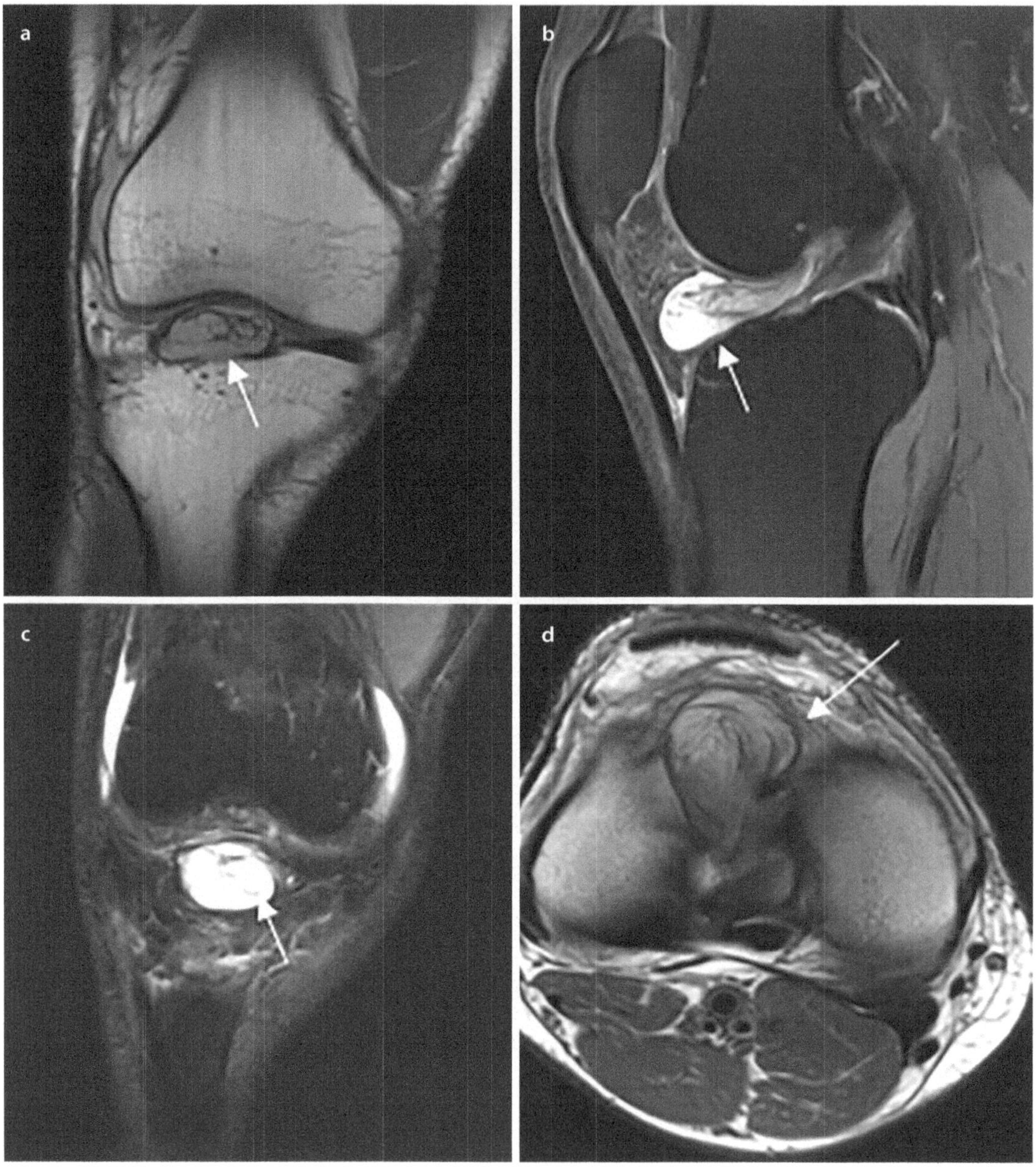

◻ MRI knee, T2-weighted coronal **a**, PDFS Sagittal **b**, coronal **c** and T2-weighted axial sequences showing a well-defined oval T2/PDFS hyperintense cyst (arrows) related to the tibial attachment of Anterior cruciate ligament (ACL), suggesting ACL ganglion cyst

Anterior Cruciate Ligament Ganglion Cyst

An anterior cruciate ligament (ACL) ganglion cyst is a benign, fluid-filled lesion arising from the synovial tissue surrounding the ACL. These cysts are uncommon, often incidental findings on MRI, but can cause pain or mechanical symptoms if large.

Location and Appearance

1. Intra-ligamentous: Within the ACL fibres (mimicking a mucoid degeneration).
2. Juxta-ligamentous: Adjacent to the ACL, often near the tibial insertion.

Clinical Presentation

1. Asymptomatic (Most Common): Found incidentally during imaging for other knee issues.
2. Symptomatic Cases (Rare): Anterior knee pain (worse with extension); Stiffness or limited ROM (due to mechanical impingement); "Clicking" or "locking" (if cyst encroaches the intercondylar notch).

MRI Characteristics (Diagnostic Clues)

1. Well-defined, lobulated fluid signal (hyperintense on T2/PDFS, hypointense on T1).
2. No internal enhancement (distinguishes from solid tumours).
3. May cause a mass effect on the ACL (mimicking a tear).

Management Options

Conservative or image-guided drainage or arthroscopic excision.

Prognosis and Complications

1. Excellent outcomes after arthroscopic removal (low recurrence if fully excised).
2. Risk of ACL injury if cyst is large and weakens the ligament (rare).

Suggested Reading

AlGhamdi YS, Mahmoud BM, AlBlaui SM, Altaraman KK, Alhumam KE, AlSinan IA, AlHossan AM. A ganglion cyst in the anterior cruciate ligament of a 13-year-old boy. Cureus. 2023;15(4):e37692.

Vaishya R, Esin Issa A, Agarwal AK, Vijay V. Anterior cruciate ligament ganglion cyst and mucoid degeneration: a review. Cureus. 2017;9(9):e1682.

Case 2

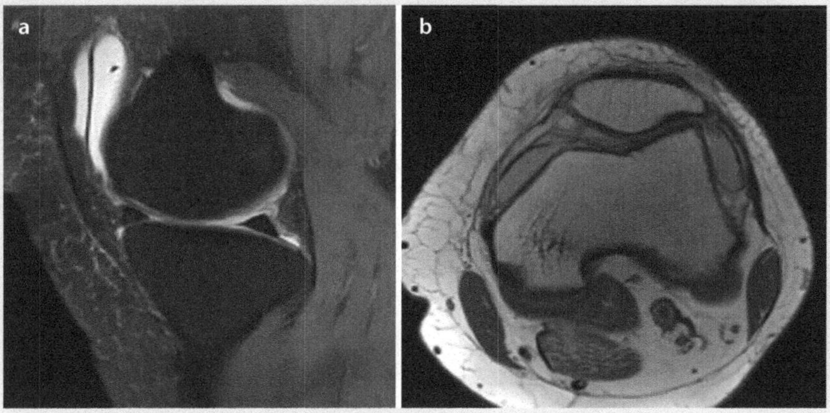

A 33-year-old female with pain and swelling in the knee joint

S. Saran et al., *101 Knee Imaging Case Series*, 101 MSK Imaging 1,
https://doi.org/10.1007/978-3-032-21567-3_2

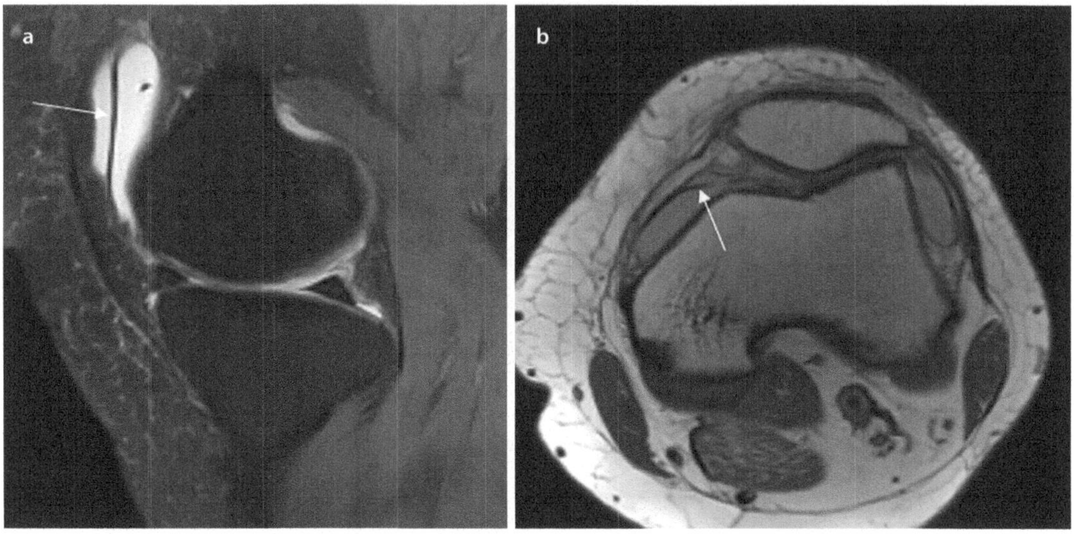

▪ MRI knee, PDFS weighted sagittal **a** and T2 weighted axial **b**, sequences showing mild suprapatellar joint effusion with a linear hypointense band traversing the suprapatellar recess, suggesting suprapatellar plica (arrows)

Suprapatellar Plica – Definition and Embryology

- A suprapatellar plica (also known as a plica synovialis suprapatellaris or superior plica) is a normal, synovial fold remnant of embryonic development within the knee joint.
- During fetal development, the knee is divided into three compartments by synovial membranes. These membranes typically involute before birth. A plica is a persistence of these membranes postnatally.
- It arises from the suprapatellar pouch and courses distally along the anterior femur, attaching to the synovium surrounding the patella.
- A common anatomical variant, present in a significant portion of the population (often asymptomatic).

Classification

The Zidorn classification categorises suprapatellar plicae into four types based on their structure:
- Type I: A complete septum that fully separates the knee joint from the suprapatellar bursa, allowing no communication.
- Type II: A perforated septum with one or more holes (called porta) that allow fluid to pass between the joint and the bursa.
- Type III: A small, arched fold of tissue (plica), most commonly found on the medial side.
- Type IV: Complete absence of a suprapatellar plica.

Pathophysiology (Plica Syndrome)

- The plica itself is not pathological. It becomes a source of pain, known as plica syndrome, when it is inflamed, thickened, or fibrotic due to:
  - Direct trauma: A blow to the anterior knee.
  - Repetitive stress/overuse: activities involving extensive knee flexion and extension (e.g., cycling, running, stair climbing).
  - Secondary inflammation: concurrent intra-articular pathology (e.g., meniscal tear, chondral defect) can cause general synovitis that irritates the plica.
  - The inflamed, stiff plica can then snap over the femoral condyle during knee motion, causing pain, a sensation of snapping, and potentially leading to chondromalacia.

Clinical Presentation

- Anterior knee pain, often medial to the patella.
- Pain with activity (especially knee flexion), prolonged sitting ("movie sign"), or stair climbing.
- Palpable, tender cord: A thickened, tender band may be felt on physical exam.
- Snapping or clicking sensation during knee flexion and extension.
- Symptoms can closely resemble patellofemoral pain syndrome or a medial meniscal tear.

Imaging Findings

- MRI
  - Best seen on sagittal and axial T2-weighted or PD-weighted images as a thin, curvilinear low-signal structure (synovial tissue) within the high-signal fluid in the suprapatellar pouch.
  - Signs of pathology: a plica is considered pathological if it appears thickened (>2 mm); associated with bone marrow oedema on the medial aspect of the trochlea or medial femoral condyle (from impingement); and surrounded by fluid, indicating inflammation.
- Ultrasound
  - Can dynamically visualise the plica as a hypoechoic band snapping over the bony contour during knee movement.

Management

- Conservative
  - Activity modification: avoid activities that provoke symptoms (e.g., deep squats).

- Physical therapy: the cornerstone of treatment.
- Strengthening: Vastus medialis obliquus (VMO) and core/hip stabilizers.
- NSAIDs: For pain and inflammation control.
- Corticosteroid Injection: An ultrasound-guided injection into the plica or surrounding area can provide significant diagnostic and therapeutic relief by breaking the cycle of inflammation.

- Surgical management (arthroscopic resection)
  - Persistent symptoms that fail 3–6 months of conservative management.
  - Mechanical symptoms (catching, locking) due to a thickened plica.
  - Arthroscopic finding of a fibrotic, impinging plica causing chondral damage.
  - Procedure: Arthroscopic plica resection (plicaectomy).

Key difference between different knee plicae is summarised in the table below:

Feature	Medial patellar plica	Infrapatellar plica	Suprapatellar plica	Lateral patellar plica
Prevalence	~72% (arthroscopic)	~86% (arthroscopic)	~87% (arthroscopic), up to 89% (autopsy)	Least common: ~1–3% (up to 20% in some studies)
Anatomical course	From the medial joint capsule, it courses down to the infrapatellar fat pad.	Runs anterior to the ACL, through the infrapatellar fat pad, to the inferior patella.	Courses from the femur to the quadriceps tendon, separating the joint from the suprapatellar bursa.	From the lateral joint capsule to the infrapatellar fat pad.
Clinical significance	Most frequently symptomatic. It can snap over the medial femoral trochlea, causing pain and cartilage damage.	Usually asymptomatic. Rarely injured directly, causing pain and a locking sensation.	Usually asymptomatic. It can cause compartmentalisation, trapping fluid or loose bodies in the suprapatellar bursa.	Rarely symptomatic. It can cause lateral pain and snapping if inflamed.

Suggested Reading

García-valtuille R, Abascal F, Cerezal L, et al. Anatomy and MR imaging appearances of synovial plicae of the knee. Radiographics. 2002;22(4):775–84.

Hodge JC, Ghelman B, O'Brien SJ, et al. Synovial plicae and chondromalacia patellae: correlation of results of CT arthrography with results of arthroscopy. Radiology. 1993;186(3):827–31.

Case 3

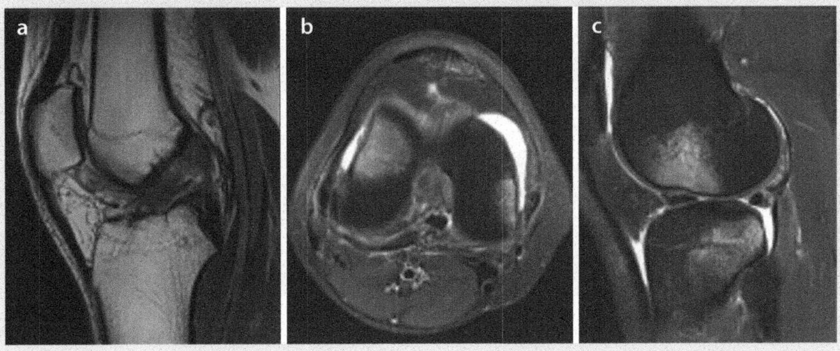

▪ A 28-year-old female with a history of twisting knee injury

S. Saran et al., *101 Knee Imaging Case Series*, 101 MSK Imaging 1,
https://doi.org/10.1007/978-3-032-21567-3_3

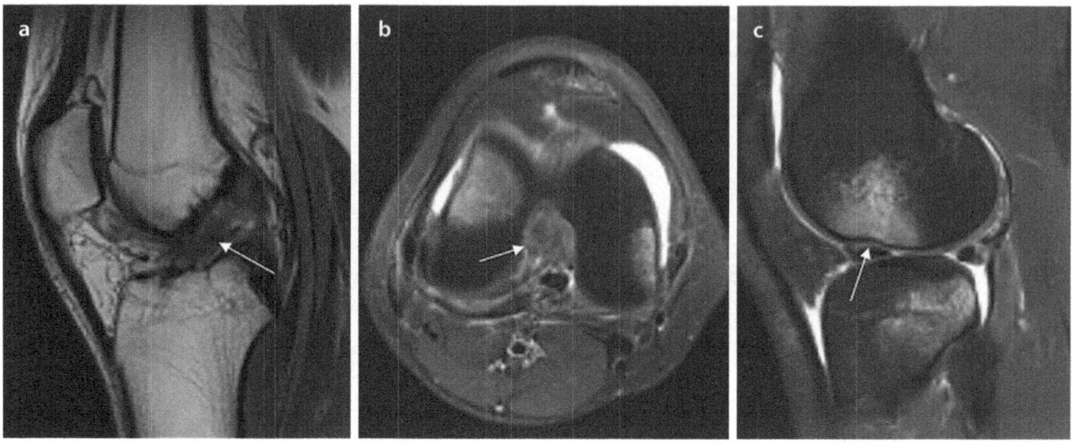

■ MRI knee, PD sagittal **a**, PDFS axial **b** and sagittal **c** showing full-thickness anterior cruciate ligament (ACL) tear (arrows in **a** and **b**) with classic pivot shift pattern of contusion, i.e., oedema of the lateral femoral condyle and posterolateral tibial plateau with notch sign (arrow in **c**)

Complete ACL Tear with Classic Pivot Shift Pattern of Contusion

- Key imaging findings of ACL tear include discontinuity of ACL fibres on T2-weighted or PD sequences, increased signal intensity within the ligament, indicating oedema/rupture and the empty notch sign (absence of normal ACL in the intercondylar notch). Secondary signs include anterior tibial translation (>7 mm on sagittal images) and an uncovered posterior horn of the lateral meniscus (due to anterior subluxation).
- Classic bone contusion pattern (lateral compartment)/"Kissing Contusions": results from anterior tibial translation & pivot-shift injury (valgus + internal rotation). It involves:
  - Lateral femoral condyle (midportion, near sulcus terminalis) with deepening of notch.
  - Posterolateral tibial plateau (opposing injury from tibial impact).
- The (deep) lateral femoral notch sign describes a depression on the lateral femoral condyle at the terminal sulcus, a junction between the weight-bearing tibial articular surface and the patellar articular surface of the femoral condyle. A notch depth of 1.5 mm is shown as a useful additional sign of a torn ACL.
- Prognostic indicator: Severe contusions correlate with higher-grade instability.

Suggested Reading

Baessler AM, Buchman JM, Witte DA, Spence DD, Throckmorton TW, Brolin TJ, Azar FM, Bernholt DL. Skeletally immature patients with classic anterior cruciate ligament bone bruise patterns have a higher likelihood of having an intact anterior cruciate ligament compared with skeletally mature patients. J Pediatr Orthop. 2023;43(1):13–7.

Cobby MJ, Schweitzer ME, Resnick D. The deep lateral femoral notch: an indirect sign of a torn anterior cruciate ligament. Radiology. 1992;184(3):855–8.

Sanders TG, Medynski MA, Feller JF, Lawhorn KW. Bone contusion patterns of the knee at MR imaging: footprint of the mechanism of injury. Radiographics. 2000;20 Spec No:S135–51.

Case 4

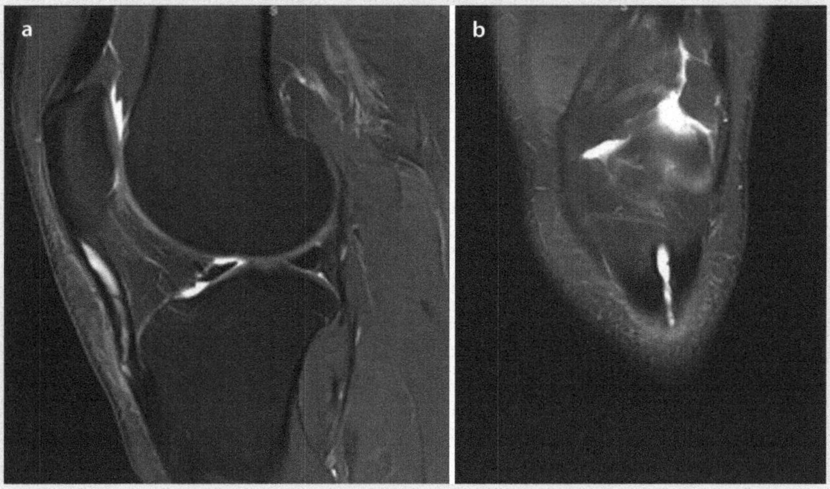

◘ A 20-year-old athlete presented with a chief complaint of persistent anterior knee pain that had progressively worsened over the past 2–3 months

S. Saran et al., *101 Knee Imaging Case Series*, 101 MSK Imaging 1,
https://doi.org/10.1007/978-3-032-21567-3_4

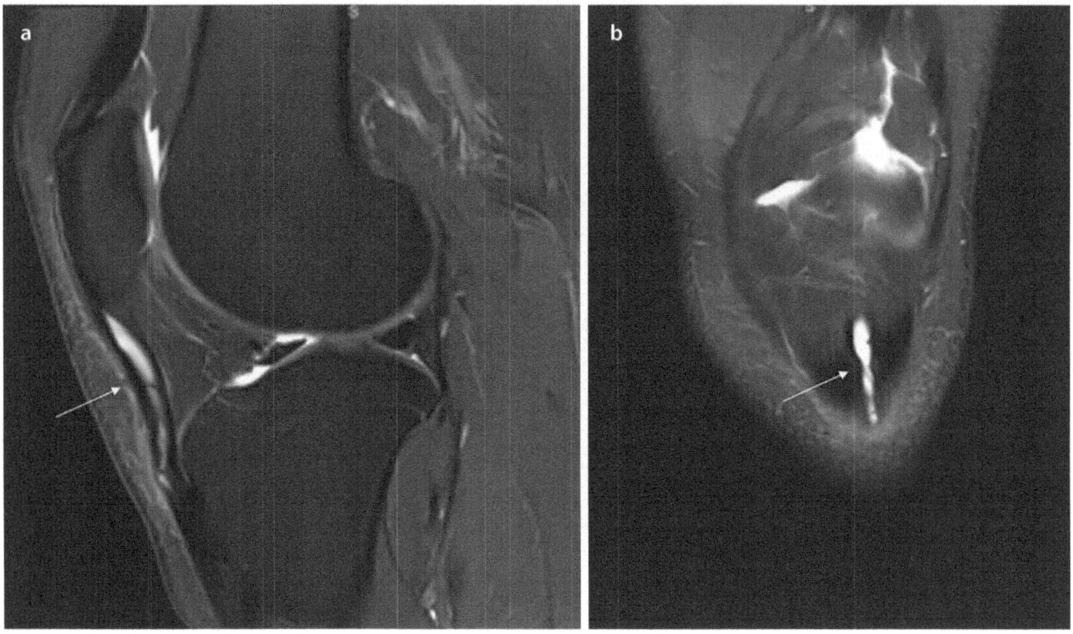

■ The MRI scan revealed a well-defined, linear-shaped cystic lesion (arrows) located within the substance of the patellar tendon. The cyst exhibited hyperintensity on PDFS sagittal sequence **a** and coronal **b**, indicating a high-water content, which is a characteristic feature of ganglionic cysts. Importantly, there are no visible septations or solid components within the cyst, suggesting a homogeneous fluid-filled structure. There is evidence of a partial tear of a few fibres of the patellar tendon

Intratendinous Ganglionic Cyst of the Patellar Tendon

Definition and Pathophysiology

- An intratendinous ganglionic cyst is a non-neoplastic, fluid-filled cyst that forms within the substance of a tendon. When it occurs in the patellar tendon, it is a rare cause of anterior knee pain.
- Pathogenesis: The exact cause is unknown, but the leading theory is mucoid degeneration or a focal flaw in the tendon's collagen matrix that allows synovial-like fluid to accumulate. It is not a true ganglion cyst, which is typically connected to a joint or tendon sheath.

Clinical Presentation

- Anterior Knee Pain: Localised, activity-related pain, often exacerbated by jumping, kneeling, or stair climbing.
- Clinically, it can be very difficult to distinguish from patellar tendinosis ("Jumper's Knee"), which is a more common degenerative condition.

Imaging Findings

- Ultrasound
  - A well-defined, anechoic or hypoechoic oval or round lesion within the tendon fibres, which shows posterior acoustic enhancement and no internal blood flow, confirming its cystic nature.
  - The surrounding tendon may appear normal or show adjacent tendinosis.
- MRI
  - MRI provides an exquisitely detailed demonstration of the relationship between the cyst and the entire tendon.
  - T1-Weighted: Well-circumscribed, homogeneously low-signal lesion within the tendon.
  - T2-Weighted/PDFS/STIR: Markedly hyperintense, confirming its fluid content.
  - Margins: Sharp, non-infiltrative borders. The surrounding tendon may exhibit an intermediate T2 signal if tendinosis is present.

Differential Diagnosis

- Patellar tendinosis ("jumper's knee"): The main differential. Appears as tendon thickening and fusiform, intermediate signal on T2 (rather than a well-defined, bright cyst). On ultrasound, it is hypoechoic but not purely cystic.
- Partial-thickness patellar tendon tear: A focal, fluid-signal defect extending from the tendon surface.
- Hoffa's fat pad impingement/cyst: Pain and mass located deeper, behind the patellar tendon.
- Osgood-Schlatter Disease: In adolescents, involves the tibial tubercle attachment of the patellar tendon with associated bone fragmentation.

Management

- Conservative management with image-guided intervention
  - Activity modification: avoid activities that provoke symptoms (e.g., jumping, deep squats).

  - Physical therapy: eccentric strengthening exercises are the cornerstone of treatment for patellar tendinopathy and can help manage symptoms related to the cyst.
  - Ultrasound-guided aspiration & corticosteroid injection. It often provides excellent short-term relief, but recurrence is common because the underlying defect in the tendon matrix remains.
  - Ultrasound-guided fenestration/decompression: A minimally invasive option where the cyst wall is repeatedly punctured with a needle to decompress it and stimulate a healing response.
- Surgical Intervention
  - Persistent, disabling pain after 3–6 months of failed conservative and image-guided care.
  - Arthroscopic or open excision: The definitive treatment. The surgeon identifies the cyst, incises the tendon longitudinally, and completely excises the cyst and its wall. The tendon is then repaired.

Suggested Reading

Botchu R, Bharath A, Uhiara O, Davies M, James S. Iatrogenic intratendinous ganglion cyst of the extensor digitorum tendon following intravenous cannulation. J Ultrasound. 2018;21(4):329–31.

Jose J, O'Donnell K, Lesniak B. Symptomatic intratendinous ganglion cyst of the patellar tendon. Orthopedics. 2011;34(2).

Venati U, Rahul BN, Damayanthi Y, Botchu R. Unusual etiology of anterior knee pain in a young athlete engaged in chronic jumping exercises: the intratendinous ganglionic cyst of the patellar tendon. Indian J Musculoskelet Radiol. 2024;6:65–9.

Case 5

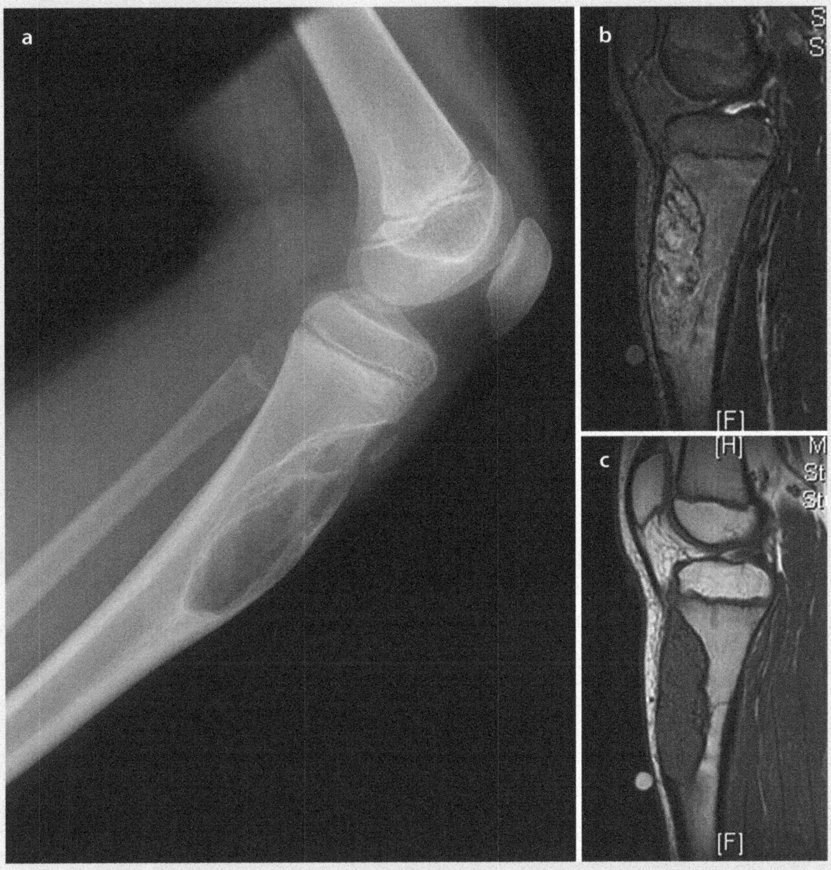

A 13-year-old female presented with long-standing progressive pain and bony swelling in the right leg

S. Saran et al., *101 Knee Imaging Case Series*, 101 MSK Imaging 1,
https://doi.org/10.1007/978-3-032-21567-3_5

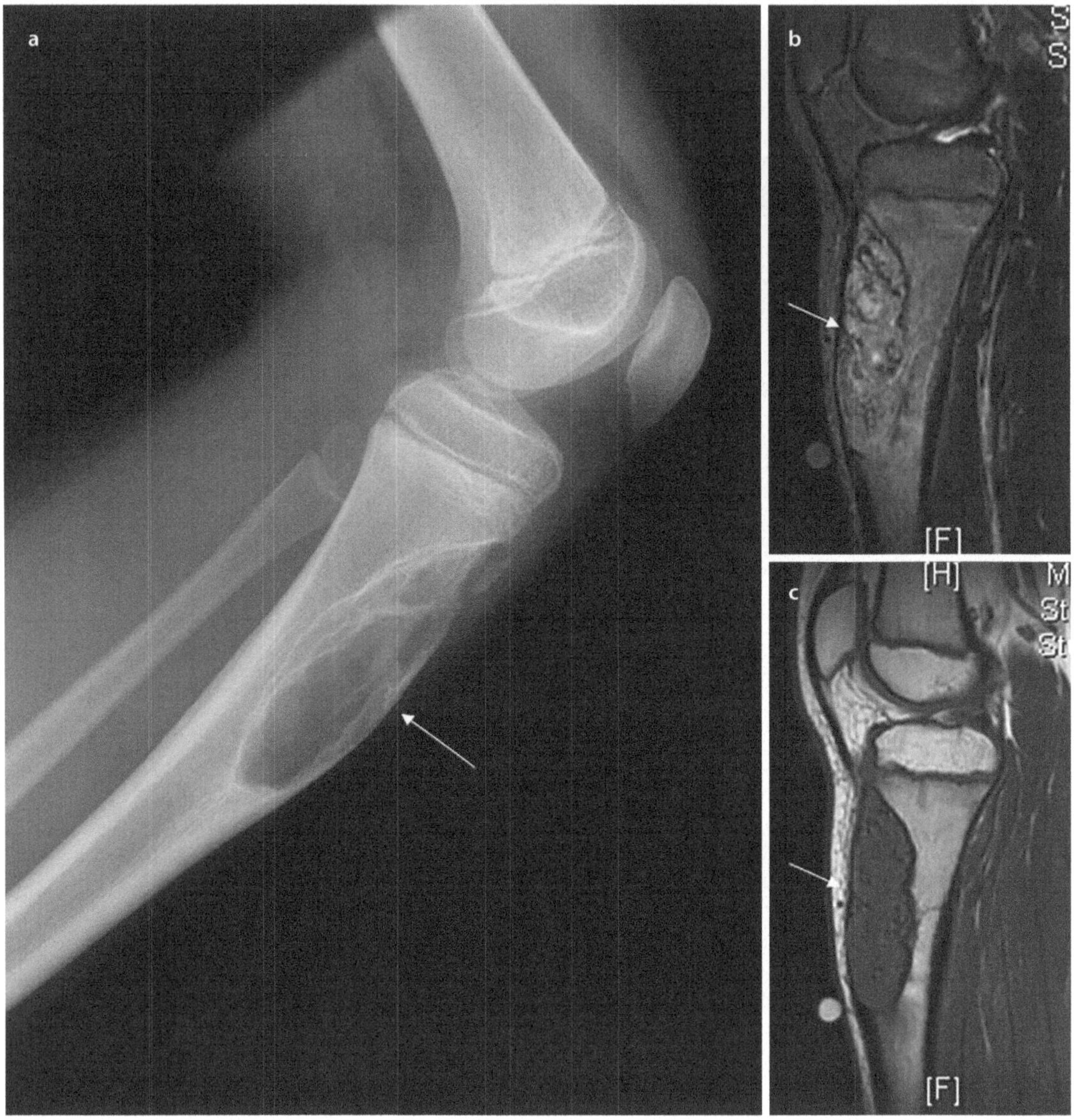

▣ Radiograph lateral view **a** shows the presence of a well-defined lobulated eccentric osteolytic lesion (arrow) in the proximal tibial anterior cortical region with a sclerotic rim and internal pseudotrabeculation. MRI sagittal STIR (**b**) and T1 (**c**) shows the lesion (arrows) as heterogeneously hypointense. Imaging findings suggest the possibility of a Chondromyxoid fibroma. Differentials include non-ossifying fibroma (NOF) and fibrous dysplasia

Chondromyxoid Fibroma

Definition and Pathophysiology

- Chondromyxoid Fibroma (CMF) is a rare, benign bone tumour characterised by its lobulated growth pattern and a unique histologic composition of chondroid, myxoid, and fibrous tissue. Despite its name, it is a distinct entity and not a variant of chondrosarcoma. It typically arises in the

metaphyseal region of long bones, with the proximal tibia being a common site.
- CMF is benign and does not metastasise. However, it can be locally aggressive, causing progressive bone destruction and expansion, which can lead to pain and a risk of pathological fracture.

Clinical Features

- Demographics: Most common in adolescents and young adults (second-third decades of life).
- Location: Predilection for the long bones, especially the proximal tibia (a very common site). It is typically eccentrically located in the metaphysis.
- Symptoms:
  - Insidious onset of mild, localised pain and swelling over several months to years.
  - Pain may be mechanical due to cortical thinning and bone weakening.
  - A palpable, firm mass may be present.
  - Pathological fracture is a potential complication but is less common than in other benign bone tumours.

Imaging Findings

- Radiography
  - Eccentric, lytic lesion.
  - Sclerotic margins: often has a thin rim of sclerotic bone, indicating its slow growth.
  - Lobulated & expansile: the lesion frequently has a scalloped, lobulated border and may cause mild expansion or thinning of the overlying cortex.
  - No mineralized matrix: unlike other cartilaginous tumours (e.g., enchondroma), it typically does not show internal calcifications.
- MRI
  - Lobulated morphology: clearly demonstrates the multilobulated internal architecture of the tumour.
  - T2 hyperintensity: the myxoid and chondroid components are markedly hyperintense on T2-weighted images. Fibrous components are hypointense.
  - Peripheral enhancement: post-contrast images often show characteristic enhancement around the periphery of the lobules and in the septations, with variable central enhancement.
  - It can show surrounding bone marrow oedema.

Management

- Pre-operative planning: Accurate diagnosis is crucial. A biopsy is often required to confirm CMF and rule out its malignant mimics.
- The standard treatment is aggressive curettage followed by bone grafting.
- En bloc resection is considered for large, recurrent lesions.

Suggested Reading

Gowda PC, Dunlap RH, Ahlawat S, Gross JM, Morris CD, Lyons GR. Recurrent chondromyxoid fibroma of the distal femur treated with percutaneous cryoablation. Skeletal Radiol. 2023;52(12):2497–501.

Zhong J, Si L, Geng J, Xing Y, Hu Y, Jiao Q, Zhang H, Yao W. Chondromyxoid fibroma-like osteosarcoma: a case series and literature review. BMC Musculoskelet Disord. 2020;21(1):53.

Case 6

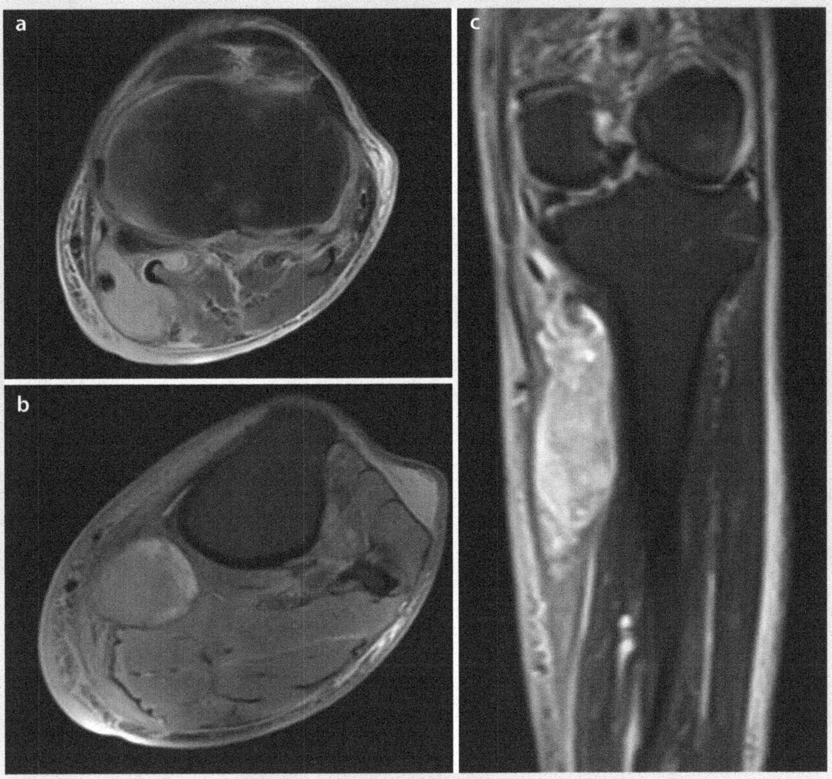

An 88-year-old male presented with severe calf pain and swelling

S. Saran et al., *101 Knee Imaging Case Series*, 101 MSK Imaging 1,
https://doi.org/10.1007/978-3-032-21567-3_6

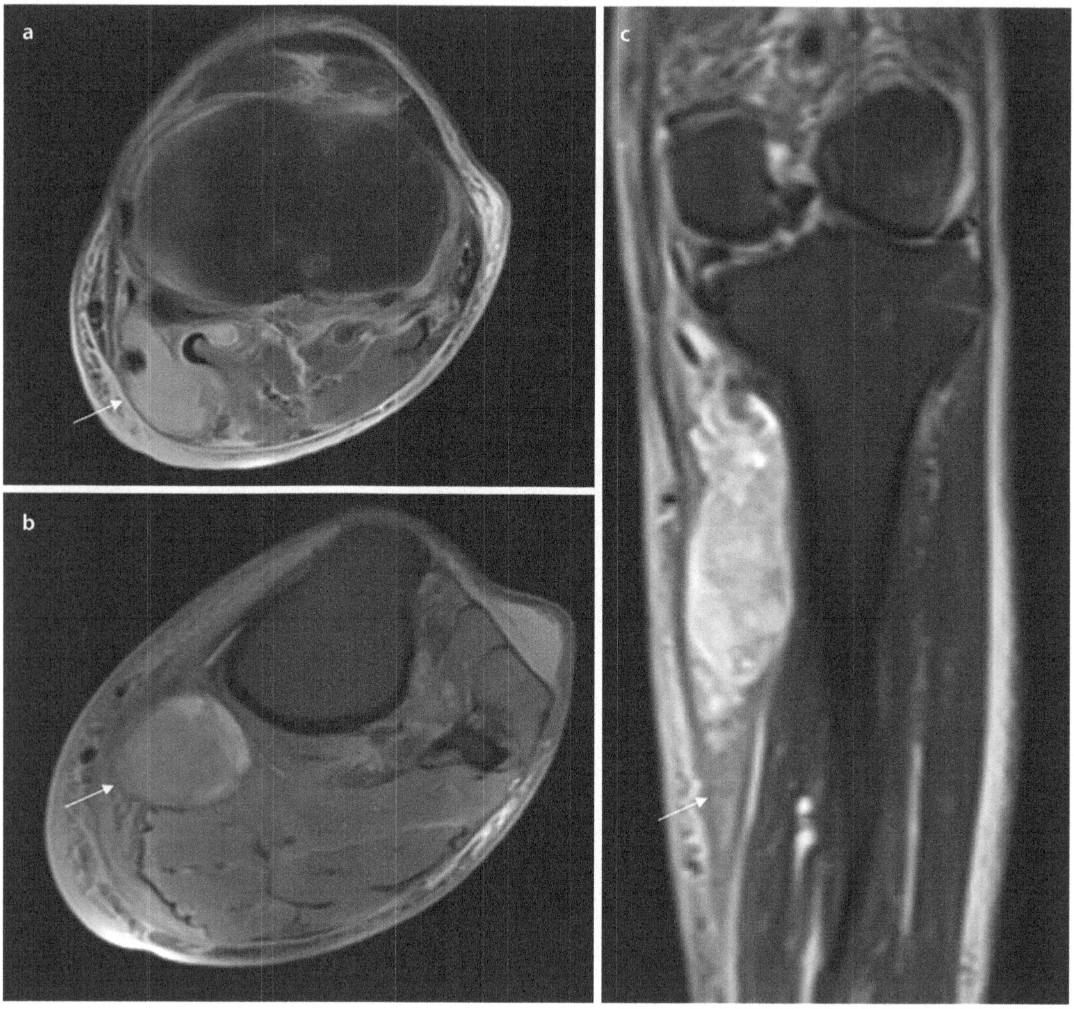

■ MRI knee axial PDFS weighted sequences **a** and **b** show the presence of a well-defined cystic lesion (arrows) in the popliteal fossa localised between the tendons of semimembranosus and medial head of gastrocnemius, suggestive of Baker's cyst. Coronal PDFS weighted sequence **c** shows extension of the cyst caudally in the proximal leg with a pointed tip (arrow) and soft tissue oedema suggestive of Baker's cyst rupture

Baker's Cyst Rupture

Definition and Pathophysiology

- A Baker's cyst rupture occurs when the fluid-filled sac in the popliteal fossa ruptures, leading to leakage of synovial fluid into the calf. This is not a true cyst but a posterior extension of the knee joint capsule, often communicating with the joint via a valve-like mechanism.
- Anatomy: Typically arises between the medial head of the gastrocnemius and the semimembranosus tendon.

- Incidental or secondary to an intra-articular pathology that causes chronic joint effusion, such as osteoarthritis, rheumatoid arthritis and other inflammatory arthropathies.

Clinical Presentation

- The classic presentation is the acute, sudden onset of sharp, intense pain in the popliteal fossa and proximal calf and can mimic a deep vein thrombosis (DVT), a critical distinction to make.
- Swelling & bruising.

Imaging Findings

Imaging is crucial to confirm the diagnosis and rule out DVT or other pathologies.

- Ultrasound
  - Confirms rupture: shows a collapsed, sac-like structure in the popliteal fossa with fluid tracking down between the gastrocnemius and soleus muscles.
  - Doppler: essential to rule out DVT by confirming venous patency.
  - Can identify the underlying cause (e.g., joint effusion, meniscal tear).
- MRI
  - MRI exquisitely demonstrates the extent of fluid leakage and the underlying intra-articular pathology.
  - T2-Weighted / STIR: Shows a "track" or "flame-shaped" area of hyperintense fluid signal dissecting caudally from the popliteal fossa into the subcutaneous tissues of the proximal calf, deep to the gastrocnemius.
  - Associated findings: Will almost always reveal the underlying cause, such as a meniscal tear, cartilage loss, or synovitis.

Differential Diagnosis

- Deep Vein Thrombosis (DVT): The most important mimic. Requires Doppler ultrasound to exclude.
- Calf muscle tear (e.g., plantaris or gastrocnemius rupture—"Tennis Leg"): Pain is typically more focal to the muscle belly.

Management

- Acute phase management
  - PRICE Protocol: Protection, Rest, Ice, Compression, Elevation.
  - NSAIDs: For pain and inflammation control.
  - Reassurance: Educating the patient that the bruising and swelling are expected and will resolve.
- Management of the underlying cause
  - This is the key to preventing recurrence.
  - Intra-articular corticosteroid injection: can be highly effective in reducing the synovitis and effusion that feeds the cyst.
  - Physical therapy: to address muscle weakness and improve joint biomechanics.
- Surgical intervention for the cyst
  - Cyst excision: reserved for rare cases of persistent, symptomatic cysts that fail conservative management and where the primary intra-articular pathology has been addressed.

Suggested Reading

Balik MS, Turan A, Celik FB. Is there a relationship between three-dimensionally measured Baker's cyst volume and knee pathologies? Eurasian J Med. 2019;51(1):64–9.

Irismetov ME, Tursunov KK, Khudayberdiev KT, Tursunova MA, Roitblat Y. Diagnostics and surgical treatment of ruptured Baker's cysts: a prospective study. J Clin Orthop Trauma. 2024;58:102792.

Kim DK, Lee KC, Kim JK, Kim T. Assessment of imaging factors associated with Baker's cyst rupture on knee MRI. J Belg Soc Radiol. 2023;107(1):77.

Case 7

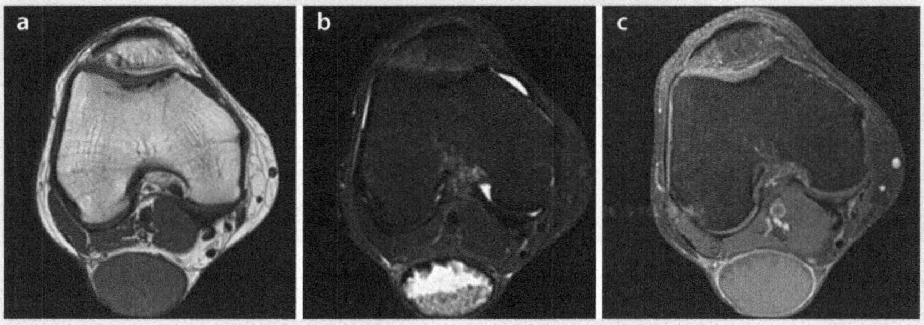

A 37-year-old female presented with a firm swelling in the popliteal region

S. Saran et al., *101 Knee Imaging Case Series*, 101 MSK Imaging 1,
https://doi.org/10.1007/978-3-032-21567-3_7

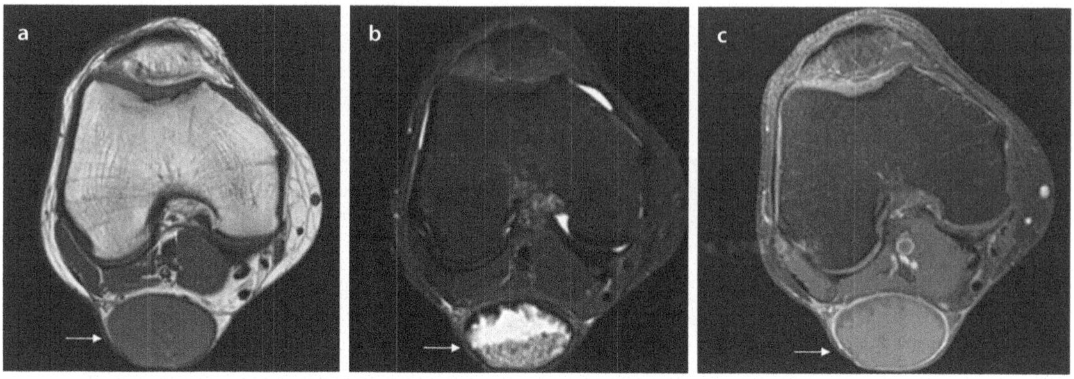

■ MRI **a**–**c** shows a well-defined oval-shaped lesion in the subcutaneous plane in the popliteal region (arrows). The lesion appears hypointense on T1-weighted **a** sequence and hyperintense on T2-weighted fat-suppressed sequence **b** with debris in the dependent region. The lesion shows thin enhancement of the wall on post-contrast T1-weighted sequence **c**. MRI findings are indicative of an epidermal inclusion cyst

Epidermal Inclusion Cyst (EIC)

Definition and Pathophysiology

- An epidermal inclusion cyst (also known as an epidermoid cyst) is a common, benign cutaneous cyst that results from the traumatic implantation of epidermal elements into the dermis or subcutis. It is lined by stratified squamous epithelium and filled with keratinaceous debris.
- It is firmly attached to the skin, often with a visible punctum (a small opening), and is mobile over deeper structures.

Clinical Presentation

- Symptoms
  - A slow-growing, round, firm, and mobile subcutaneous nodule.
  - Typically asymptomatic unless complicated.
  - The overlying skin may be normal or may have a central punctum.
- Complications
  - Inflammation/Infection: This is the most common reason for seeking medical attention.
  - Rupture: Leakage of keratin into the surrounding tissue causes a severe foreign-body inflammatory reaction, leading to significant pain, swelling, and cellulitis.
  - Foul-smelling discharge may be present if the punctum is open.

Imaging Findings

- Ultrasound
  - A well-defined, oval or round, hypoechoic mass in the subcutaneous fat, just deep to the dermis.
  - It may show internal echoes or a "pseudotestis" appearance due to the lamellated keratin debris.
  - There may be acoustic enhancement.
  - No internal vascularity on Doppler.
  - If ruptured/inflamed: The margins become ill-defined, and there is increased surrounding vascularity and oedema.
- MRI
  - T1-Weighted: The cyst is typically isointense or slightly hyperintense to muscle. The high signal is due to the lipid content in keratin and debris.
  - T2-Weighted / STIR: The cyst is heterogeneously hyperintense. It may show lamellated concentric rings ("onion ring" appearance) representing layers of keratin or dependent keratin debris.
  - Diffusion-Weighted Imaging (DWI): Often shows restricted diffusion, a key feature that helps distinguish it from a simple cyst. This is due to the dense, organised keratin content.
  - T1-Weighted post-contrast: The thin cyst wall may enhance, especially if inflamed. The central contents do not enhance.

Differential Diagnosis

- Baker's cyst: The most common cyst in the popliteal fossa. It is a deep cyst arising from the knee joint, located between the semimembranosus and medial gastrocnemius tendons. It is not in the subcutaneous tissue.
- Pilomatrixoma: A benign tumour of hair follicle matrix cells, often calcified, and more common in children.
- Lipoma: A soft, mobile subcutaneous mass that follows fat signal on all MRI sequences.
- Ganglion cyst: A myxoid-containing cyst, often associated with a joint or tendon sheath. It typically has a very high, homogeneous T2 signal, unlike the heterogeneous EIC.
- Soft tissue sarcoma: A solid, enhancing mass, not a cyst. Any solid, vascularized component warrants further investigation.

Management

- No treatment is necessary if the cyst is not symptomatic.
- Management of inflamed/infected cyst:
  - Warm compresses.
  - Oral antibiotics (e.g., cephalexin) if cellulitis is present.
  - Incision and drainage: provides immediate relief for a painful, abscessed cyst. However, this is not curative, and the cyst will recur.
  - Complete excision.

Suggested Reading

Kim HK, Kim SM, Lee SH, Racadio JM, Shin MJ. Subcutaneous epidermal inclusion cysts: ultrasound (US) and MR imaging findings. Skeletal Radiol. 2011;40(11):1415–9.

Pressney I, Khoo M, Hargunani R, Saifuddin A. Description of the MRI and ultrasound imaging features of giant epidermal cysts. Br J Radiol. 2020;93(1114):20200413.

Case 8

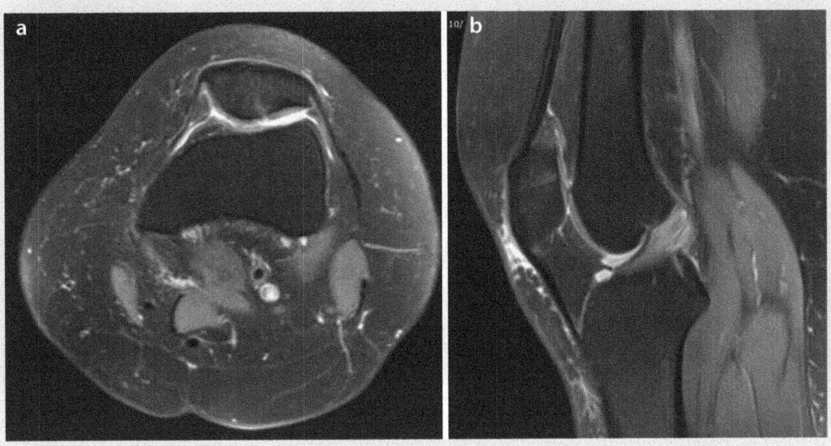

▪ A 32-year-old female presented with anterior knee pain on walking and climbing stairs

S. Saran et al., *101 Knee Imaging Case Series*, 101 MSK Imaging 1,
https://doi.org/10.1007/978-3-032-21567-3_8

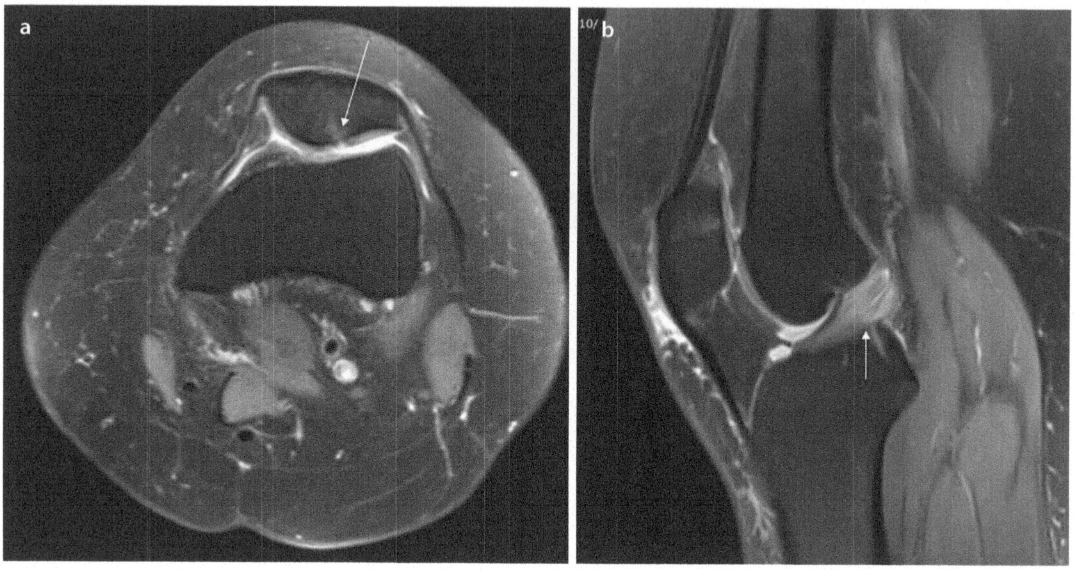

■ MRI knee, axial PDFS weighted axial sequence **a** shows the presence of a full-thickness cartilage defect involving the medial facet of patella with the presence of subchondral marrow oedema (arrow). It is grade 4 as per the modified Outerbridge grading of chondromalacia. Sagittal PDFS weighted sequence **b** shows the presence of mucoid degeneration of ACL (arrow)

Chondromalacia Patellae

Definition and Pathophysiology

- Chondromalacia patellae is a condition characterised by softening, fraying, and degeneration of the articular cartilage of the patella. It represents a common cause of anterior knee pain, particularly in young athletes.
- Mechanism: It results from abnormal patellar tracking and excessive pressure on the patellofemoral joint.

Clinical Presentation

- Demographics: Common in adolescents and young adults, especially athletes involved in running and jumping sports. More prevalent in females.
- Symptoms:
  - Anterior knee pain: a dull, aching pain behind or around the patella, exacerbated by activities that load the patellofemoral joint (e.g., climbing stairs, squatting, running, or prolonged sitting with knees bent—the “movie sign”).
  - Crepitus: a grating or crunching feeling when moving the knee.

- Pseudolocking: a transient sensation of the knee "catching", not due to a true mechanical block.
- Mild swelling: occasional mild effusion.

Grading System (Modified Outerbridge Classification)

The modified Outerbridge grading system for chondromalacia is a 5-level scale (0–4) used to assess cartilage damage, adapted from the original to include MRI findings.

- Grade 0: Normal cartilage.
- Grade 1: Softening and swelling of the cartilage, which may involve a focal area of increased signal intensity on an MRI but appears architecturally intact.
- Grade 2: Partial-thickness defects, characterised by surface fraying, blistering, or fragmentation, without reaching the subchondral bone.
- Grade 3: Deeper partial-thickness defects, with fissures or ulcerations that extend to or expose the subchondral bone.
- Grade 4: Full-thickness cartilage loss, with exposed subchondral bone, which may include underlying bone marrow oedema.

Imaging Findings

While clinical diagnosis is key, imaging, particularly MRI, is the gold standard for confirmation and staging.

- Radiography
  - Often normal in early stages.
  - May show indirect signs like patella alta (high-riding patella) or tilt.
  - In advanced cases, joint space narrowing and subchondral sclerosis may be visible.
- MRI
  - MRI directly visualises the articular cartilage and is essential for grading.
  - Subchondral bone marrow oedema. Common in grade III/IV.
  - Patellar malalignment: shallow trochlear groove, patellar tilt, or subluxation.

Differential Diagnosis

- Patellofemoral pain syndrome (PFPS): a clinical diagnosis of pain without specific cartilage damage on imaging.
- Patellar tendinopathy ("jumper's knee"): pain localised to the inferior pole of the patella or the patellar tendon.

- Plica syndrome: pain from a thickened synovial fold, often medial to the patella.
- Osgood-Schlatter disease: pain and tenderness at the tibial tuberosity in adolescents.
- Patellofemoral osteoarthritis: the end stage of chondromalacia, typically in older adults.

Management

Treatment is primarily conservative and focuses on correcting biomechanical imbalances.

- Conservative management (first-line)
  - Activity modification: avoid activities that provoke pain (e.g., deep squats, prolonged kneeling).
  - Physical therapy.
  - NSAIDs: For short-term pain and inflammation control.
  - Patellar taping/bracing: to temporarily improve alignment and reduce pain.
- Surgical intervention (for refractory cases)
  - Indications: failure of 6–12 months of conservative management with significant mechanical symptoms or high-grade cartilage lesions.
  - Arthroscopic debridement: shaving of frayed cartilage to smooth the surface.
  - Lateral retinacular release: to relieve excessive lateral pull on the patella.
  - Cartilage restoration procedures: for focal, high-grade defects in young patients (e.g., microfracture, autologous chondrocyte Implantation (ACI), Osteochondral Autograft Transfer (OATS)).
  - Realignment procedures (e.g., tibial tubercle osteotomy): for severe malalignment.

Suggested Reading

Kim JN, Park HJ, Choi YG, Kim MS. Patellar height measured on radiographs and MR imaging and its relationship with chondromalacia patella. J Clin Ultrasound. 2025.

Masroori Z, Haseli S, Abbaspour E, Pouramini A, Azhideh A, Fathi M, Kafi F, Chalian M. Patellar non-traumatic pathologies: a pictorial review of radiologic findings. Diagnostics (Basel). 2024;14(24):2828.

Süner U, Çilengir AH, Bulut T, Gürsoy M, Önder Y, Mete BD. Association of patellofemoral malalignment with early trochlear and patellar chondromalacia: a prospective T2* mapping study. Diagn Interv Radiol. 2025.

Case 9

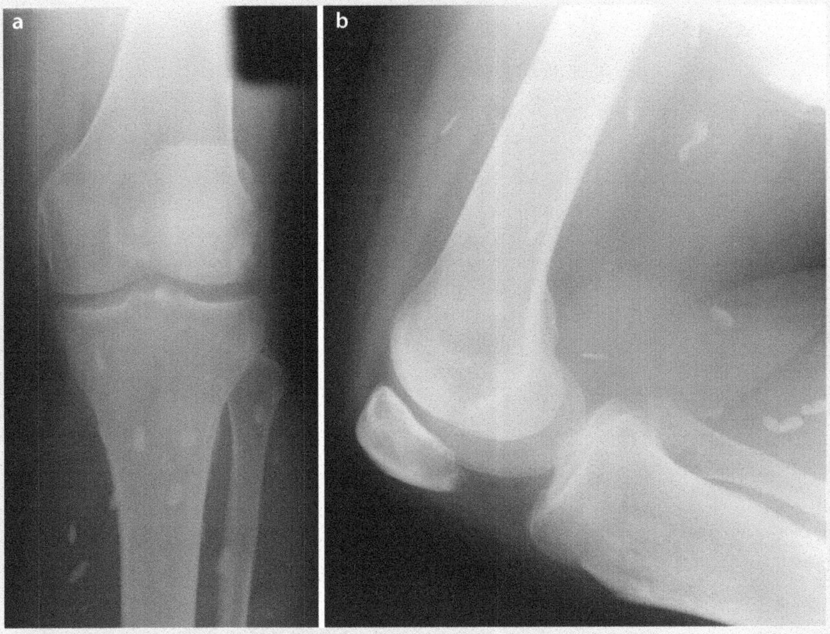

A 45-year-old male presented with mild pain in the right knee

S. Saran et al., *101 Knee Imaging Case Series*, 101 MSK Imaging 1,
https://doi.org/10.1007/978-3-032-21567-3_9

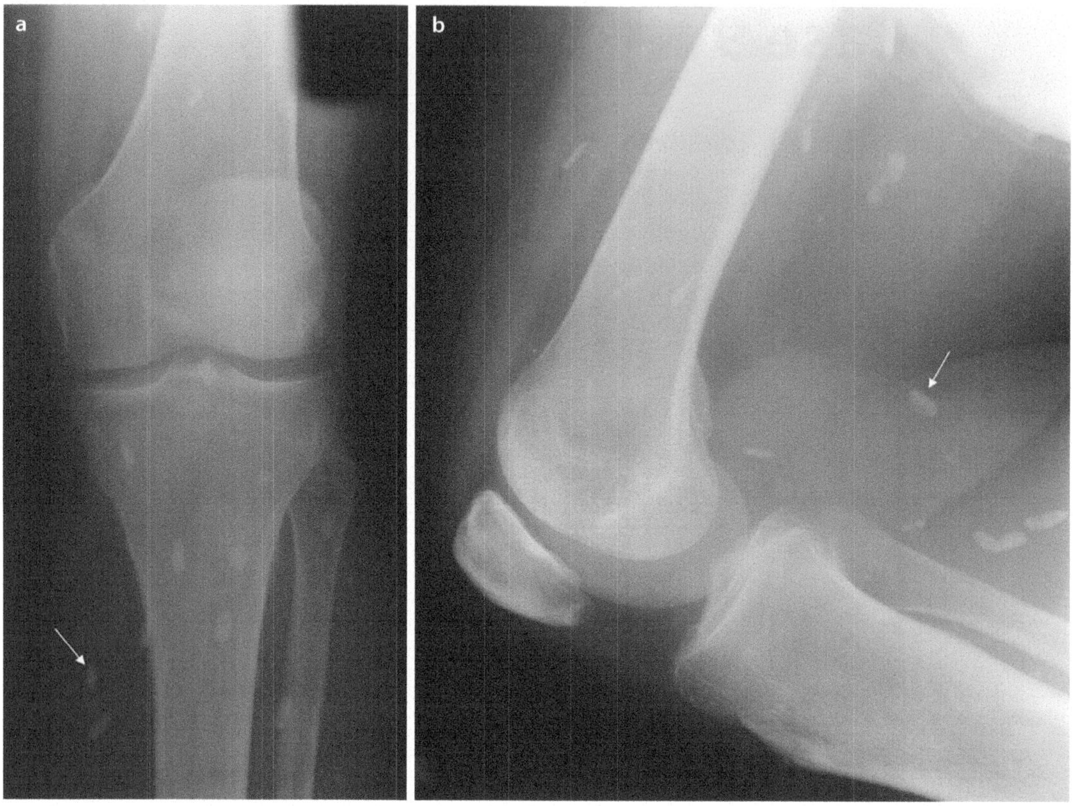

Radiographs **a** (anteroposterior) and **b** (lateral) of the knee joint show oblong calcific specks (arrows) diffusely scattered in the soft tissue surrounding the knee joint. Radiographic features are characteristic of musculoskeletal cysticercosis. These calcific specks are also known as rice-grain calcification due to their oblong shape

Musculoskeletal Cysticercosis

Definition and Pathophysiology

- Musculoskeletal cysticercosis is a parasitic infection caused by the larval stage (cysticerci) of the pork tapeworm, Taenia solium. It occurs when humans ingest tapeworm eggs from contaminated food or water, acting as an accidental intermediate host.
- Life cycle in muscles:
  - Ingestion: Embryonated eggs or proglottids are ingested.
  - Hatching & invasion: eggs hatch in the intestine, releasing oncospheres that penetrate the gut wall, enter the bloodstream, and disseminate throughout the body.
  - Encystment: The larvae lodge in tissues, including skeletal muscle, and develop into cysticerci—fluid-filled vesicles containing a single invaginated scolex.

- Phases: The cysts go through viable, degenerative, and calcified phases, each with distinct clinical and imaging findings.

Clinical Presentation

- Demographics: Endemic in regions with poor sanitation (Latin America, sub-Saharan Africa, parts of Asia). In non-endemic areas, it is seen in immigrants or travellers.
- Symptoms:
  - Asymptomatic: the most common presentation, discovered incidentally.
  - Palpable nodules: multiple, small, mobile, and painless subcutaneous or intramuscular nodules.
  - Myalgia and muscle weakness: rarely, if there is a significant inflammatory response to degenerating cysts ("pseudohypertrophic myositis").
  - Acute myositis: can mimic polymyositis, with pain, swelling, and fever.

Imaging Findings

- Radiography
  - Multiple, small, oval or cigar-shaped calcifications aligned with the direction of muscle fibres ("rice grain" or "snowstorm" appearance).
  - This is a feature of the dead, calcified cyst stage, which occurs years after initial infection.
- Ultrasound
  - Viable cyst: appears as a well-defined, anechoic (fluid-filled), oval cyst with an eccentric, hyperechoic nodule representing the scolex ("hole-with-dot" sign). There is minimal surrounding inflammation.
  - Degenerating cyst: the cyst becomes heterogeneous, the wall thickens, and there is surrounding inflammatory oedema.
  - Calcified cyst: shows a hyperechoic focus with posterior acoustic shadowing.
- MRI
  - MRI exquisitely demonstrates the cyst morphology and the host inflammatory response.
  - T1-Weighted: Cyst fluid is hypointense. The scolex appears as an eccentric isointense nodule within the cyst.
  - T2-Weighted / STIR: Cyst fluid is markedly hyperintense. The scolex is a small, low-signal dot within the bright fluid ("hole-with-dot" sign). Minimal surrounding oedema.
  - T1-Weighted post-contrast: The cyst wall and scolex enhance, especially during the degenerative phase. The fluid content does not enhance.

Differential Diagnosis

- Other parasitic infections (e.g., trichinosis): cause myositis but lack the discrete cystic lesions with a scolex.
- Pyomyositis/abscess: a bacterial infection presenting as a single, large, complex fluid collection with significant surrounding cellulitis and systemic symptoms.
- Soft tissue tumours (e.g., myxoma, haemangioma): typically solitary lesions without the characteristic scolex.
- Hydatid disease: larger cysts, often with daughter cysts, and no scolex.
- Multiple calcified lesions: old trauma (myositis ossificans), dermatomyositis, or scleroderma can cause calcifications but lack the specific morphology.

Management

- Treatment depends on the location of the cysts and the clinical symptoms.
- Asymptomatic muscular disease:
  - No treatment is necessary. The cysts are dead or will eventually die and calcify. Anti-parasitic drugs are not indicated as they can incite a severe inflammatory reaction in the muscle.
- Symptomatic or active disease:
  - Analgesics: For pain from myositis.
  - Corticosteroids (e.g., prednisone): used to control the inflammatory response, especially if anti-parasitic therapy is initiated for concurrent neurocysticercosis.
  - Anti-parasitic drugs (albendazole or praziquantel): use is controversial for isolated muscular disease. They are typically reserved for cases with concurrent neurocysticercosis or severe, progressive symptoms. Must be administered with corticosteroids to mitigate the inflammatory reaction to dying cysts.

Suggested Reading

Meena D, Gupta M, Jain VK, Arya RK. Isolated intramuscular cysticercosis: clinicopathological features, diagnosis and management - a review. J Clin Orthop Trauma. 2016;7(Suppl 2):243–9.

Thapa S, Lamichhane N, Joshi S. Isolated cysticercosis of sternocleidomastoid muscle: role of ultrasonography. Case Rep Infect Dis. 2021;2021:7102416.

Case 10

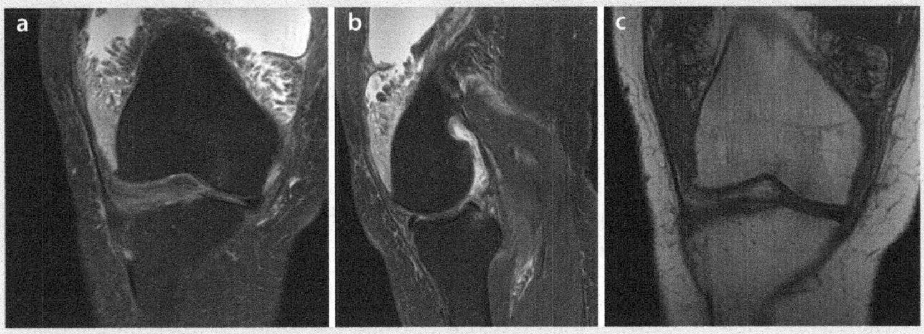

A 39-year-old male with a history of knee pain and swelling

S. Saran et al., *101 Knee Imaging Case Series*, 101 MSK Imaging 1,
https://doi.org/10.1007/978-3-032-21567-3_10

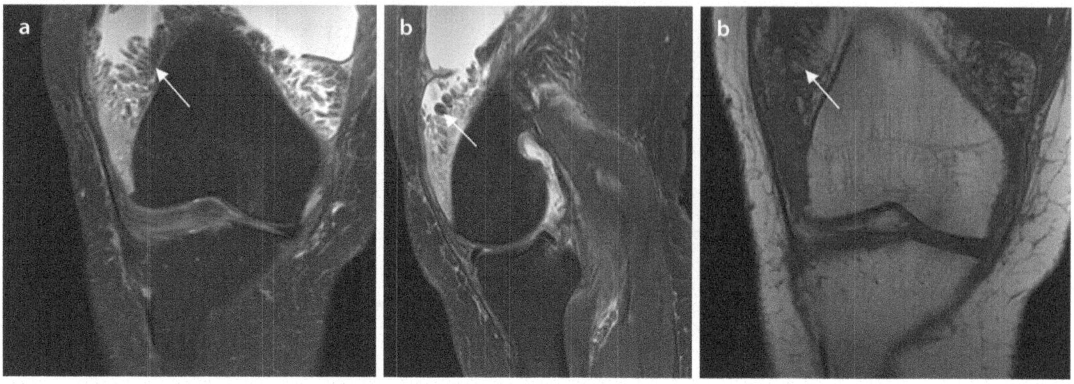

MRI knee, PDFS weighted coronal **a**, sagittal **b**, and T1 weighted coronal sequence **c**, showing moderate joint effusion extending into the suprapatellar joint recess with frond-like synovial thickening showing fat signal intensities (arrows) suggestive of Lipoma arborescens. It is most commonly associated with chronic arthropathy, either degenerative or inflammatory

Lipoma Arborescens – Definition

Lipoma arborescens (LA) is a rare, benign intra-articular lesion characterised by diffuse villous proliferation of the synovial membrane due to non-neoplastic fatty infiltration. The term arborescens (Latin for "tree-like") describes its frond-like appearance.

Pathophysiology

- Synovial hyperplasia with fat deposition: The synovium undergoes villous transformation with replacement of subsynovial connective tissue by mature adipocytes.
- Chronic inflammation & mechanical stress: Often associated with degenerative joint disease (e.g., osteoarthritis) or chronic synovitis, suggesting a reactive rather than neoplastic process.
- No malignant potential: Unlike synovial lipoma, LA is not a true tumour but rather a metaplastic synovial proliferation.

Clinical Features

- Slow-growing, typically monoarticular (most commonly the knee).
- Painless joint swelling (effusion) with possible mechanical symptoms (stiffness, restricted motion).
- No trauma-related instability (differentiates from ligament/meniscal injuries).

MRI Findings

- "Villous fatty proliferation": Frond-like synovial projections with fat signal intensity (hyperintense on T1, suppresses on fat-saturated sequences).
- Associated joint effusion & possible degenerative changes (e.g., osteoarthritis).

Management

- Conservative (if asymptomatic):
- Monitoring, NSAIDs, or joint aspiration for symptomatic relief.
- Surgical synovectomy (definitive treatment):
- Arthroscopic or open synovectomy for recurrent effusions or mechanical symptoms.
- Low recurrence rate after complete resection.

Suggested Reading

Bora N, Parihar P, Raj N, Shetty N, Nunna B. Lipoma arborescens where MRI is a boon. Cureus. 2023;15:e39212.

Li M, Ding L, Nie Q, Jiang Z. Lipoma arborescens in a 22-year-old male: a case report. Medicine (Baltimore). 2024;103(49):e40801.

Theermann R, Ohlmeier M, Hartwig CH, et al. Lipoma arborescens—uncommon diagnosis for joint swelling: case report and review of the literature. Z Orthop Unfall. 2020;158:618–24.

Case 11

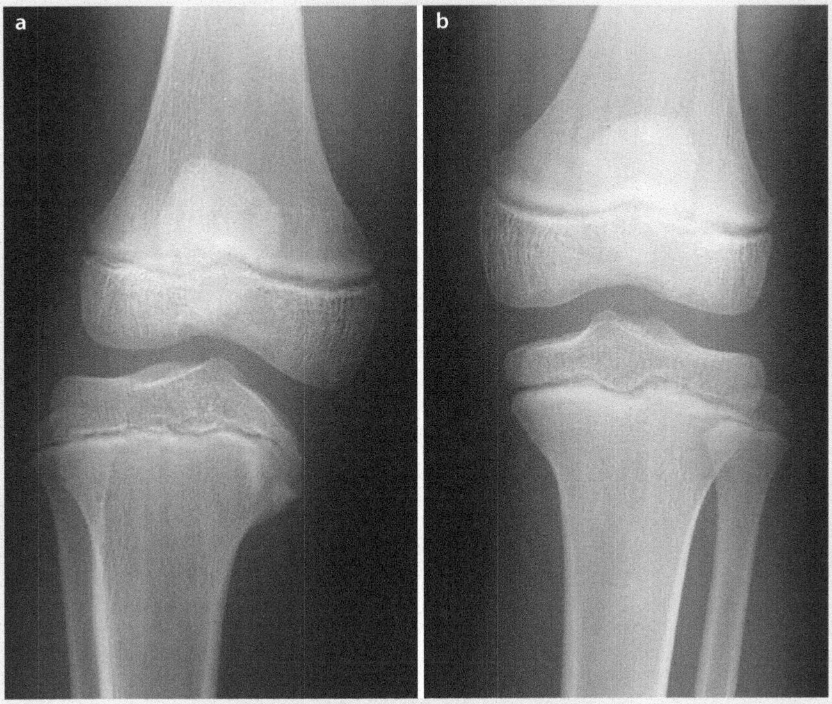

◘ A paediatric patient presented with a complaint of noticeable and worsening "bowing" of his right knee

S. Saran et al., *101 Knee Imaging Case Series*, 101 MSK Imaging 1,
https://doi.org/10.1007/978-3-032-21567-3_11

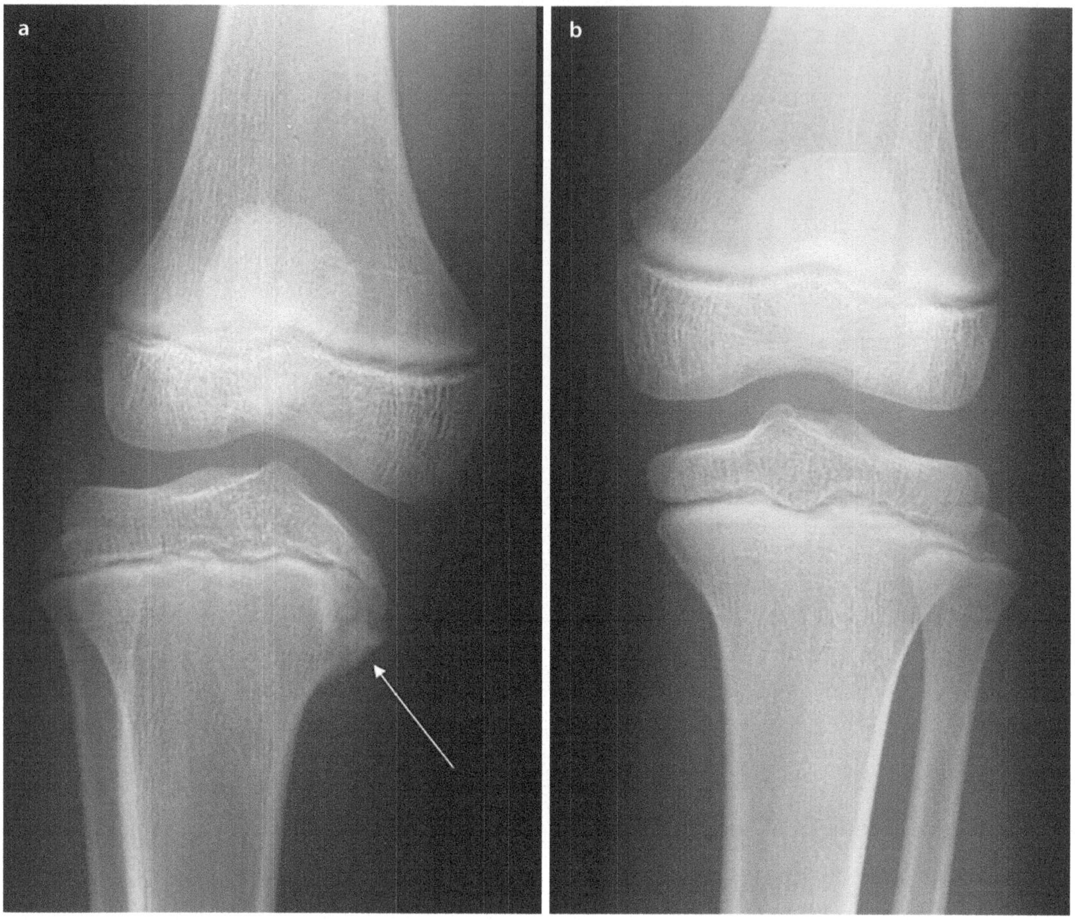

■ Radiograph of right knee **a** shows proximal tibial varus deformity with "beaking" of the medial metaphysis and flattening of the medial part of the tibial epiphysis (arrow). Contralateral knee is normal **b**. The diagnosis is Blount's disease (tibia vara)

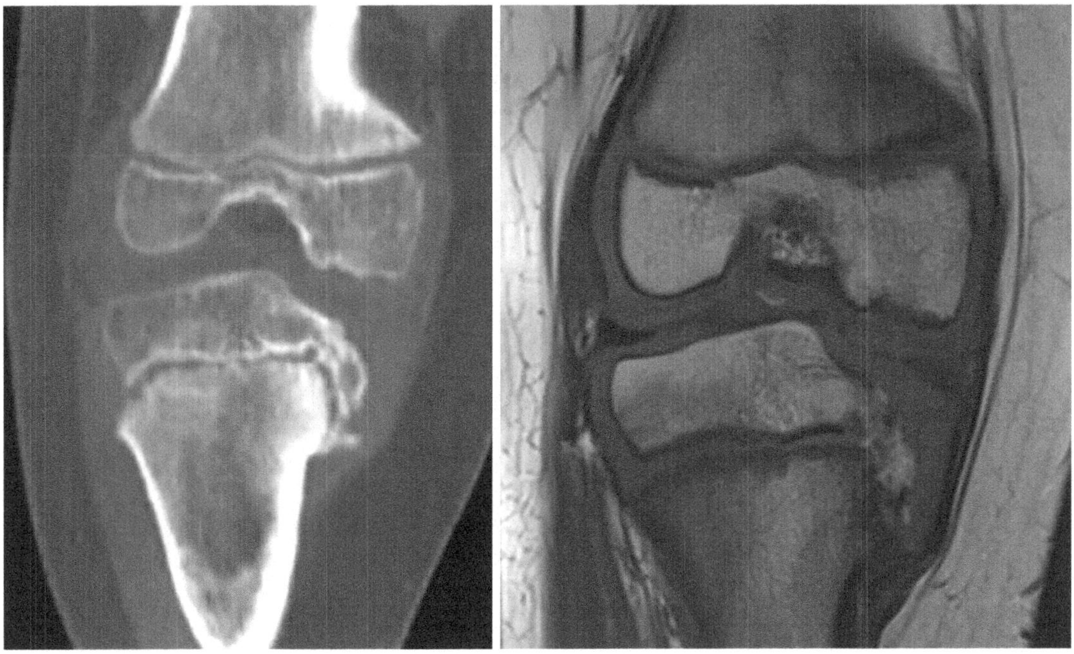

Companion case: A 7-year-old male with Blount's disease

Blount's Disease (Tibia Vara)

Definition and Pathophysiology

- Blount's disease is a growth disorder of the proximal tibia that results in a progressive varus deformity and internal tibial torsion. It is caused by a disturbance in the function of the medial portion of the proximal tibial physis.
- The medial physis experiences repetitive compressive forces that inhibit its normal growth, while the lateral physis continues to grow normally. This asymmetrical growth leads to the characteristic bowing and twisting of the leg.

Classification

Blount's disease is classified by the age of onset, which correlates with severity and prognosis.

- Infantile Blount's disease (age 1–3 years)
  - Most common form.
  - Usually bilateral (~60–80% of cases).
  - Presents after the child begins walking.
  - Has a greater potential for progression and deformity if untreated.

- Juvenile Blount's disease (age 4–10 years)
  - Less common.
  - Often unilateral.
  - Thought to be due to underlying physiological bowing that fails to resolve and is exacerbated by obesity.
- Adolescent Blount's disease (age 11+ years)
  - Typically unilateral.
  - Strongly associated with obesity.
  - The deformity is often less severe than the infantile form but is symptomatic.

Clinical Presentation

- Visible deformity: progressive, often painful, bowing of one or both legs.
- Physiological bowing is common in toddlers, is usually symmetrical, and resolves spontaneously by age 3–4. Blount's disease is progressive and worsens over time.

Imaging Findings

- Radiography
  - Weight-bearing radiographs of both legs are essential for diagnosis and staging.
  - Proximal tibial varus.
  - Sharp medial bowing: the angulation is localised to the proximal tibia.
  - "Beaking" of the medial metaphysis: a downward and medial projection of the bone.
  - Widening and irregularity of the medial physis: the growth plate appears ragged and sloped.
  - Medial epiphyseal wedging: the medial part of the tibial epiphysis appears smaller and more densely sclerotic than the lateral part.
- Langenskiöld classification (for infantile form)
  - This system stages the disease based on radiographic changes and predicts prognosis. It progresses from Stage I (mild metaphyseal beaking) to Stage VI (severe epiphyseal deformation and a bony bridge across the medial physis).

Management

Treatment is based on the patient's age and the severity of the deformity.

- Conservative management
  - Indication: For children under 3 years old with early-stage (Langenskiöld I-II) disease.

  - Treatment: knee-ankle-foot orthosis or a specially designed brace that unloads the medial physis.
  - Success rate: Bracing is most effective when initiated early; success rates drop significantly after age 4 or in advanced stages.
- Surgical intervention
  - Surgery is required for most children who do not respond to bracing, present late, or have advanced disease.
  - For younger children (age 4–10) with open physis- proximal tibial osteotomy with fibular osteotomy.
  - For adolescents or children with a physeal bar: a physeal bar resection with more complex osteotomy.
  - In severe cases or near skeletal maturity, a hemiplateau elevation may be needed to correct the depressed medial joint line.

Suggested Reading

Chkili S, Simoni P. Blount disease. J Belg Soc Radiol. 2021;105(1):51.

S DMTS, Taqi M, De Leucio A. Blount disease. 2024 Jan 9. In: StatPearls [Internet]. Treasure Island (FL): StatPearls Publishing; 2025.

Taksande A, Kumar A, Vilhekar K, Chaurasiya S. Infantile blount disease: a case report. Malays Fam Physician. 2009;4(1):30–2.

Case 12

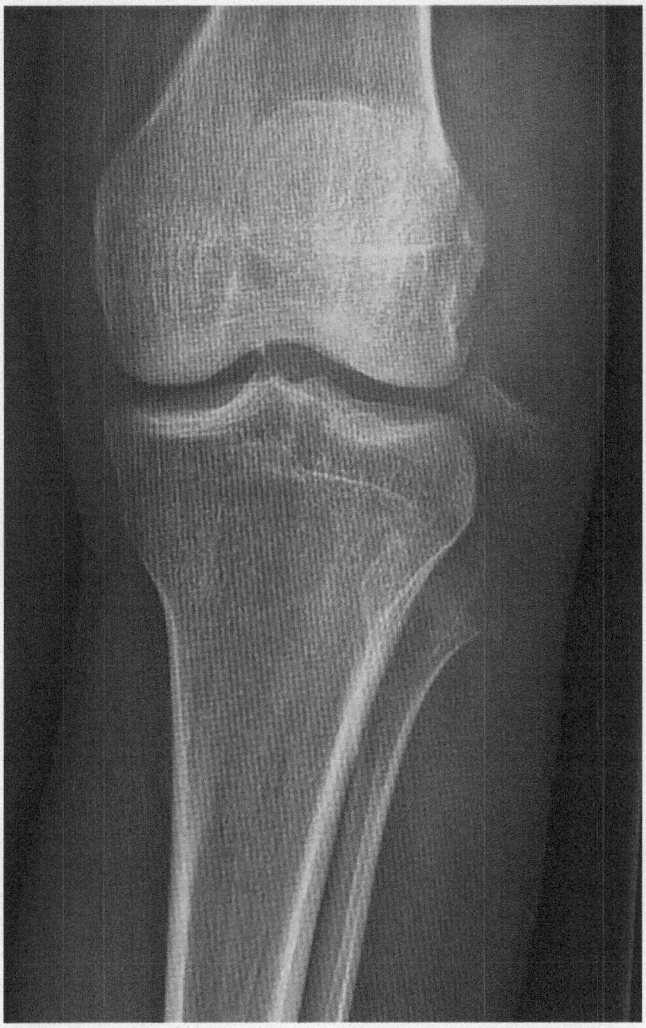

A 27-year-old male with knee trauma

S. Saran et al., *101 Knee Imaging Case Series*, 101 MSK Imaging 1,
https://doi.org/10.1007/978-3-032-21567-3_12

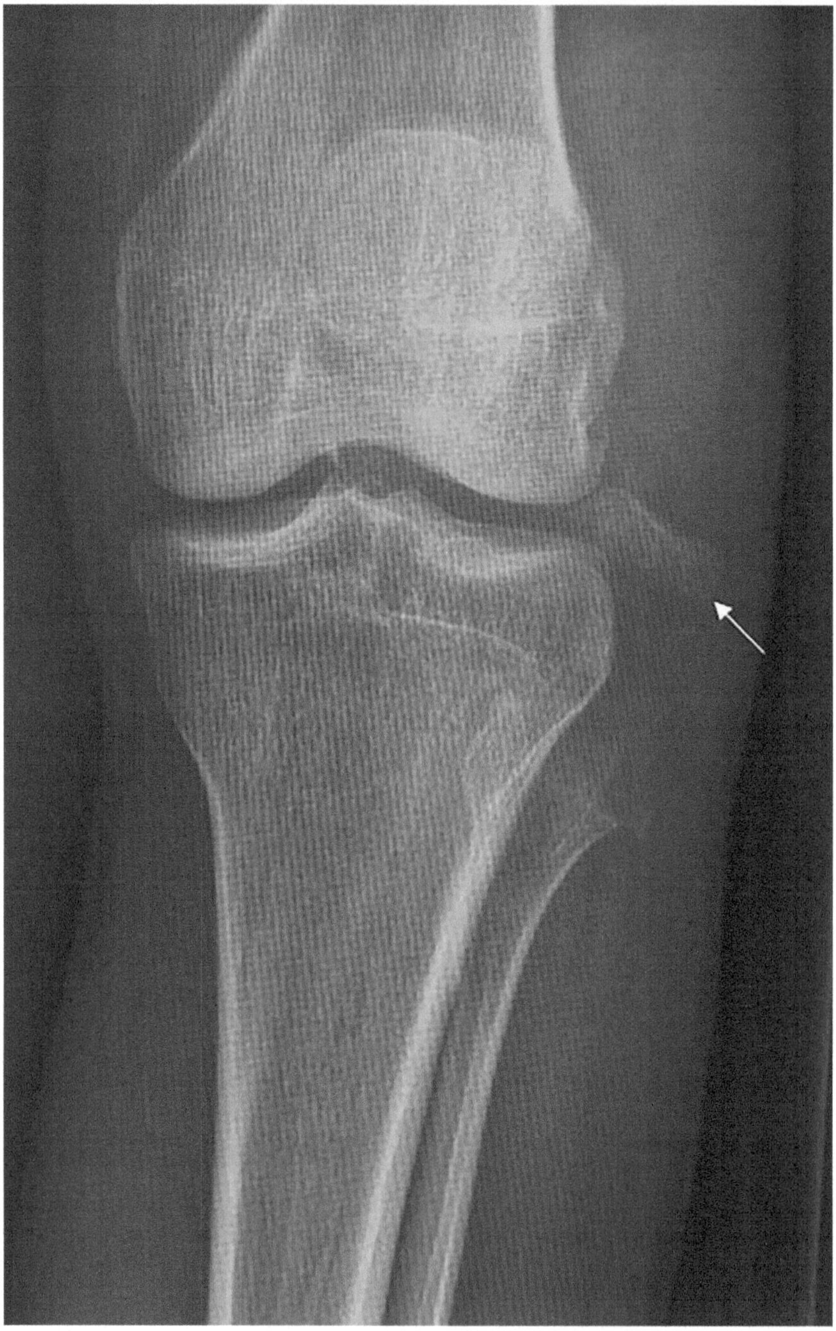

■ Radiograph (anteroposterior) shows the presence of a displaced avulsion fracture involving the fibular head and styloid process (arrow)

Fibular Head and Styloid Avulsion Fracture

Definition and Pathophysiology

- An avulsion fracture of the fibular head or styloid process is a bony injury where a fragment of the proximal fibula is torn away by the tensile force of an attached ligament or tendon. It is not a primary bone injury but rather a signifier of severe ligamentous disruption.
- Caused by the avulsion of the fibular collateral ligament (FCL), biceps femoris tendon, and/or the popliteofibular ligament. This is a hallmark of a posterolateral corner (PLC) injury.
- This fracture is a critical clue to a major destabilising knee injury, often involving multiple ligaments. It is commonly seen in knee dislocations or multi-ligament knee injuries, even if the dislocation has spontaneously reduced.
- Mechanism of Injury: High-energy trauma (e.g., motor vehicle accident, sports injury) involving a combined hyperextension and varus (bowlegged) force, often with external rotation of the tibia.

Clinical Presentation

- Acute pain and tenderness directly over the proximal fibula.
- Instability: Patients may report a sense of the knee "giving way", particularly with lateral or posterolateral thrust.
- Neurological deficit: High risk of injury to the common peroneal nerve, which courses around the fibular neck. This can cause foot drop and numbness in the dorsum of the foot.
- "The Fracture is the Tip of the Iceberg": The small bony avulsion often belies the extensive soft tissue damage to the posterolateral corner structures.

Imaging Findings

- Radiography
  - A small, often subtle, fleck of bone avulsed from the tip of the fibular styloid.
  - The "Arcuate Sign" is a specific term for an avulsed fragment from the apex of the fibular styloid, resembling the arcuate complex.

- MRI
  - Confirms the avulsion: Shows the bony fragment and the attached ligament (e.g., FCL, popliteofibular ligament).
  - Routinely reveals concurrent injuries such as ACL and/or PCL tears, meniscal tears, and bone bruises.

Management

Management is focused on restoring knee stability, which often requires addressing the fractured fragment and the torn ligaments.

- Initial management:
  - Immobilisation in a knee brace or hinged knee immobiliser.
  - Strict non-weight-bearing.
  - Neurological assessment to evaluate for common peroneal nerve injury.
- Surgical management: standard of care
  - Open Reduction and Internal Fixation (ORIF): The avulsed bone fragment, along with its attached ligaments, is surgically reduced and fixed back to the fibula using a screw, suture anchor, or tension band construct. This effectively repairs the posterolateral corner structures.
  - Addressing associated injuries: Concurrent ACL or PCL tears are typically reconstructed in the same setting.

Suggested Reading

Lee CH, Tan CF, Kim O, Suh KJ, Yao MS, Chan WP, Wu JS. Osseous injury associated with ligamentous tear of the knee. Can Assoc Radiol. 2016;67(4):379–86.

Spadafore S, Khodaee M. Avulsion fracture of the proximal fibula (arcuate sign) in a young woman. BMJ Case Rep. 2020;13(9):e237368.

Case 13

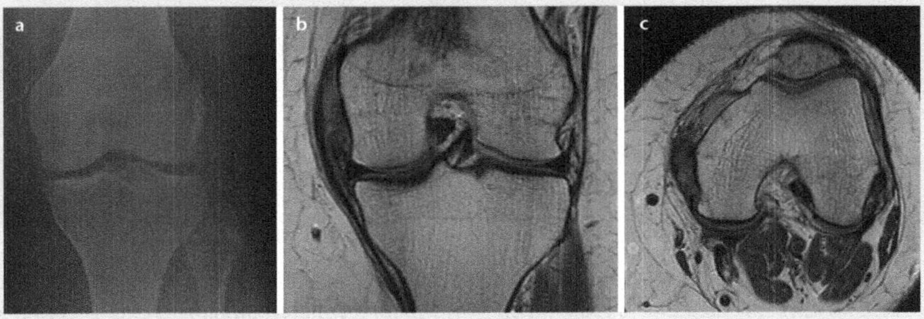

A 50-year-old male with pain along the medial aspect of the knee joint

S. Saran et al., *101 Knee Imaging Case Series*, 101 MSK Imaging 1,
https://doi.org/10.1007/978-3-032-21567-3_13

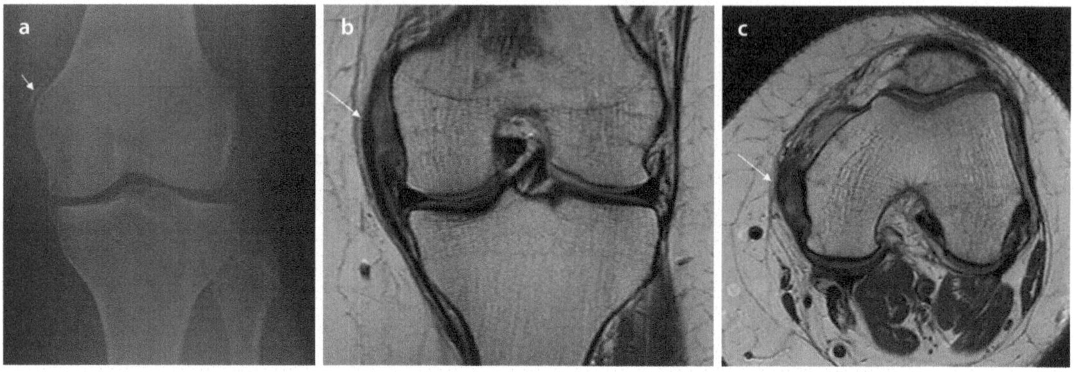

■ Anteroposterior radiograph **a** showing well-defined linear calcification (arrow) along the medial femoral condyle at the expected location of the femoral attachment of the medial collateral ligament (MCL). MRI knee, T2-weighted coronal **b** and axial **c** sequences showing femoral attachment of MCL as thickened and showing amorphous signal intensities (arrows). Imaging findings are of a Pellegrini-Stieda lesion

Pellegrini-Stieda Lesion – Definition and Pathophysiology

- A Pellegrini-Stieda lesion refers to post-traumatic calcification or ossification at the femoral attachment of the medial collateral ligament (MCL). It is a specific radiographic finding and a potential complication of an MCL injury.
- It occurs following an MCL sprain or tear, typically from a valgus force on the knee.
- Trauma causing haemorrhage and damage at the MCL's femoral origin. This leads to metaplasia of the local hematoma and damaged connective tissue. Further dystrophic calcification or heterotopic ossification (the formation of bone in soft tissue) at the injury site occurs.

Clinical Presentation

- Previous knee injury (often weeks to months prior) with a mechanism consistent with an MCL sprain.
- Persistent pain and tenderness over the medial femoral epicondyle.
- Palpable firmness or a bony hard mass at the proximal MCL attachment. Pain may be elicited with valgus stress testing.

Imaging Findings

- Radiography
  - A curvilinear, linear, or flame-shaped opacity projecting superior and posterior to the medial femoral epicondyle.
  - Not visible acutely. Calcification typically appears 2–4 weeks post-injury and matures over several months.
  - Best seen on an anteroposterior view of the knee.
- MRI
  - Acute phase: shows the underlying MCL tear (ligament thickening, oedema, discontinuity) and soft tissue haemorrhage.
  - Chronic phase: shows the calcific/ossific focus as a signal void (dark on all sequences) at the femoral attachment.
  - MRI plays a crucial role in evaluating for associated injuries (e.g., ACL tear, meniscal tears, "hidden" lesions like the MCL bursa we discussed), which are common.
- Ultrasound
- Can show the hyperechoic calcific focus with posterior acoustic shadowing at the MCL origin

Management

- Conservative
  - Bracing: hinged knee brace to protect against valgus stress.
  - Physical therapy: focused on restoring the range of motion and strengthening dynamic stabilisers.
- Image-guided intervention
  - Extracorporeal shockwave therapy (ESWT): Can be used to break down calcifications and alleviate pain.
  - Barbotage (US-guided needling & lavage): Under ultrasound guidance, a needle is used to fragment and aspirate the calcific deposit, often combined with a corticosteroid injection. This can provide significant symptomatic relief.

Suggested Reading

Somford MP, Lorusso L, Porro A, Van Loon C, Eygendaal D. The Pellegrini–Stieda lesion dissected historically. J Knee Surg. 2018;31(06):562–7.

Somford MP, Janssen RP, Meijer D, Roeling TA, Brown JC, Eygendaal D. The Pellegrini–Stieda Lesion of the knee: an anatomical and radiological review. J Knee Surg. 2019;32(07):637–41.

Case 14

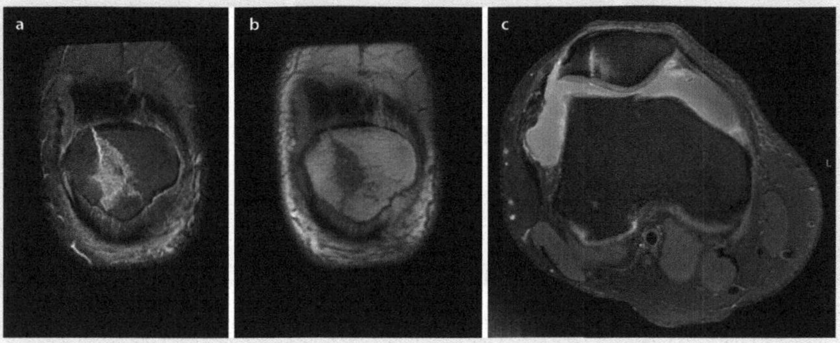

A 23-year-old male presented with severe pain in the anterior aspect of knee joint with rapid onset of swelling

S. Saran et al., *101 Knee Imaging Case Series*, 101 MSK Imaging 1, https://doi.org/10.1007/978-3-032-21567-3_14

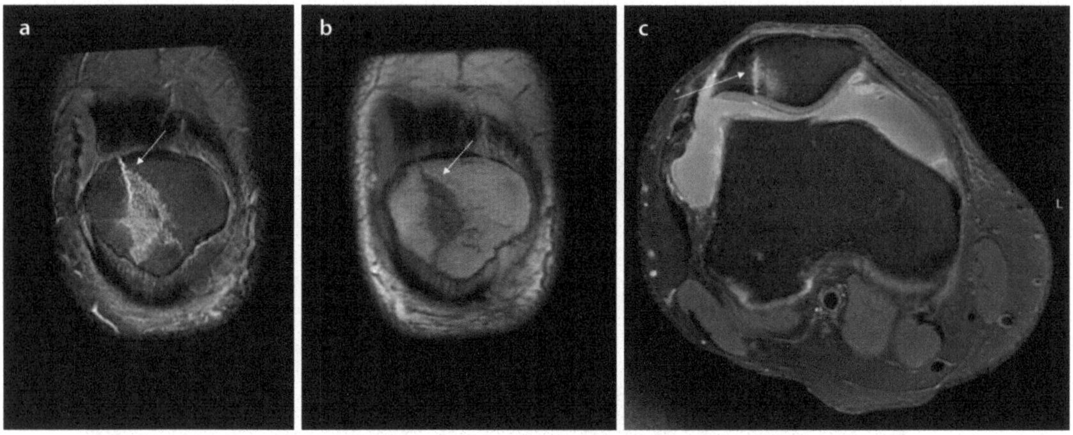

◘ MRI knee (PDFS coronal **a**, T1 coronal **b** and PDFS axial **c**) shows the presence of a vertical fracture line (arrows) traversing through the patella, in keeping with a patellar fracture. Associated joint effusion is also seen

Patellar Fracture

Definition and Pathophysiology

- A patellar fracture is a break in the patella, a critical sesamoid bone embedded within the quadriceps tendon. It functions to increase the leverage of the extensor mechanism. These fractures are significant as they disrupt the knee's primary extensor apparatus.
- Mechanism:
  - Direct trauma: a direct blow to the patella (e.g., dashboard injury in a car accident, fall directly onto the knee). Often causes stellate or comminuted fractures.
  - Indirect trauma: a sudden, forceful contraction of the quadriceps against a fixed load (e.g., catching a fall, misstep). This typically causes transverse fractures with disruption of the medial and lateral retinacula.
  - Combined: a combination of both direct and indirect forces.

Clinical Presentation

- History: Acute trauma followed by immediate pain and inability to use the leg.
- Symptoms & signs:
  - Severe anterior knee pain and swelling.
  - Palpable defect: a noticeable gap may be felt between the fracture fragments.

  - Functional loss: Inability to actively extend the knee or perform a straight leg raise. This indicates disruption of the extensor mechanism.
  - Tenderness and ecchymosis over the patella.

Classification

- Transverse (~50%): A horizontal fracture line, often displaced.
- Comminuted/Stellate (~30–35%): Multiple fracture fragments.
- Vertical/Polar: A fracture through the upper or lower pole.
- Osteochondral: A fracture involving the articular cartilage surface.

Imaging Findings

- Radiography
  - Anteroposterior (AP), lateral, and skyline view. Assesses fracture displacement, comminution, and integrity of the articular surface.
  - A visible fracture line is often visible.
  - Patella alta: a high-riding patella on the lateral view suggests a transverse fracture with superior pole displacement due to quadriceps pull.
  - Patella baja: a low-riding patella suggests a superior pole fracture or quadriceps tendon rupture.
- Computed Tomography
  - Used for complex, comminuted, or osteochondral fractures to better delineate the fracture pattern and articular surface involvement for pre-operative planning.
- MRI
  - Rarely needed for acute fracture diagnosis but excellent for evaluating associated injuries like quadriceps or patellar tendon rupture and meniscal or ligamentous injuries (e.g., ACL tear from the same trauma).

Differential Diagnosis

- Bipartite/Multipartite Patella: A normal developmental variant with smooth, rounded edges and no history of acute trauma. Bipartite patella is an unfused ossification centre which can mimic a fracture; it is typically located in the superolateral pole with smooth, sclerotic margins.

Management

The goal is to restore the articular surface and preserve the extensor mechanism function.

- Non-surgical management (conservative)
  - Non-displaced fractures with an intact extensor mechanism (patient can perform a straight leg raise).
  - Fractures with <2–3 mm of displacement and <1–2 mm of articular step-off.
  - Immobilisation: long leg cast or knee immobiliser for 4–6 weeks.
  - Rehabilitation: gradual range-of-motion and strengthening exercises after immobilisation.
- Surgical Intervention (Open Reduction and Internal Fixation—ORIF)
  - Tension band wiring: The gold standard for transverse fractures. Uses figure-of-eight wires over the anterior surface to convert distracting forces into compressive forces at the articular surface.

Suggested Reading

Jarraya M, Diaz L, Arndt W, Roemer F, Guermazi A. Imaging of patellar fractures. Insights Imaging. 2016;8(1):49–57.

Lazaro L, Wellman D, Pardee N, et al. Effect of computerized tomography on classification and treatment plan for patellar fractures. J Orthop Trauma. 2013;27(6):336–44.

Case 15

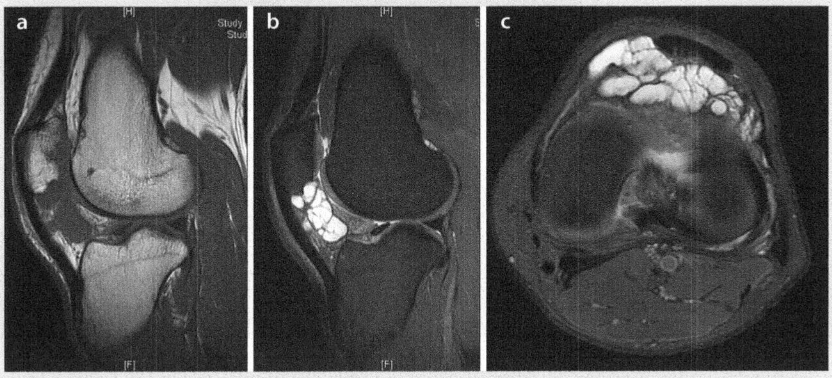

◘ A 27-year-old male presented with knee pain and swelling

S. Saran et al., *101 Knee Imaging Case Series*, 101 MSK Imaging 1,
https://doi.org/10.1007/978-3-032-21567-3_15

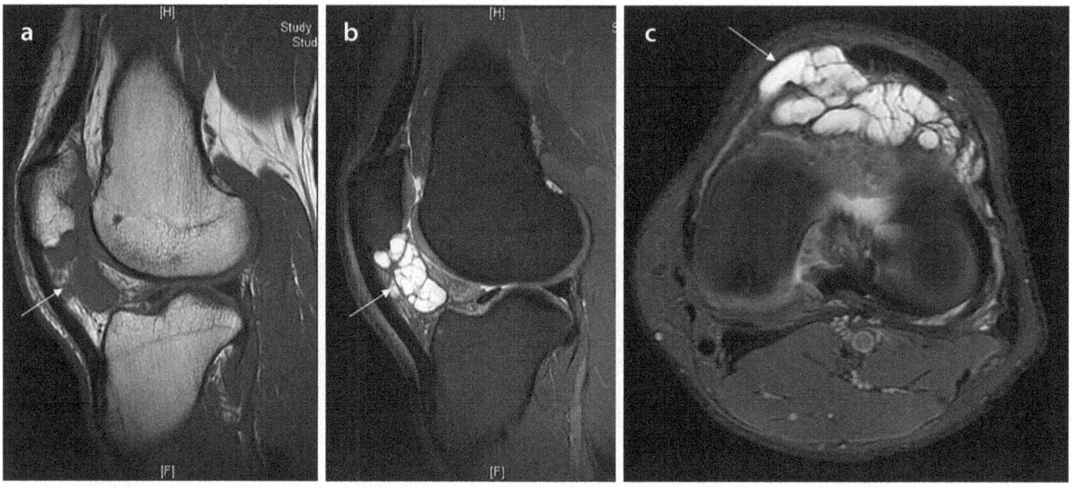

▪ MRI knee **a**–**c** shows the presence of a multiloculated cystic lesion (arrows) in the Hoffa's fat pad following fluid signals on T1-weighted sagittal **a**, PDFS weighted sagittal **b** and axial **c** sequences. appearances are of a ganglion cyst. There are pressure erosions on the adjacent patella

Ganglion Cyst of Hoffa's Fat Pad

Definition and Pathophysiology

- A ganglion cyst is a benign, non-neoplastic cyst located in and around the joint and tendon sheaths. Most commonly seen around the wrist.
- The exact cause is debated, but it is thought to arise from mucinous degeneration of connective tissue or herniation of the synovial membrane through the joint capsule or tendon sheath.
- Unlike a true synovial cyst, a ganglion cyst lacks a distinct synovial cell lining. Its wall is composed of fibrous tissue.
- The cyst is filled with thick, gelatinous, mucinous fluid rich in hyaluronic acid and other mucopolysaccharides.
- It may be associated with repetitive microtrauma, chronic irritation, or underlying joint pathology like meniscal tears or osteoarthritis. However, many cases are idiopathic.

Clinical Features

- Often discovered incidentally.
- A palpable mass may or may not be felt.
- Mechanical symptoms, like catching or locking if the cyst is large enough to impinge on surrounding structures.

Imaging Findings

- Ultrasound
  - Ganglion cysts are anechoic cystic lesions with distal acoustic enhancement, sometimes multiloculated, in close relation to a joint or tendon sheath.
- MRI findings
  - A clearly marginated cystic structure with fluid signal intensity in or around a joint with a clear or obscured connection.
  - The cyst fluid does not enhance with gadolinium contrast, though the thin wall may show mild enhancement. Absence of internal enhancement is an important differentiator from possible sarcoma.

Management

- Conservative: observation if asymptomatic.
- Ultrasound-guided corticosteroid injection into the cyst or adjacent joint can reduce inflammation and provide symptomatic relief, but the cyst may recur.
- Surgical Excision (if conservative measures fail).

Suggested Reading

Huntington LS, Talia A, Devitt BM, Batty L. Management and outcomes of proximal tibiofibular joint ganglion cysts: a systematic review. Knee. 2022;37:60–70.

Vosoughi F, Kaseb MH, Malek M, Toofan H, Mortazavi SMJ. Intra-articular ganglion cysts of the knee. JBJS Rev. 2022;10(9).

Case 16

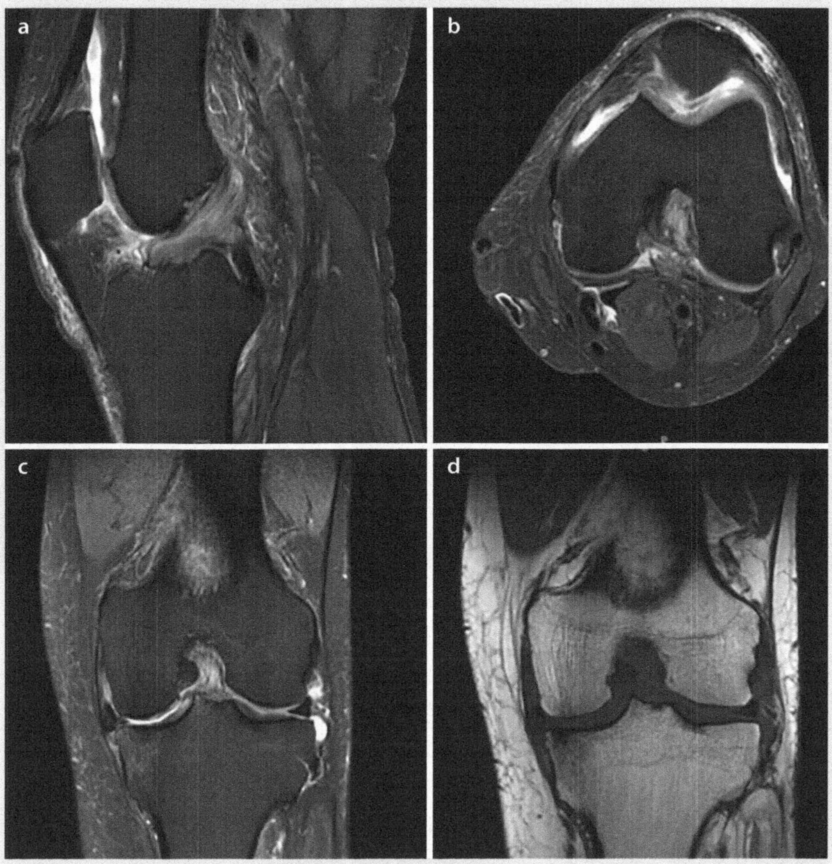

A 45-year-old male with history of knee pain

S. Saran et al., *101 Knee Imaging Case Series*, 101 MSK Imaging 1,
https://doi.org/10.1007/978-3-032-21567-3_16

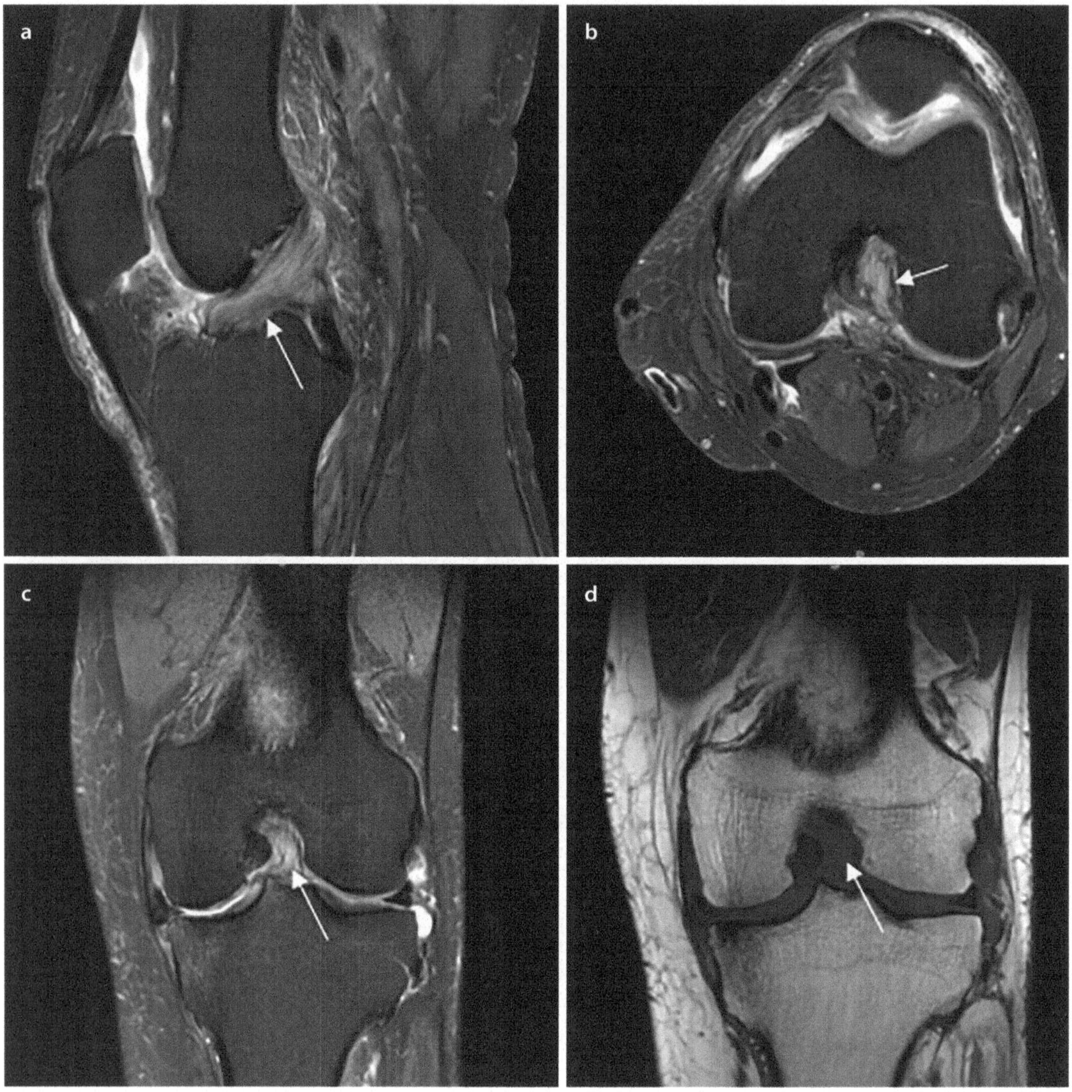

■ MRI knee, PDFS weighted sagittal **a**, axial **b**, and coronal **c**, and T1 weighted coronal sequence **d** showing homogeneous thickening of the anterior cruciate ligament (arrows) with increased signal intensity on PDFS sequence and decreased signal intensity on T1 weighted sequence with maintained fibre continuity giving celery stalk sign. appearances are of Mucoid degeneration of the ACL

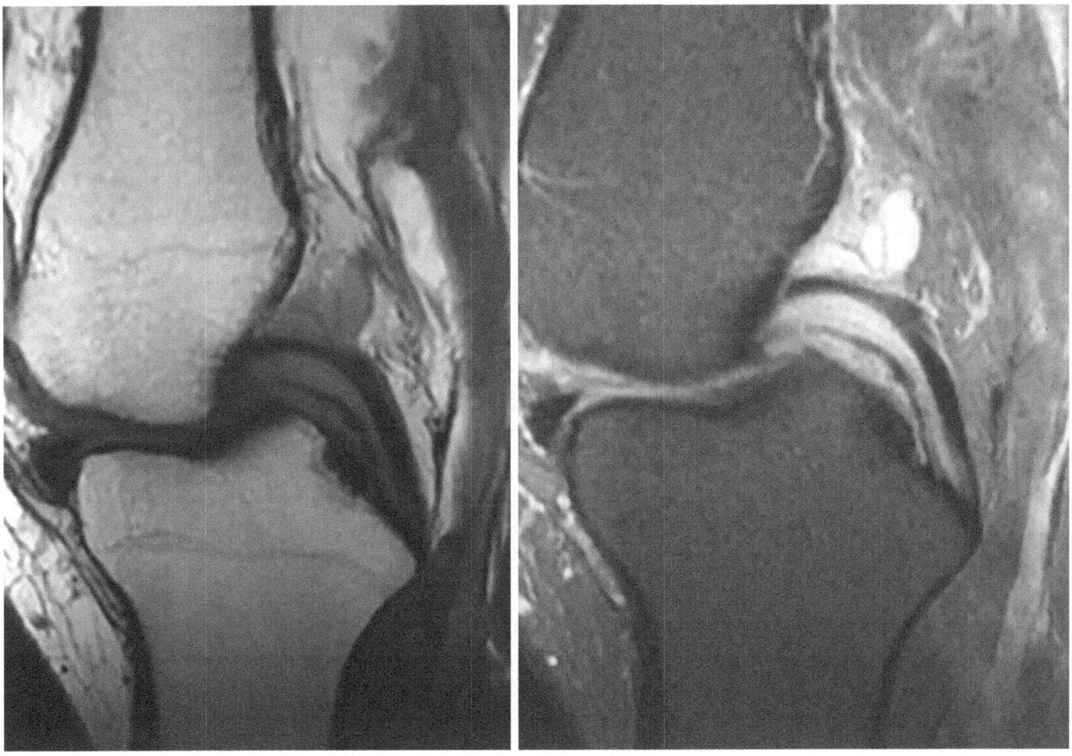

Companion case: A case of mucoid degeneration in the posterior cruciate ligament

Mucoid Degeneration of the Anterior Cruciate Ligament (ACL)

Definition and Pathophysiology

- Mucoid degeneration of the ACL is a non-neoplastic, degenerative condition characterised by the accumulation of mucoid (myxoid) material—a gelatinous substance rich in glycosaminoglycans—within the substance of the ligament. This leads to swelling and disruption of the normal collagen fibre architecture.
- Pathogenesis:
  - A degenerative process due to repetitive microtrauma and impaired mucoid substance clearance.
  - A reactive process to chronic stress or altered joint biomechanics, often associated with degenerative joint disease (osteoarthritis).
  - Synovial tissue incorporation into the ligament, producing the mucoid substance.

Clinical Presentation

- Demographics: Most common in middle-aged and older adults.
- Symptoms:
  - A deep, aching pain, often localised to the back of the knee, is a classic symptom. This is thought to be due to impingement of the enlarged ligament.
  - Pain with full knee flexion or extension.
  - Stiffness and mild swelling.

Imaging Findings

- MRI features
  - T1-Weighted: The ACL appears thickened and diffusely enlarged with intermediate signal intensity. The normal hypointense fibrillar pattern is partially or completely lost.
  - T2-Weighted/PD/STIR (fat-saturated): The ACL is diffusely hyperintense with "celery stalk sign".
  - "Celery Stalk" Sign: On sagittal images, the thickened ACL with retained longitudinal fibres surrounded by high-signal mucin resembles a stalk of celery.
  - Ganglion cyst: A discrete, fluid-signal cyst may be present within or adjacent to the ACL.
  - Osteoarthritis: Often seen as a concomitant finding, including joint space narrowing, osteophytes, and meniscal degeneration.

Management

- Treatment is primarily conservative, as the condition is not a true ligamentous insufficiency.
- Conservative management: activity modification and physical therapy.
- Image-Guided Intervention: Ultrasound-guided corticosteroid injection can provide diagnostic confirmation and significant therapeutic relief by reducing inflammation around the ligament.
- Surgical intervention (for refractory symptoms).
  - Arthroscopic debridement: The mucoid material is evacuated, and the hypertrophied ligament is partially resected or debrided to decompress the impingement.

Suggested Reading

Eustace SK, Hynes J, Byrne AO, Hurley D, Murray O, Eustace S. Percutaneous image-guided treatment of mucoid degeneration of the ACL in advanced knee osteoarthritis-Preliminary observations. Ir J Med Sci. 2024;193(3):1527–31. https://doi.org/10.1007/s11845-024-03606-8. Epub 2024 Feb 13.

Kwee RM, Hafezi-Nejad N, Roemer FW, Zikria BA, Hunter DJ, Guermazi A, Demehri S. Association of mucoid degeneration of the anterior cruciate ligament at MR imaging with medial tibiofemoral osteoarthritis progression at radiography: data from the Osteoarthritis Initiative. Radiology. 2018;287(3):912–21.

Vaishya R, Esin Issa A, Agarwal AK, Vijay V. Anterior cruciate ligament ganglion cyst and mucoid degeneration: a review. Cureus. 2017;9(9):e1682.

Case 17

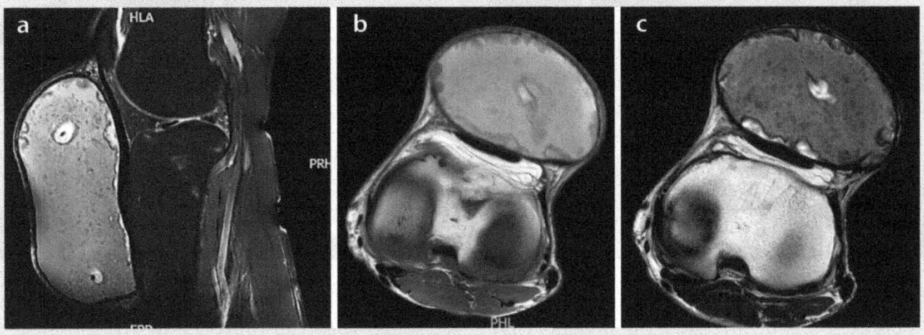

■ A 32-year-old male patient with no underlying co-morbid conditions presented with complaints of pain and swelling in the left knee for 5 years

S. Saran et al., *101 Knee Imaging Case Series*, 101 MSK Imaging 1,
https://doi.org/10.1007/978-3-032-21567-3_17

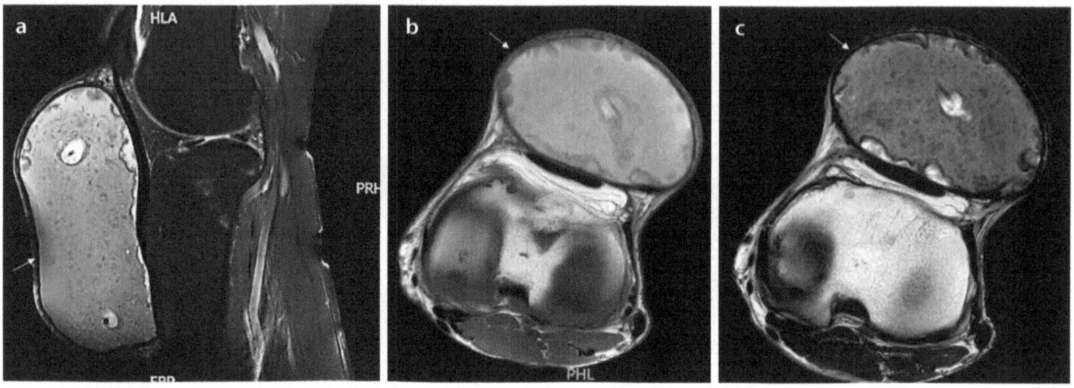

MRI knee **a**–**c** shows the presence of a large well-defined collection (arrows) in the Superficial infra-patellar region, showing increased signal intensity on sagittal PDFS sequence with the presence of hypointense areas **a**; increased signal intensity on axial T2 weighted **b** and low signal on axial T1 weighted sequences **c**. The collection extends caudally up to the proximal tibial diaphysis. The diagnosis in this case is a giant complex superficial infra-patellar bursitis

Giant Complex Superficial infra-patellar Bursitis

Definition and Pathophysiology

- Giant complex superficial infra-patellar bursitis is a severe, chronic inflammatory enlargement of the bursa, significantly exceeding the typical swelling seen in common bursitis.
- Caused by chronic, repetitive microtrauma and friction from prolonged or frequent kneeling (e.g., carpet layers, miners, grinders). This leads to inflammation, hypertrophy, and massive fluid accumulation within the bursal sac.

Clinical Presentation

- Demographics: Historically linked to specific occupational or cultural kneeling practices (e.g., "housemaid's knee", "carpet layers' knee", tribal corn grinders).
- Symptoms:
  - Large, visible swelling in the superficial infra-patellar region.
  - Pain & tenderness.
  - Restricted mobility.

Imaging Findings

- Ultrasound
  - Shows a complex, fluid-filled sac with internal septations (loculations), debris, and marked thickening of the bursal wall.

- Typically shows no internal vascularity, confirming its non-neoplastic nature (unless secondarily infected).
- MRI
  - T1-weighted: The bursal fluid is hypointense, while the thickened wall isointense to muscle.
  - T2-weighted/STIR: The fluid content is hyperintense, clearly delineating the full extent of the often multiloculated sac. The septations and fibrotic wall appear as low-signal strands.
  - T1-Weighted post-contrast: The thickened bursal wall and septa show intense enhancement, but the central fluid does not.
- Differential diagnosis
  - Septic bursitis: presents with erythema, warmth, and significant pain; requires aspiration for culture.
  - Morel-Lavallée effusion.
  - Gouty or rheumatoid arthritis (RA): Associated with systemic signs of the underlying disease; bursal fluid analysis confirms crystals (gout) or inflammatory cells (RA).
  - Sarcoma: presents as a solid, enhancing mass on imaging.
  - Soft tissue abscess: May mimic infected bursitis but is typically not confined to the classic pre-patellar location.

Management

- Conservative management
  - Activity modification: avoidance of kneeling.
  - PRICE Protocol: Protection, Rest, Ice, Compression, Elevation.
  - NSAIDs: For pain and inflammation control.
- Image-guided intervention
  - Aspiration: can be attempted but has a high recurrence rate in complex, septated bursae, as complete drainage is often impossible.
  - Corticosteroid injection: May be used after aspiration to reduce inflammation and slow recurrence.
- Surgical intervention (definitive for giant complex cases)
  - Surgery is indicated for large, symptomatic, or recurrent bursitis that fails conservative care.

Suggested Reading

Abdelghany M, Abdelrazak A, Raafat M, Fattouh E. An unusually massive hemorrhagic superficial infrapatellar Bursa excised in a one-stage procedure: case report. J Orthop Case Rep. 2023;13(8):142–6.

Maguire A, Lawrence C, Nicolai P, Rosenbloom C. Massive bilateral haemorrhagic prepatellar bursitis: a case report. Cureus. 2024;16(11):e74351.

Retal H, Cavez N, De Smet E, Abid W, Kadi R. Prepatellar Morel-Lavallée effusion mimicking a bursitis. Cureus. 2024;16(4):e59129.

Case 18

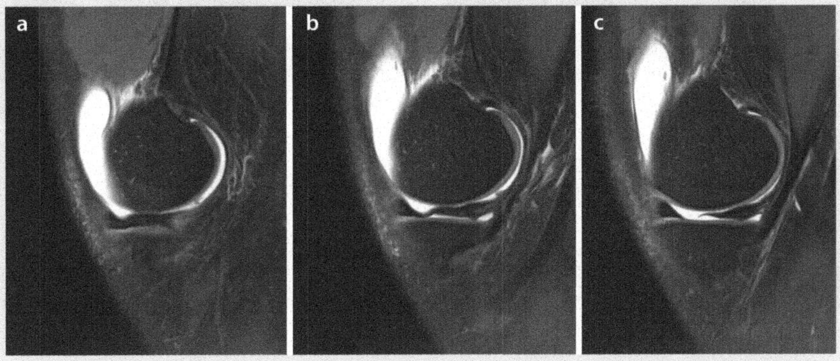

A 25-year-old female presented with pain and stiffness in the left knee joint

S. Saran et al., *101 Knee Imaging Case Series*, 101 MSK Imaging 1,
https://doi.org/10.1007/978-3-032-21567-3_18

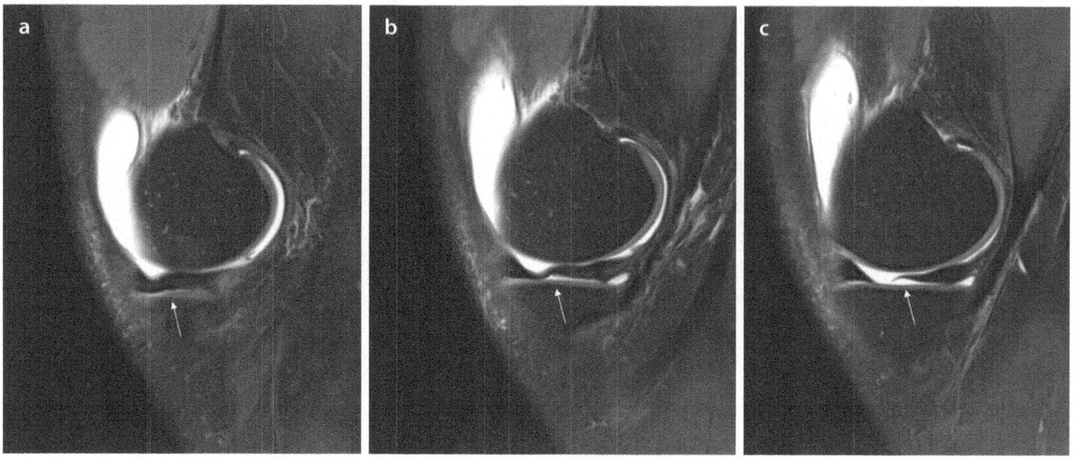

MRI PDFS weighted sagittal images **a**–**c** of the knee joint showing the medial meniscus having a kink or flounce (arrows) in its inner margin at the mid portion of the meniscus. It is a medial meniscal flounce

Meniscal Flounce

Definition and Pathophysiology

- A meniscal flounce is a normal anatomical variant characterised by a redundant, wavy, or buckled appearance of the free edge of the medial meniscus. It represents a transient, physiological folding of the meniscal tissue rather than a tear or pathological lesion.
- The flounce is thought to occur due to a combination of meniscal mobility and ligamentous tension. It is often a dynamic finding that can change or resolve with different knee positions and degrees of flexion. It is most commonly seen when the knee is imaged in extension, as the meniscus is relatively lax in this position.

Clinical Presentation

- Incidental Finding: The flounce is asymptomatic and is almost always discovered incidentally on MRI performed for other reasons (e.g., trauma, pain).
- There is no direct link between a meniscal flounce and specific patient symptoms. Any presenting pain is likely due to the primary reason for the MRI.

Imaging Findings

- MRI is the only modality that can visualise this finding. It is almost exclusively seen in the medial meniscus due to its greater inherent mobility and firm attachment to the joint capsule.
- Appearance: a smooth, undulating, "s-shaped" or sinusoidal fold at the free, inner edge of the medial meniscus.
- Signal intensity: the folded meniscus maintains its normal low signal intensity on all sequences (T1, T2, PD). There is no high signal intensity extending to the articular surface to suggest a tear.
- Dynamic nature: The flounce may appear or disappear on different MRI slices or if the knee is imaged in a different position (e.g., flexion).

Clinical Significance and Management

- "Do Not Touch" Lesion: A meniscal flounce is a normal variant and requires no treatment, follow-up, or intervention.
- The clinical management should be directed solely at the patient's actual symptoms or other pathological findings on the MRI.

Suggested Reading

Kim HJ, Ahn JM, Kim Y, Kang Y, Lee E, Lee JW, Kang HS. Association of meniscal flounce in the knee with the pattern and location of meniscal tear, concomitant ligamentous injury, amount of knee joint effusion, and flexion and rotation angles: a magnetic resonance evaluation. Skeletal Radiol. 2020;49(8):1277–84.

Yoo HJ, Ryu KN, Park JS, Jin W, Park SY, Kang HJ, Kim HS, Kwon GH. Preoperative meniscus: pitfalls and traps to avoid. Taehan Yongsang Uihakhoe Chi. 2022;83(3):582–96.

Case 19

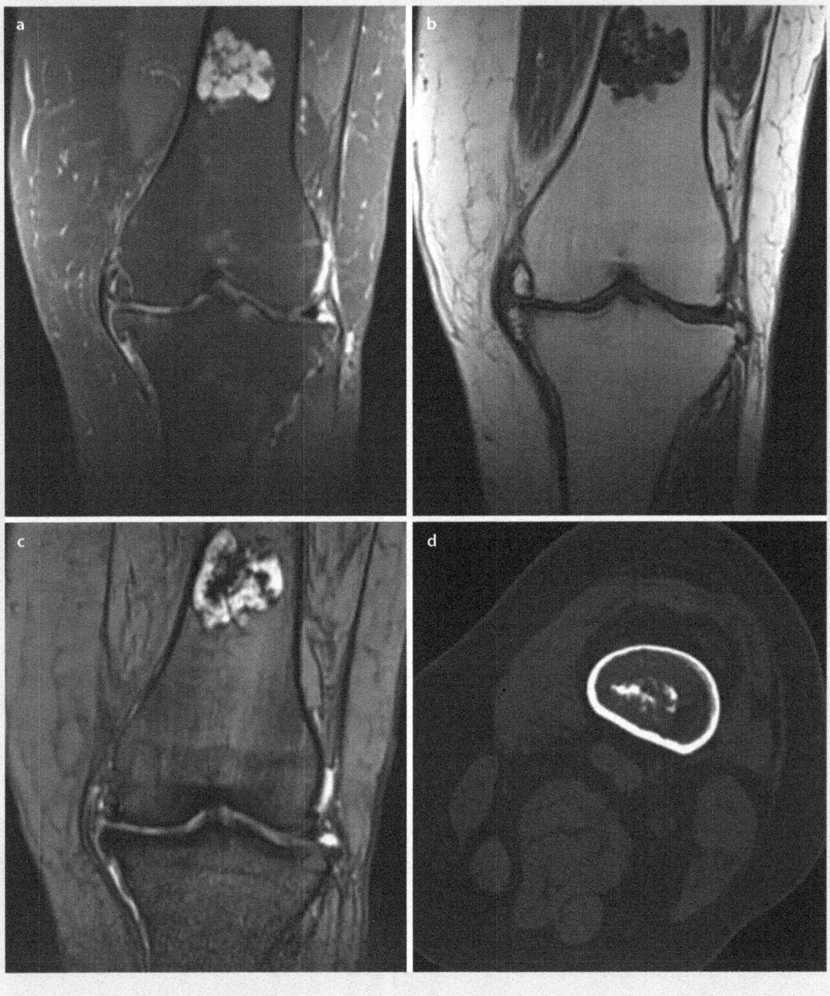

A 56-year-old male with chronic knee pain underwent an MRI of the knee

S. Saran et al., *101 Knee Imaging Case Series*, 101 MSK Imaging 1,
https://doi.org/10.1007/978-3-032-21567-3_19

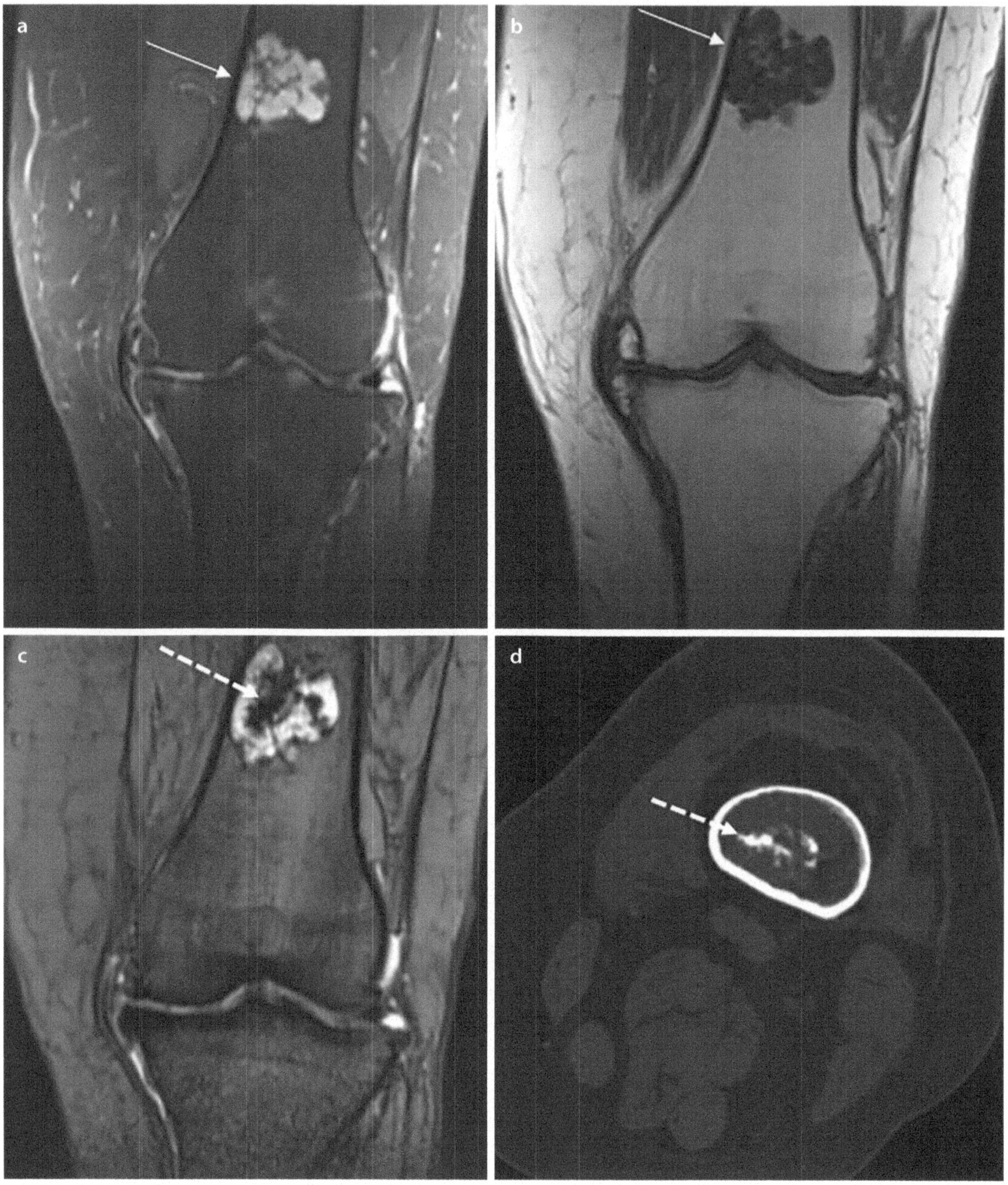

▪ MRI knee coronal images **a**–**c** shows a well-defined lobulated lesion in the medullary cavity of the distal femoral diaphysis (arrows), showing high signal intensity on PDFS weighted sequence **a** and low signal intensity on T1 weighted sequence **b**. The lesion demonstrates low signal intensity on GRE (dashed arrow in **c**), suggesting mineralisation. CT of the lesion shows areas of ring-and-arc or stippled calcifications (dashed arrow in **d**). The constellation of findings suggests the possibility of enchondroma

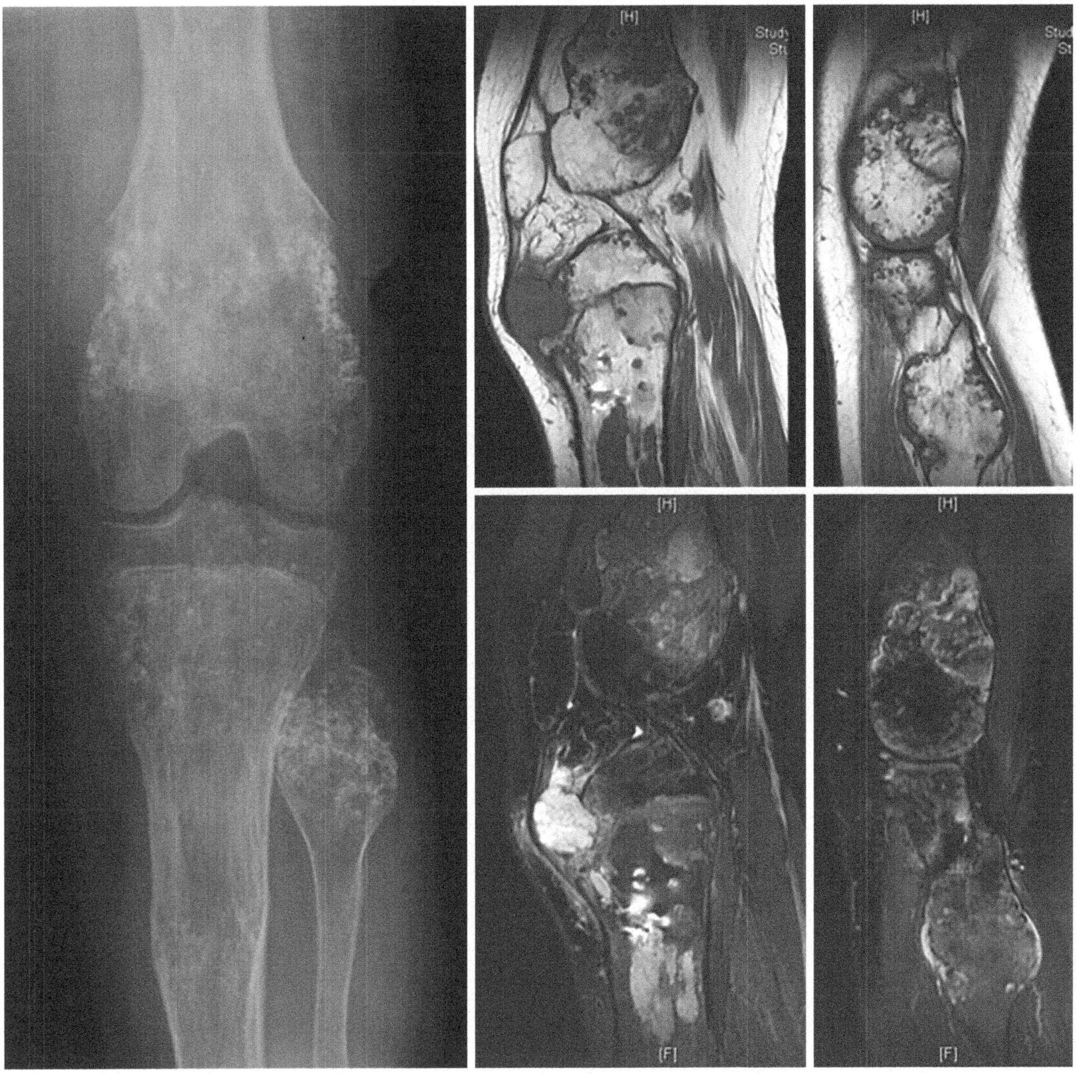

Companion case: Multiple expansile osteolytic lesions with chondroid calcifications seen in the distal femur, proximal tibia and proximal fibula, appearances are of enchondromatosis or Ollier disease

Enchondroma

Definition and Pathogenesis

- A benign, intramedullary cartilaginous tumour arising from aberrant rests of physeal cartilage. These rests fail to undergo normal endochondral ossification and persist in the metaphysis as the bone grows.
- Epidemiology: Common, constituting 12–24% of all benign bone tumors.
- Location: Most common in the metaphyses of long bones around the knee (distal femur > proximal tibia).

Clinical Presentation

- Incidental finding: The vast majority are asymptomatic and discovered incidentally on radiographs or MRIs performed for other reasons (e.g., knee pain, trauma).
- Typically, not painful unless complicated by:
  - Pathologic Fracture: Especially in small bones of the hand (less common in the femur).
  - Malignant Transformation: (Rare, <1% for solitary lesions). The presence of pain without a clear explanation is a red flag.

Imaging Findings

- Radiography/CT: often show a well-defined, lytic lesion with intralesional "ring-and-arc", "stippled", or "popcorn" calcifications (mineralised cartilage). There may be mild endosteal scalloping.
- MRI:
  - T1-weighted: lobulated, low to intermediate signal intensity mass.
  - T2-weighted/PD FS/STIR: Markedly hyperintense due to the high water content of cartilage.
  - Characteristic pattern: The classic appearance is of a lobulated, "bubbly" mass with the described signal characteristics and without aggressive features like soft tissue extension.
  - Areas of calcifications show "blooming" on GRE and low signal intensities on other sequences.

Management

- Birmingham Atypical Cartilaginous Tumour Imaging Protocol (BACTIP) is an algorithm for the MRI differentiation of central cartilaginous tumours in the proximal humerus, distal femur and proximal tibia and is primarily used for lesions that are atypical but not definitively malignant, allowing for objective monitoring instead of immediate biopsy.
- Asymptomatic, Typical Lesion: No treatment or biopsy is necessary. These are considered "leave-me-alone" lesions.
- Observation: For indeterminate lesions that don't clearly meet malignant criteria, serial imaging (e.g., X-rays or MRI annually for 2–3 years) is appropriate to document stability.
- Biopsy & surgical intervention: Indicated only for lesions with suspicious features (pain, large size, deep scalloping, oedema).

Enchondroma Versus Chondrosarcoma

Feature	Enchondroma (benign)	Concern for chondrosarcoma (malignant)
Size	Typically <4 cm	>4–5 cm
Pain	Asymptomatic (unless fractured)	Unexplained, persistent pain at the lesion site
Endosteal scalloping	Absent or mild (<2/3 of cortical thickness)	Deep scalloping (>2/3 of cortical thickness)
Cortical thinning	None or minimal	Significant, with possible cortical disruption
Perilesional oedema on MRI	Typically absent	Often present
Rapid growth	Stable over time	Documented growth on serial imaging

Suggested Reading

Davies AM, Patel A, Azzopardi C, James S, Botchu R. Birmingham atypical cartilaginous tumour imaging protocol (BACTIP) revisited. Clin Radiol. 2025;83:106837.

Deckers C, Steyvers MJ, Hannink G, Schreuder HWB, de Rooy JWJ, Van Der Geest ICM. Can MRI differentiate between atypical cartilaginous tumors and high-grade chondrosarcoma? A systematic review. Acta Orthop. 2020;91(4):471–8.

Case 20

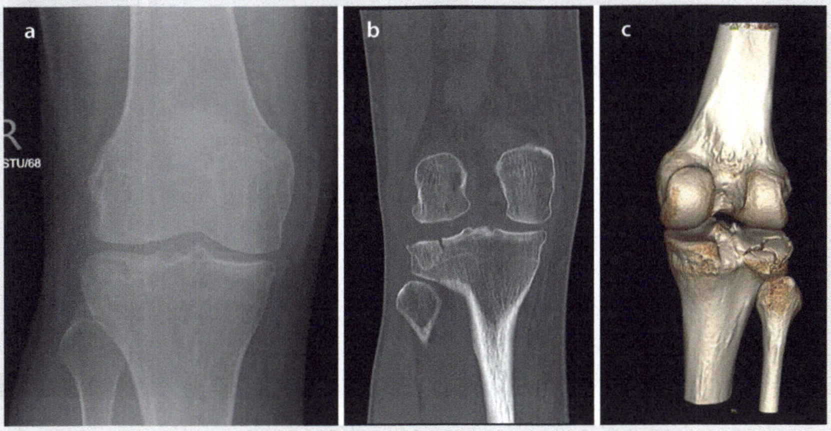

A 24-year-old male suffered a road traffic accident

S. Saran et al., *101 Knee Imaging Case Series*, 101 MSK Imaging 1,
https://doi.org/10.1007/978-3-032-21567-3_20

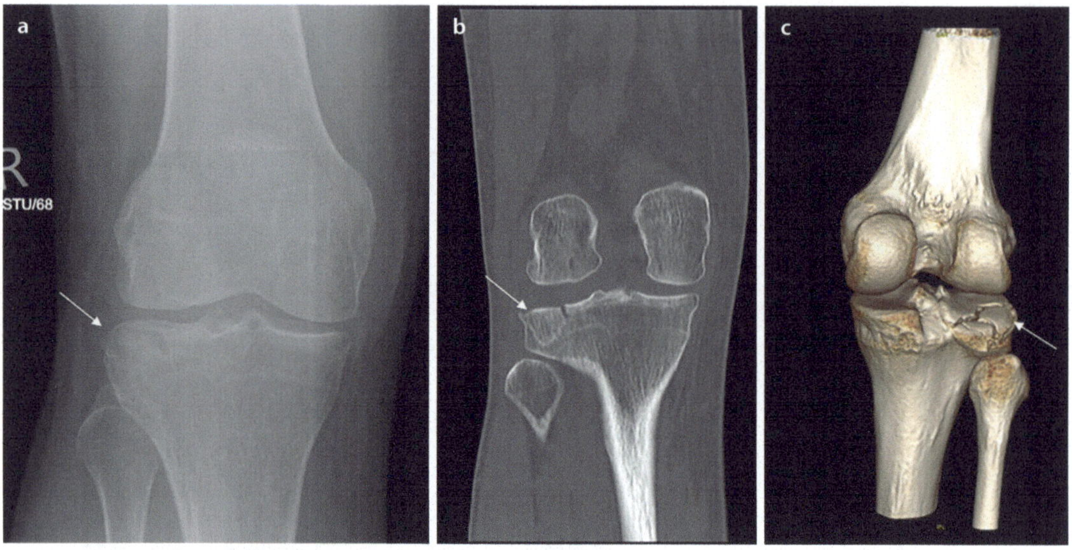

▣ Anteroposterior radiograph **a** shows a comminuted depressed fracture of the lateral tibial plateau (arrow). The fracture (arrows) is well demonstrated on coronal Computed tomography, bone window **b** and 3D volume rendered image **c**

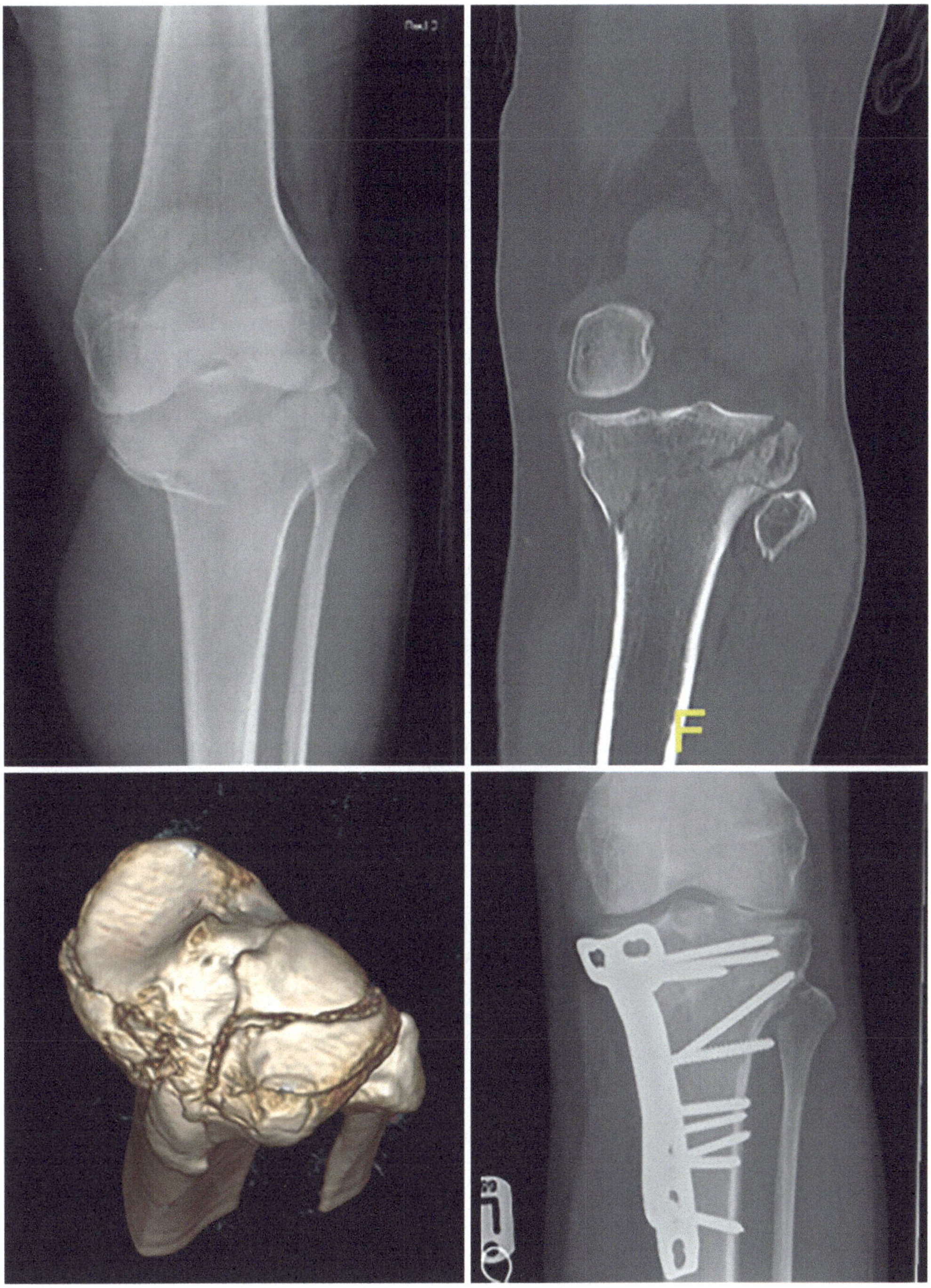

Companion case: another case of lateral tibial plateau fracture with splitting

Tibial Plateau Fracture

Definition and Pathophysiology

- A tibial plateau fracture is a break in the proximal tibia that involves the articular surface of the knee joint. This weight-bearing surface is critical for knee stability and function. These fractures range from simple, low-energy cracks to severe, comminuted (shattered) and depressed fractures.
- Axial load with varus/valgus force: The most common mechanism is a combination of an axial force (driving the femur down into the tibia) and a coronal plane stress (a bowlegged/varus or knock-kneed/valgus force). This is often seen in falls from height or motor vehicle accidents ("bumper fracture").
- Shear forces: high-energy trauma can also cause pure split fractures due to shear forces.
- Soft tissue sequelae: The high-energy force can also cause meniscal tears, ligamentous injuries, lipohemarthrosis and compartment syndrome.

Schatzker Classification

- This common classification system helps describe the fracture pattern and guide treatment.
- Type I: Pure split fracture of the lateral plateau.
- Type II: Split depression fracture of the lateral plateau.
- Type III: Pure depression fracture of the lateral plateau.
- Type IV: Fracture of the medial plateau with a split or depressed component.
- Type V: Bicondylar fracture (both medial and lateral plateaus are involved, with an intact tibial metaphysis).
- Type VI: Fracture with dissociation between the metaphysis and diaphysis.

Management

Management is based on fracture pattern, displacement, stability, and patient factors.

- Non-operative management: in non-displaced or minimally displaced (<2 mm) stable fractures, and fractures in non-ambulatory or low-demand patients.
- Surgical management: in articular step-off >2–3 mm, condylar widening >5 mm, unstable fracture patterns, open fractures, or associated neurovascular injury/compartment syndrome.

Suggested Reading

Markhardt BK, Gross JM, Monu JU. Schatzker classification of tibial plateau fractures: use of CT and MR imaging improves assessment. Radiographics. 2009;29(2):585–97.

Molenaars RJ, Mellema JJ, Doornberg JN, Kloen P. Tibial plateau fracture characteristics: computed tomography mapping of lateral, medial, and bicondylar fractures. J Bone Joint Surgery Am. 2015;97(18):1512–20.

Case 21

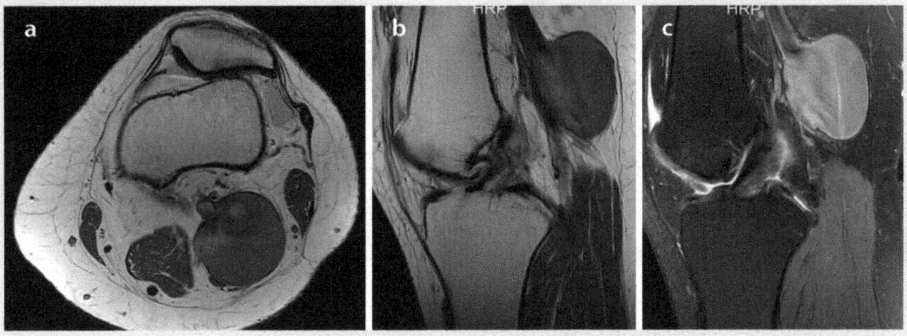

A 42-year-old female presented with soft swelling in the popliteal region

S. Saran et al., *101 Knee Imaging Case Series*, 101 MSK Imaging 1,
https://doi.org/10.1007/978-3-032-21567-3_21

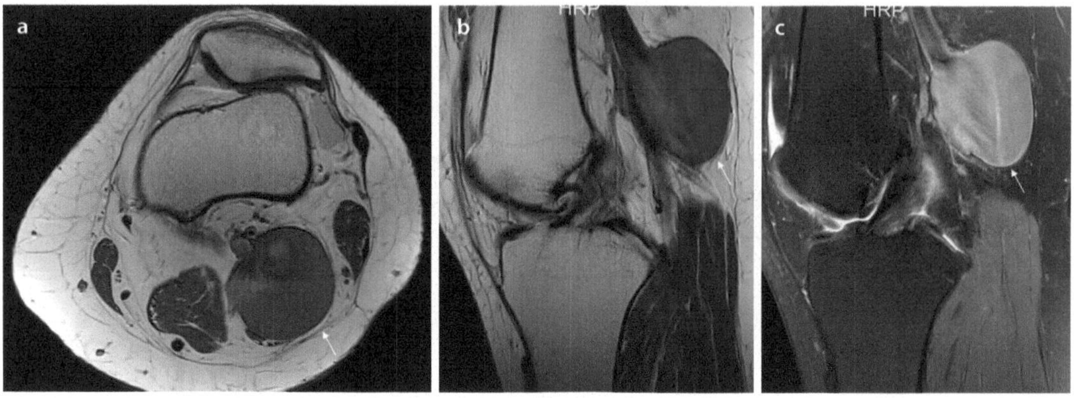

▪ MRI **a**–**c**. PD axial **a** and sagittal **b**, PDFS sagittal **c** sequences show a saccular outpouching of the popliteal vein, suggestive of a popliteal venous aneurysm (arrow)

Popliteal Venous Aneurysm

Definition and Pathophysiology

- A popliteal venous aneurysm is a focal, saccular or fusiform dilation of the popliteal vein that exceeds its normal diameter by at least 50% or has an absolute diameter typically >2.0 cm. It is a rare but potentially life-threatening condition due to its strong association with pulmonary embolism (PE).
- The wall of the aneurysm shows structural abnormalities, including thinning of the media, fragmentation of elastic fibres, and loss of smooth muscle cells. This leads to a loss of venous wall integrity and dilation. Popliteal vein aneurysms are predominantly true aneurysms involving all three layers of the venous wall.
- Unlike arterial aneurysms, the primary risk is not rupture but thromboembolism. The dilated, turbulent blood flow within the aneurysm promotes stasis and thrombus formation, which can then embolize to the lungs.

Clinical Presentation

- Asymptomatic: often discovered incidentally during imaging for other reasons.
- Symptomatic: A palpable, soft mass in the popliteal fossa that may enlarge with the Valsalva manoeuvre. There may be a sensation of fullness or discomfort behind the knee.
- The most dreaded presentation can be a pulmonary embolism (sudden onset dyspnoea, chest pain) without a clear source of DVT in the calf.
- Local complications from mass effect on the tibial nerve (paresthesia) or popliteal artery (claudication).

Imaging Findings

- Diagnosis is primarily made with duplex ultrasound, with other modalities used for confirmation and surgical planning.
- Duplex ultrasound: Shows a focal, hypoechoic outpouching from the popliteal vein. It may be saccular (with a narrow neck) or fusiform (spindle-shaped dilation of the entire circumference). Doppler confirms the structure is venous and demonstrates turbulent or swirling flow within the aneurysm.
- Spectral Doppler: May show phasic flow (confirming it is not arterial) and can demonstrate the communication with the main vein.
- Intraluminal thrombus must be ruled out.
- CT venography or MR venography: Excellent for confirming the diagnosis, defining the precise anatomy, and assessing for thrombus.

Differential Diagnosis

- Baker's (popliteal) cyst: The most common mass in the popliteal fossa. It is a synovial cyst arising from the knee joint, does not communicate with the vasculature, and shows no flow on Doppler.
- Popliteal artery aneurysm: More common than venous aneurysms. It is pulsatile and shows arterial waveform on Doppler.
- Venous varix/tortuosity: A tortuous vein can mimic an aneurysm but lacks the focal, saccular dilation.

Management

- Due to the high risk of pulmonary embolism, surgical repair is the standard of care for most popliteal venous aneurysms.
- Indications:
  - All symptomatic aneurysms (especially those with prior PE).
  - Asymptomatic aneurysms >2.0 cm in diameter.
  - Aneurysms with intraluminal thrombus.

Suggested Reading

Musa J, Rahman M, Saliaj K, Siddik AB, Khadra R, Guy A, Aliu Q, Madani K, Kola I, Ceka E. Popliteal vein aneurysm in a teenager with knee swelling. Radiol Case Rep. 2021;16(6):1410–9.

Norimatsu T, Aramoto H. Surgical repair for popliteal venous aneurysm causing severe or recurrent pulmonary thromboembolism: three case reports. Ann Vasc Dis. 2015;8(1):56–8.

Case 22

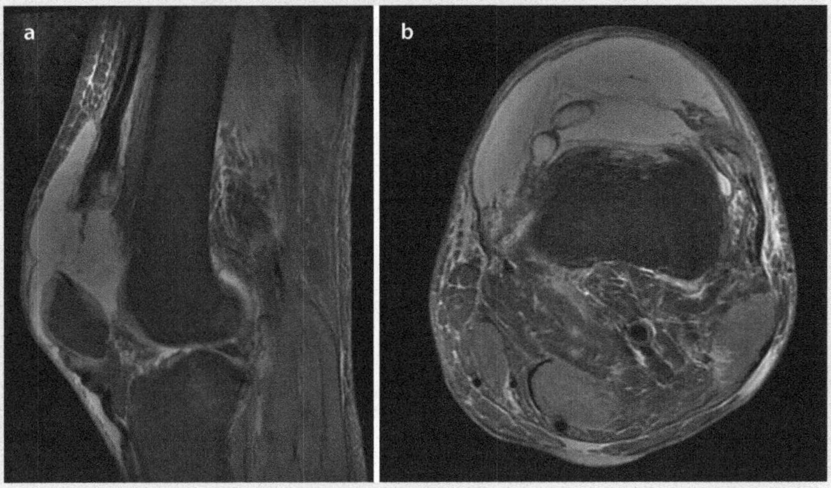

■ A 55-year-old diabetic male presented with acute pain, swelling, and an inability to actively extend the knee, following an audible pop

S. Saran et al., *101 Knee Imaging Case Series*, 101 MSK Imaging 1,
https://doi.org/10.1007/978-3-032-21567-3_22

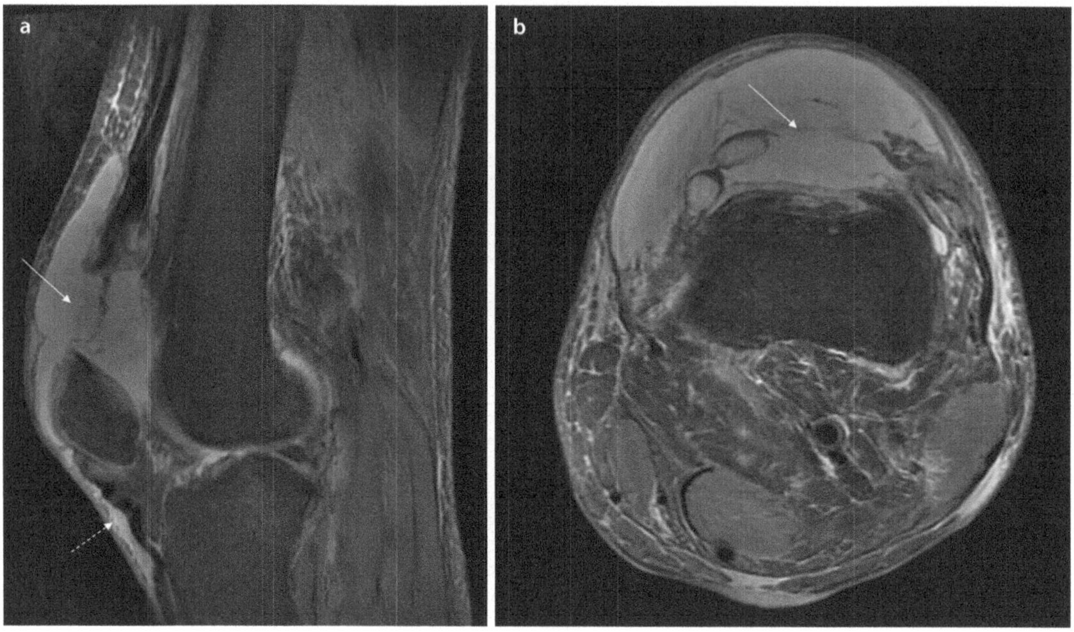

■ MRI knee, PDFS sagittal **a** and axial **b** shows the presence of a full-thickness tear involving the distal quadriceps tendon at the patellar attachment (arrow in **a** and **b**) with Patella Baja and curling of the patellar tendon (dashed arrow). Diagnosis is complete quadriceps tendon rupture

Quadriceps Tendon Rupture

Definition and Pathophysiology

- Mechanism: Typically caused by a sudden, forceful eccentric contraction of the quadriceps (the muscle contracts while it is being stretched), often with the foot planted and the knee partially flexed. This commonly occurs during a fall, a misstep, or during athletic activity.
- This injury severely compromises the knee's extensor mechanism, leading to an inability to actively straighten the leg.
- The rupture usually occurs at the osteotendinous junction, the relatively hypovascular zone just proximal to the patellar insertion. It can be partial or complete.

Risk Factors

- Age >40, systemic diseases (e.g., diabetes mellitus, renal disease, rheumatoid arthritis), corticosteroid or fluoroquinolone use, and local steroid injections.

Clinical Presentation

- History: A traumatic event often accompanied by a sensation of a "pop" or "tearing" in the front of the knee, followed by immediate pain and swelling.
- Symptoms:
  - Inability to actively extend the knee or hold the leg in a straightened position against gravity.
  - Severe pain and swelling superior to the patella.

Physical Exam Findings

- Palpable suprapatellar gap: a tender, palpable depression proximal to the superior pole of the patella.
- Low-riding patella (patella baja).
- Large hemarthrosis.
- Positive straight leg raise test: the patient is unable to lift the heel off the bed while keeping the knee straight.

Imaging Findings

- Radiography
  - Patella Baja: The patella is positioned abnormally low. This is assessed using indices like the Insall-Salvati ratio.
  - Soft tissue swelling: Seen superior to the patella.
  - Radiographs are crucial to rule out a patellar fracture, which can present with similar symptoms.
- Ultrasound (excellent for point-of-care diagnosis)
  - A hypoechoic (fluid-filled) gap between the torn tendon ends.
  - Retraction of the proximal tendon stump.
  - Non-visualisation of the normal fibrillar tendon architecture at the rupture site.
  - Dynamic imaging: can visualise the torn tendon ends and the gap in real-time. Can also assess for a hematoma.
- MRI
  - MRI provides the most comprehensive evaluation, confirming the diagnosis, characterising the tear's extent, and assessing for associated injuries.
  - T2-weighted/STIR (fat-saturated): Fluid signal filling the gap between the torn tendon and patella.
  - Patella Baja with curling of the patellar tendon.

Differential Diagnosis

- Patellar fracture: Also presents with inability to extend the knee, but the defect is palpable over the patella bone itself, and the fracture is visible on imaging.
- Patellar tendon rupture: Presents similarly, but the defect is palpable below the patella with patella alta.

Management

- Complete ruptures require prompt surgical repair to restore extensor mechanism function and achieve optimal outcomes.
- Surgical intervention: ideally performed within 1–2 weeks of injury to facilitate a primary repair before the tendon retracts and becomes scarred.
- Chronic ruptures may require tendon grafts or allografts due to tendon retraction and poor tissue quality.
- Post-operative rehabilitation is prolonged and carefully staged to protect the repair while preventing stiffness.

Suggested Reading

Alkhatatba M, Anaqreh Y, Essa SB, Alma'aiteh A, Ziad Audat H, Obeidat N, Ahmed M. Bilateral spontaneous quadriceps tendon rupture: a case report and literature review. SICOT J. 2023;9:31.

Falkowski AL, Jacobson JA, Hirschmann MT, Kalia V. MR imaging of the quadriceps femoris tendon: distal tear characterization and clinical significance of rupture types. Eur Radiol. 2021;31(10):7674–83.

Case 23

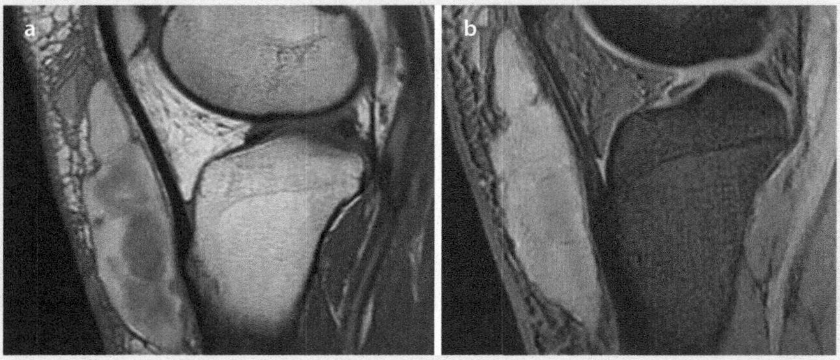

▪ A 26-year-old male presented with compressible swelling in the extensor aspect of the knee joint

S. Saran et al., *101 Knee Imaging Case Series*, 101 MSK Imaging 1,
https://doi.org/10.1007/978-3-032-21567-3_23

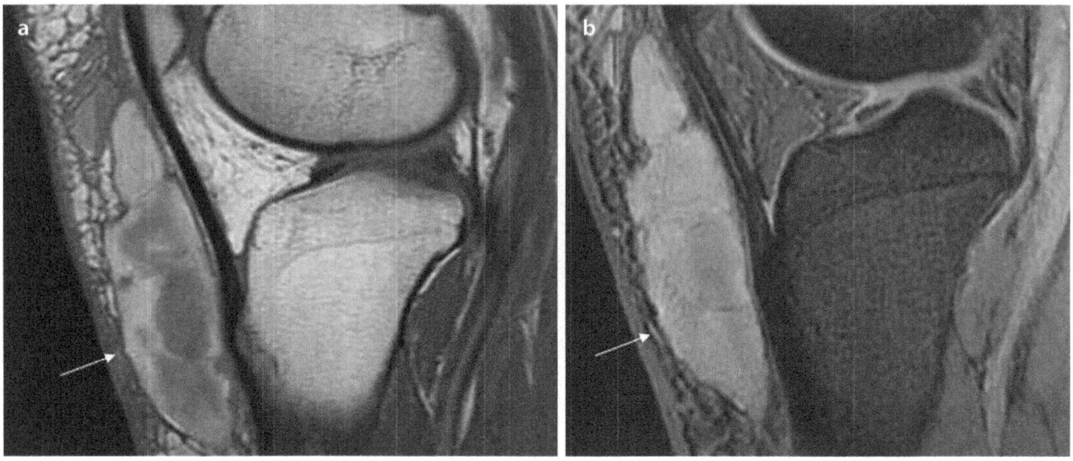

MRI knee, T1-weighted sagittal **a** and sagittal GRE **b** sequences showing a well-defined collection (arrows) in the superficial infra-patellar region with hyperintensity on T1-weighted sequences, suggesting blood products and peripheral linear hypointensity on GRE sequence, suggesting hemosiderin deposits. Findings are of haemorrhagic superficial infrapatellar bursitis

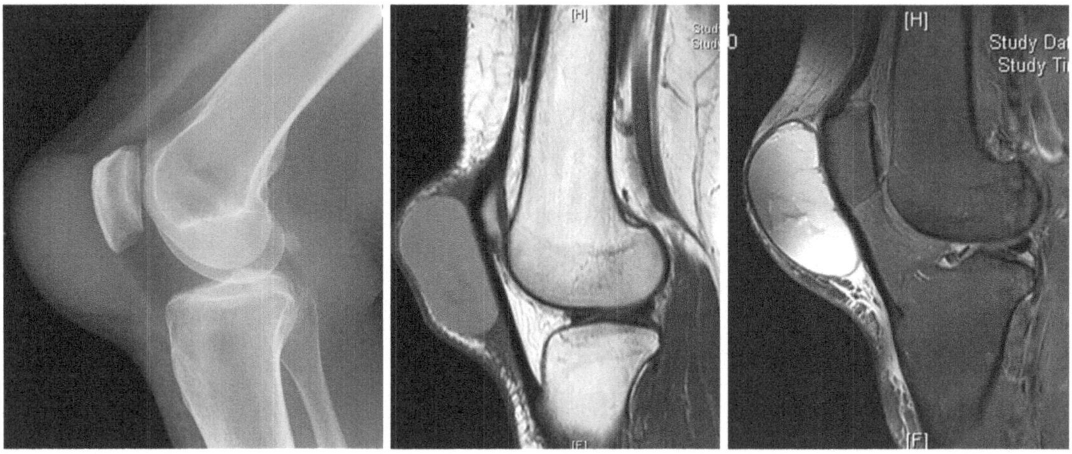

Companion case: Another case of Pre-patellar bursitis

Haemorrhagic Superficial Infrapatellar Bursitis

Definition and Pathophysiology

- Haemorrhagic superficial infrapatellar bursitis is the inflammation and bleeding into the superficial infrapatellar bursa. This bursa is located superficially, between the skin and the distal part of the patellar tendon.
- Mechanism: Typically caused by direct trauma or repetitive friction to the anterior knee, specifically over the patellar tendon area.

- At-risk activities: also known as "vicar's knee" or "clergyman's knee", it is common in occupations or activities that involve prolonged/repetitive kneeling on hard surfaces (e.g., carpet layers, plumbers, miners, wrestlers).

Clinical Presentation

- Symptoms develop rapidly after a specific traumatic event or after a period of repetitive kneeling.
- Localised, tender swelling directly over the patellar tendon, below the patella.
- A soft, fluctuant, and often bruised (ecchymotic) swelling.
- Pain is exacerbated by kneeling, squatting, or palpation. Knee flexion is often limited by pain and swelling.

Imaging Findings

- Ultrasound.
  - Shows a fluid-filled, compressible bursal sac with internal low-level echoes (complex fluid representing blood products).
  - Doppler may show hyperaemia (increased blood flow) in the surrounding soft tissues, indicating active inflammation.
- MRI: Reserved for cases where the diagnosis is unclear or to rule out other pathology (e.g., patellar tendon tear, deep infrapatellar bursitis).
  - T1-weighted: The haemorrhagic fluid may appear heterogeneously hyperintense due to the presence of methemoglobin.
  - T2-weighted/STIR: The bursal fluid is hyperintense, and there is often surrounding soft tissue oedema.

Management

- Conservative
  - Activity modification: Avoid kneeling and any activities that cause direct pressure on the area. Use knee pads if kneeling is unavoidable.
  - NSAIDs: To reduce pain and inflammation.
  - Aspiration: If the bursa is very large and tense, ultrasound-guided aspiration can provide significant symptomatic relief. However, there is a high risk of recurrence if the provoking activity continues.
  - After aspiration, a small dose of corticosteroid can be injected into the bursa under ultrasound guidance to reduce inflammation and prevent re-accumulation.

- Advanced intervention
  - Bursectomy: Surgical excision of the bursa is only considered for chronic, recurrent, and refractory cases that fail all other treatments.

Differential Diagnosis: Morel-Lavallée Lesion

Feature	Haemorrhagic superficial infrapatellar bursitis	Morel-Lavallée lesion
Anatomy	Inflammation of the superficial infrapatellar bursa, a known anatomical structure.	A closed degloving soft-tissue injury, a pathological potential space, not a natural bursa.
Mechanism of injury	Direct, repetitive trauma or acute blow to the front of the knee (e.g., kneeling, "housemaid's knee").	Shearing force from a tangential, high-energy impact (e.g., MVC, fall from height, sports collision).
Pathophysiology	Trauma causes bleeding into the bursal sac, leading to acute inflammation.	Shearing force separates the hypodermis (subcutaneous fat) from the underlying fascia, disrupting blood vessels. Blood and lymph collect in this new cavity.
Location	Very specific: Directly over the tibial tuberosity or inferior patellar tendon.	Less specific: Can occur anywhere shearing forces happen. Common sites: Greater trochanter, thigh, lumbosacral region. Around the knee, it's often on the superolateral aspect (above and outside the patella).
Clinical presentation	Localised, tender, fluctuant swelling directly over the knee bump (tibial tubercle). Pain worsens with kneeling or palpation.	A large, soft, fluctuant, often painless swelling that may develop days or weeks after the initial trauma. Skin may show signs of trauma (bruising, abrasions) or feel numb (paresthesia).
Imaging (ultrasound/ MRI)	Shows a fluid-filled, distended bursal sac with internal echoes suggesting blood, located in the classic superficial infrapatellar position.	Shows a fluid collection (often heterogeneous) in a fusiform or lenticular shape between the subcutaneous fat and the deep fascia.

Suggested Reading

Abdelghany M, Abdelrazak A, Raafat M, Fattouh E. An unusually massive hemorrhagic superficial infrapatellar Bursa excised in a one-stage procedure: case report. J Orthop Case Rep. 2023;13(8):142–6.

Diviti S, Gupta N, Hooda K, Sharma K, Lo L. Morel-Lavallee lesions-review of pathophysiology, clinical findings, imaging findings and management. J Clin Diagn Res. 2017;11(4):TE01–4.

Khodaee M. Common superficial bursitis. Am Fam Physician. 2017;95:224–31.

Stahnke M, Mangham DC, Davies AM. Calcific haemorrhagic bursitis anterior to the knee mimicking a soft tissue sarcoma: report of two cases. Skeletal Radiol. 2004;33(6):363–6.

Case 24

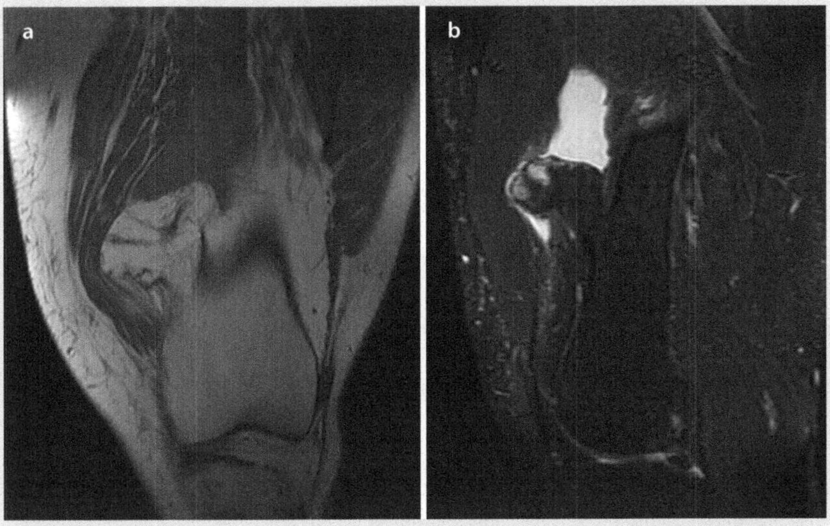

A 23-year-old male presented with a bony hard swelling in the anteromedial aspect of the distal thigh

S. Saran et al., *101 Knee Imaging Case Series*, 101 MSK Imaging 1,
https://doi.org/10.1007/978-3-032-21567-3_24

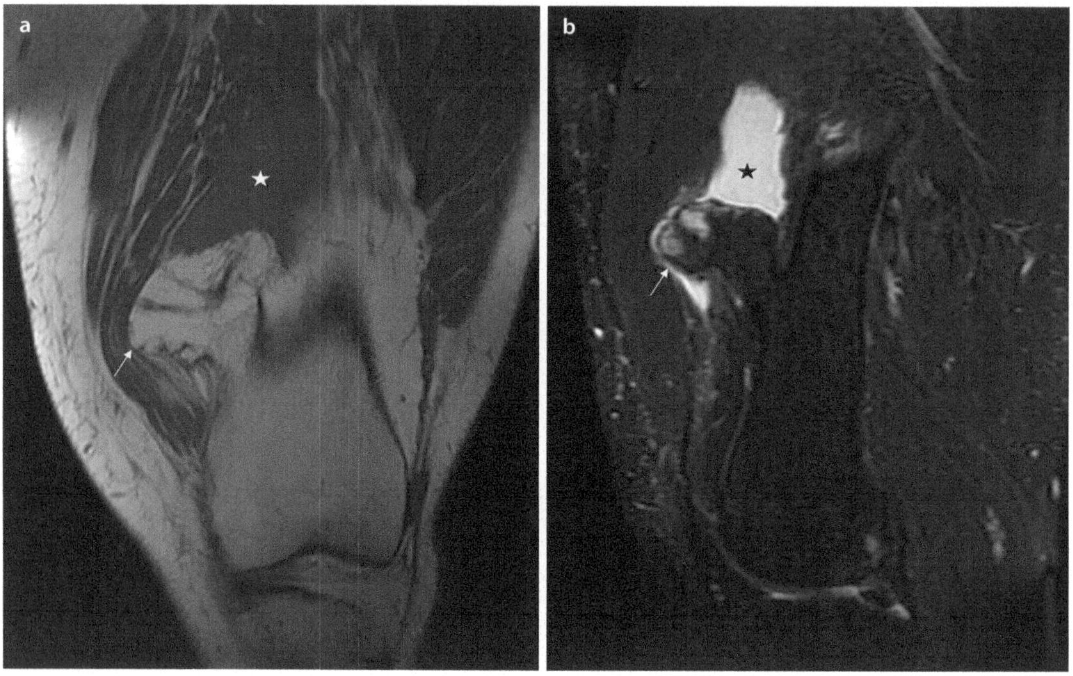

▣ MRI T1 coronal **a** and STIR sagittal **b** shows the presence of a pedunculated bony outgrowth (exostosis) arising from the anteromedial aspect of the distal femur with continuity of cortex and medulla (arrow) and presence of an overlying thin cartilage cap. Note is also made of the presence of a fluid collection (star) adjacent to the lesion. The diagnosis is pedunculated osteochondroma/exostosis with overlying bursitis

Pedunculated Osteochondroma with Overlying Bursitis

Definition and Pathophysiology

- This condition involves a benign bone tumour (osteochondroma) with a stalk-like ("pedunculated") morphology that causes mechanical irritation, leading to the inflammatory formation of a bursa (bursitis) over its tip.

Clinical Presentation

- Demographics: most common in children and adolescents (age 10–20), as osteochondromas develop and grow during skeletal maturation.
- Symptoms:
  - The osteochondroma itself is often asymptomatic and discovered incidentally.
  - The development of bursitis causes a new, often tender, soft swelling over the bony prominence.

  - Palpable mass: a firm, fixed bony mass (the exostosis) with a softer, fluctuant component on top (the bursa).
  - Common locations: areas where osteochondromas are common and prone to irritation, such as the distal femur, proximal tibia, and proximal humerus.

Imaging Findings

- Radiography.
  - Pedunculated Osteochondroma: Appears as a bony outgrowth with a slender stalk (peduncle) projecting away from the parent bone. The cortex of the osteochondroma flows seamlessly into the cortex of the host bone, and the trabecular bone (medulla) of the osteochondroma is continuous with the medullary canal of the host bone.
- Ultrasound: can demonstrate the hypoechoic cartilage cap and overlying bursitis.
- MRI.
  - MRI is the best modality for visualising the inflamed bursa and assessing the cartilage cap, which is crucial for ruling out malignant transformation.
  - A fluid-signal bursal sac positioned directly over the tip of the osteochondroma.
  - A thin (<1.5–2 cm in adults), smooth cartilage cap.

Differential Diagnosis

- Malignant transformation to chondrosarcoma: The most critical differential. Red flags include: a thickened cartilage cap >2 cm in adults, destructive bone changes, an ill-defined surface, and a large soft tissue mass with scattered/flocculent calcifications. The bursitis itself is a benign finding and should not be mistaken for a malignant soft tissue mass.

Management

- Image-guided intervention
  - Ultrasound-guided aspiration & corticosteroid injection: Aspiration of the bursal fluid followed by a corticosteroid injection can provide significant symptomatic relief. However, recurrence is common as the underlying mechanical cause (the osteochondroma) remains.
- Surgical intervention (definitive treatment)
  - Indications:
    - Persistent, painful bursitis refractory to conservative care.

– Neurological or vascular impingement by the osteochondroma.
– Suspicion of malignant transformation.
– Procedure: surgical excision of the osteochondroma.

Suggested Reading

Fang ZW, Zhang HT, Li X, Guo YF, Yu SQ. Imaging features of reactive bursitis secondary to osteochondroma. Jpn J Radiol. 2022;40(7):712–21.
Maras Ozdemır Z, Karakaplan M, Kahraman AS, Karadag N. Adventitious bursitis overlying an osteochondroma of the humerus facing the thoracic wall. Case Rep Radiol. 2013;2013:939372.

Case 25

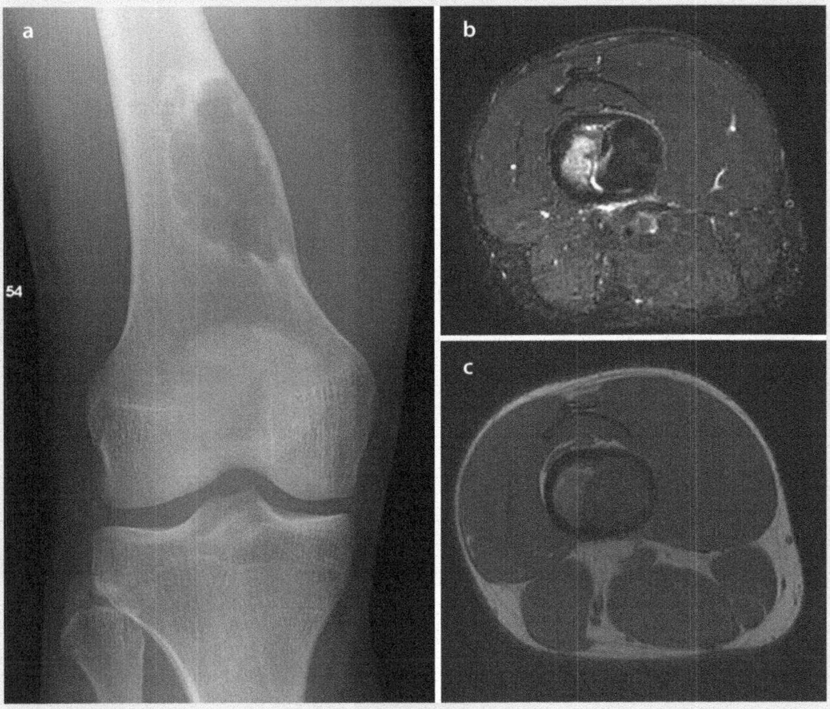

A 25-year-old male with pain in the distal thigh

S. Saran et al., *101 Knee Imaging Case Series*, 101 MSK Imaging 1,
https://doi.org/10.1007/978-3-032-21567-3_25

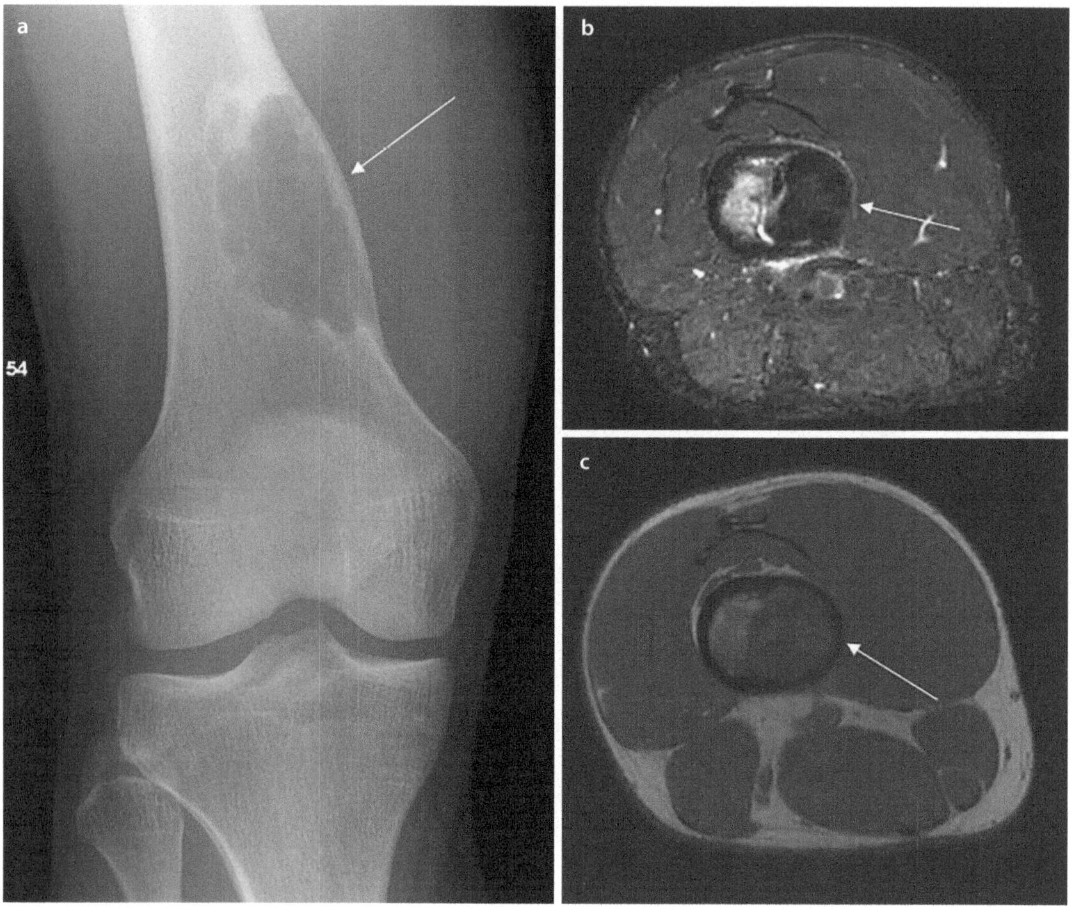

■ Anteroposterior radiograph **a** showing a bubbly osteolytic lesion (arrow) in the distal femoral diaphysis and metaphysis with sharp sclerotic margins and absence of any internal mineralisation or matrix. MRI T2 fat-saturated axial **b** and T1 weighted axial sequence **c** showing lesion (arrows) appearing predominantly hypointense without any cystic components. There is no obvious cortical breach. Imaging findings are of a benign lesion, appearance are of a non-ossifying fibroma (NOF)

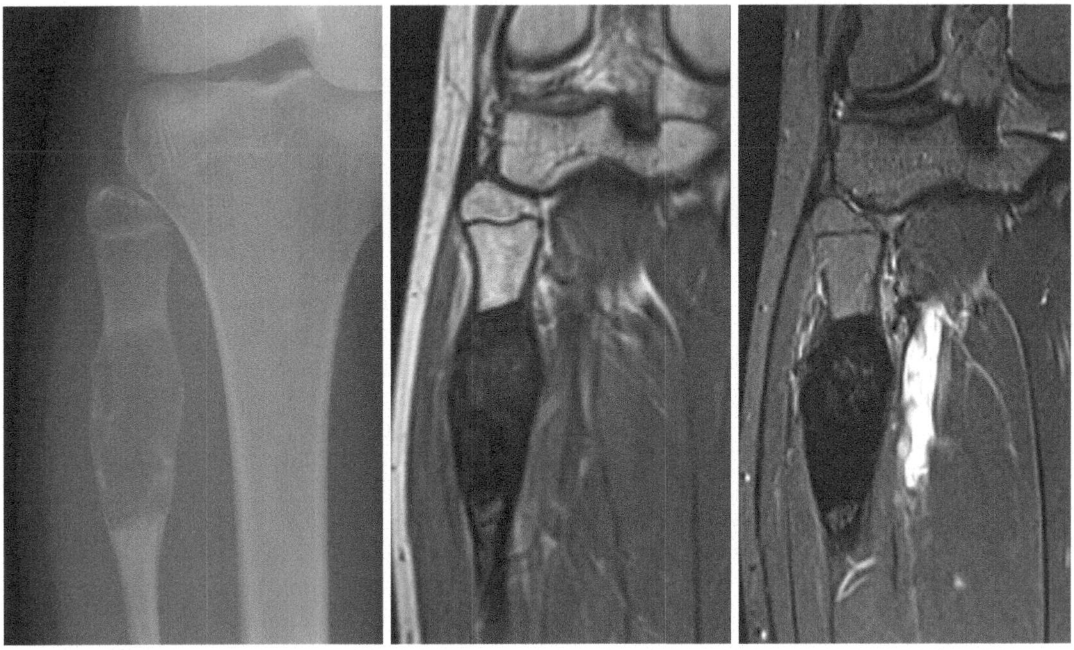

Companion case: Another case of NOF in fibular diaphysis

Non-ossifying Fibroma

Definition and Pathophysiology

- A non-ossifying fibroma (NOF) is a common, benign, fibrous bone lesion that is considered a developmental defect rather than a true tumour. It is essentially a larger version of a fibrous cortical defect (FCD).
- Likely arises from a developmental defect at the physis (growth plate) where proliferating fibroblasts fail to undergo normal ossification.
- Location: Almost exclusively in the metaphysis of long bones, most commonly around the knee (distal femur, proximal tibia).

Clinical Presentation

- Age: most common in children and adolescents (age 5–20 years).
- Asymptomatic (>99% of cases): discovered incidentally on x-rays taken for other reasons (e.g., trauma).
- Pain or pathologic fracture: rarely, a very large lesion (>50% of the bone diameter) can weaken the bone, leading to pain or a fracture after minor trauma.

- It is a "leave-me-alone" lesion. It is asymptomatic, has absolutely no malignant potential, and typically spontaneously regresses (heals by ossifying from the periphery inward) over several years as the skeleton matures.

Imaging Findings

- Radiography
  - Lucent with a well-defined, sclerotic, scalloped margin. Multiloculated or "bubbly" appearance (internal trabeculations). Expansion and thinning of the overlying cortex are common.
  - Healing phase: Gradual filling in with bone, starting from the periphery, eventually becoming sclerotic or normal-appearing bone.
- MRI
  - T1-weighted: Hypointense.
  - T2-weighted: Variable, but often hypointense due to its fibrous content and hemosiderin deposits.

Management

- Observation (standard of care)
  - Asymptomatic lesions require no treatment.
  - Patient and family education is crucial to alleviate anxiety.
- Management of pathologic fracture
  - If a fracture occurs through the lesion, it is typically treated with cast immobilisation.
  - The fracture almost always heals, and the healing process often stimulates ossification and resolution of the NOF itself.
- Surgical intervention
  - A lesion at very high risk for fracture.
  - Persistent pain.
  - A lesion that continues to grow after skeletal maturity (atypical behaviour).
  - Curettage followed by bone grafting can be done.

Suggested Reading

Kato H, Kawaguchi M, Miyase R, Iwashima K, Nagano A, Matsuo M. Comparison of MRI findings among osteofibrous dysplasia, fibrous dysplasia, and nonossifying fibroma of the long bone. Indian J Radiol Imaging. 2023;33(2):150–6. https://doi.org/10.1055/s-0042-1760363.

Rammanohar J, Zhang C, Thahir A, Krkovic M. Imaging of non-ossifying fibromas: a case series. Cureus. 2021;13(3):e14102. https://doi.org/10.7759/cureus.14102.

Case 26

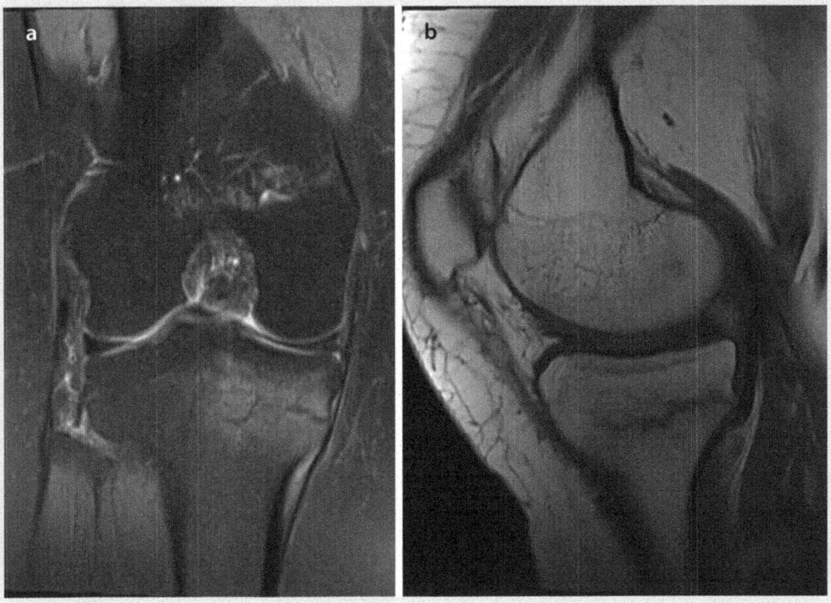

A 35-year-old female presented with persistent pain on the medial aspect of knee joint

S. Saran et al., *101 Knee Imaging Case Series*, 101 MSK Imaging 1,
https://doi.org/10.1007/978-3-032-21567-3_26

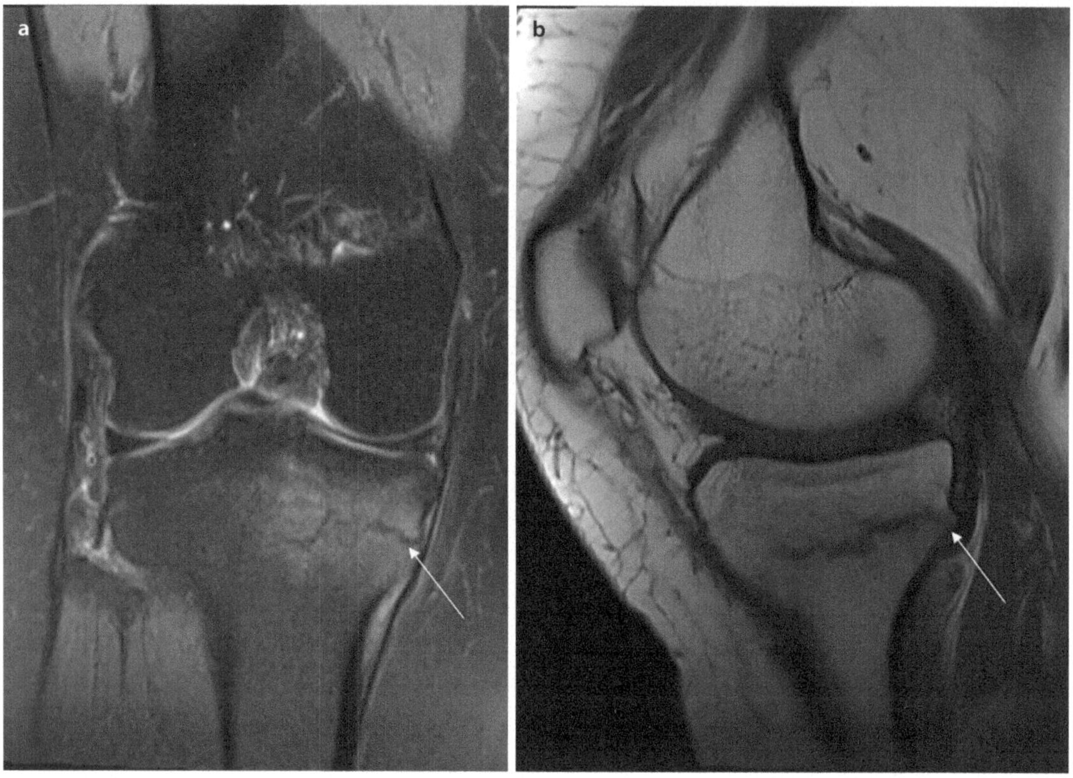

▪ MRI knee PDFS coronal **a** and T1 sagittal **b** shows the presence of a linear hypointense fracture line (arrows) traversing the medial tibial metaphysis with adjacent marrow edema. Without the presence of a history of significant trauma, this indicates the presence of stress/insufficiency fracture

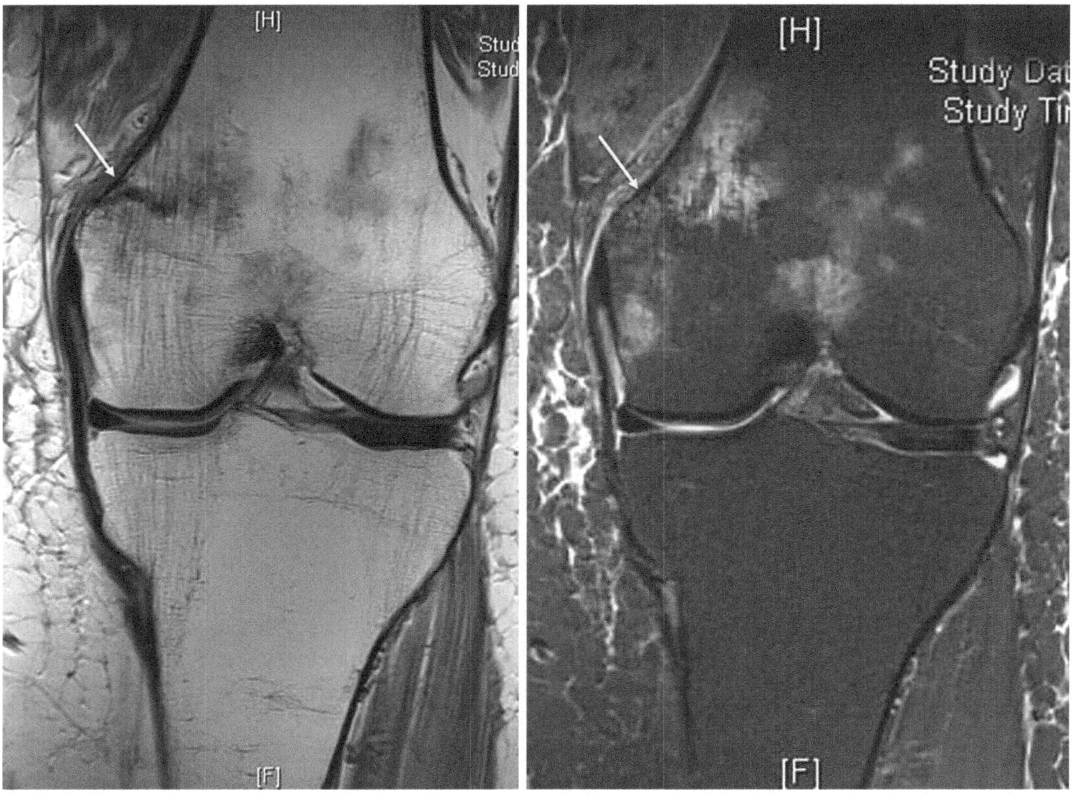

Companion case: Stress fracture in the medial femoral condyle (arrows)

Stress/Insufficiency Fracture

Definition and Pathophysiology

- A stress fracture is an overuse injury resulting from abnormal, repetitive stress on normal bone, while an insufficiency fracture results from normal stress applied to weakened, deficient bone. The medial tibial metaphysis is a common location, particularly for insufficiency fractures in older adults.
- Mechanism:
  - Stress fracture: cyclical loading from activities like running, marching, or jumping exceeds the bone's remodelling capacity, leading to microdamage accumulation and eventual cortical break.
  - Insufficiency fracture: minimal trauma or daily activities cause a fracture in bone with compromised elastic resistance, most commonly due to osteoporosis. Other causes include osteomalacia, rheumatoid arthritis, and radiation therapy.

Clinical Presentation

- Stress fracture: young, active individuals (athletes, military recruits).
- Insufficiency fracture: older, postmenopausal women; patients with comorbidities causing bone weakness.
- Symptoms:
  - Insidious onset of pain, localised to the proximal medial tibia.
  - Pain is activity-related (stress fracture) or may occur at rest (insufficiency fracture).
  - Focal tenderness to palpation over the fracture site.
  - Minimal soft tissue swelling.

Imaging Findings

Imaging appearance varies with the stage of healing.

- Radiography (often normal in early stages)
  - Early findings (2–8 weeks): may be normal or show subtle "grey cortex" sign and periosteal reaction (solid, smooth).
  - Late findings:
    - Focal linear sclerosis perpendicular to the cortex (representing healing callus).
    - A faint fracture line may become visible.
- MRI
  - MRI is exquisitely sensitive for detecting bone marrow oedema and the fracture line long before it is visible on radiograph.
  - T1-Weighted: A discrete, low-signal intensity line surrounded by more diffuse, ill-defined low-signal marrow oedema.
  - Fat-saturated T2-weighted/STIR: The fracture line remains a low-signal line. The surrounding bone marrow shows extensive, confluent high signal intensity oedema. Periosteal oedema is often present.
- Bone scan
  - Shows intense, focal linear uptake ("hot spot") at the fracture site.
  - Lacks the specificity of MRI.

Differential Diagnosis

- Medial tibial stress syndrome ("shin splints").
- Osteoid Osteoma: A benign bone tumour causing intense night pain relieved by NSAIDs. CT shows a radiolucent nidus, often with central mineralisation.

- Osteomyelitis: Clinical signs of infection (fever, erythema). MRI may show a Brodie's abscess, cortical destruction, and a sinus tract.

Management

Treatment is primarily conservative, focusing on offloading the bone to allow healing.

- Conservative management
  - Activity modification: the cornerstone of treatment.
  - Stress fracture: complete rest from the inciting activity for 6–8 weeks. Cross-training with non-impact exercises (swimming, cycling).
  - Insufficiency fracture: reduce impact activities; use assistive devices (cane, walker) for protected weight-bearing.
- Pharmacological
  - Address underlying cause: Calcium, Vitamin D, and Bisphosphonates for osteoporotic insufficiency fractures.
  - Analgesics.
- Physical therapy: For gait training, strengthening of supporting musculature, and gradual return to activity
- Surgical intervention (rare)
  - Indications:
    - Non-union after prolonged conservative treatment.
    - Displaced fracture.
    - Progression to complete fracture.
  - Procedure: Intramedullary nailing to stabilise the tibia.

Suggested Reading

Prasad N, Murray JM, Kumar D, Davies SG. Insufficiency fracture of the tibial plateau: an often missed diagnosis. Acta Orthop Belg. 2006;72(5):587–91.

Sauhta R, Makkar D. Proximal tibia fractures in osteoporosis. Indian J Orthop. 2025;59(3):326–45. https://doi.org/10.1007/s43465-025-01337-1.

Case 27

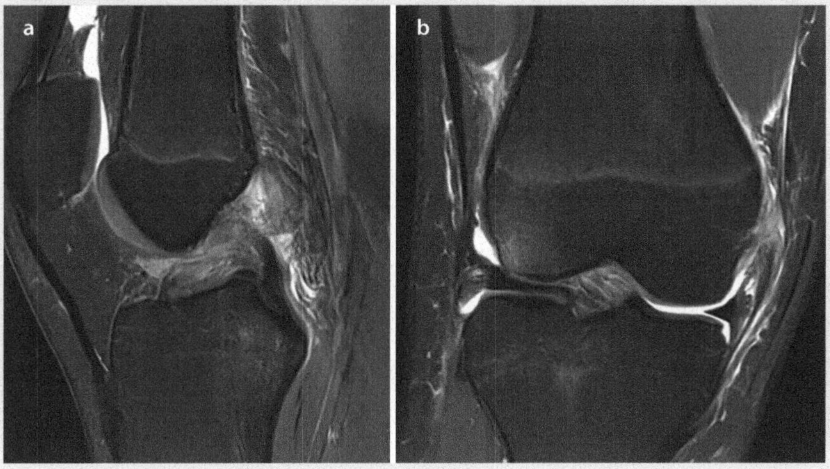

◘ A 22-year-old male with a history of knee trauma

S. Saran et al., *101 Knee Imaging Case Series*, 101 MSK Imaging 1,
https://doi.org/10.1007/978-3-032-21567-3_27

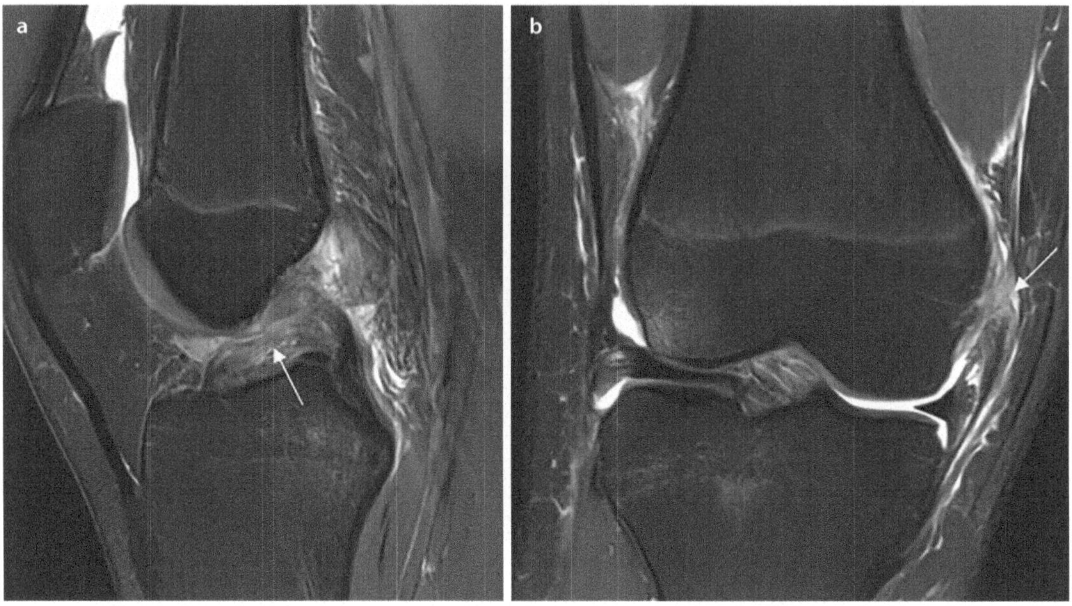

MRI knee sagittal PDFS **a** and coronal PDFS **b** images showing amorphously increased signal intensity in the anterior cruciate ligament (ACL) with laxity of fibres (arrow in **a**), suggesting near-complete thickness ACL tear. There is high-grade partial thickness tear of the femoral attachment of the superficial part of medial collateral ligament (MCL) (arrow in **b**)

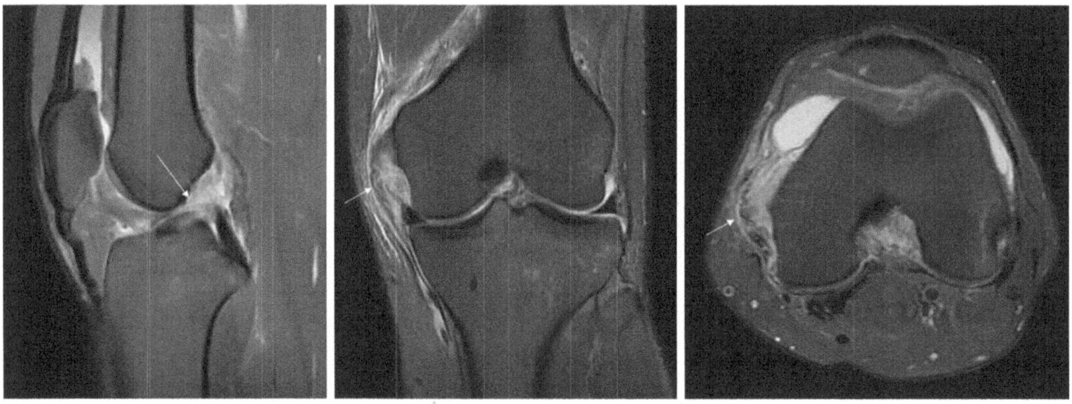

Companion case: A 24-year-old male with knee trauma. MRI shows the presence of a complete ACL tear (long arrow) along with a high-grade tear of the femoral component of the superficial MCL and meniscofemoral ligament (short arrow)

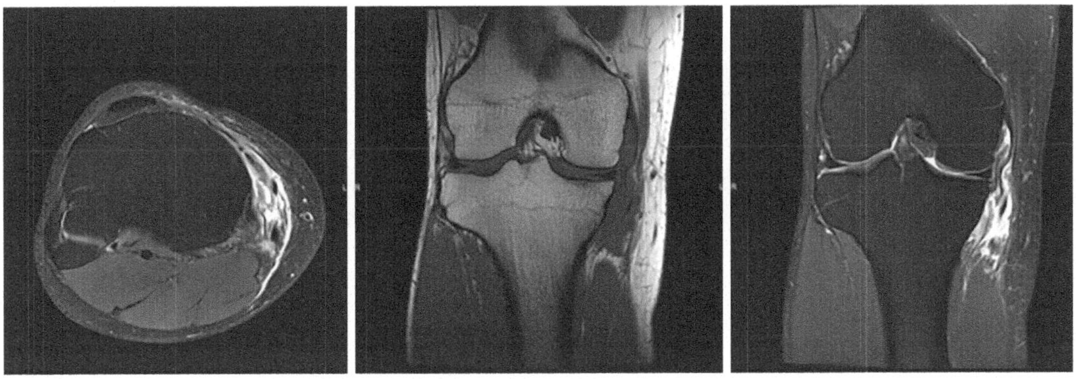

Companion case: A case of an isolated grade III distal MCL tear at the tibial attachment

Combined Anterior Cruciate Ligament (ACL) and High-Grade Medial Collateral Ligament (MCL) Tear (Multi-ligament Knee Injury)

Definition and Pathophysiology

- This is a severe knee injury involving the disruption of two of the knee's primary stabilisers: a complete tear of the Anterior Cruciate Ligament (ACL) and a high-grade (Grade II or III) tear of the Medial Collateral Ligament (MCL). This combination is often referred to as part of the "Unhappy Triad" (O'Donoghue's Triad), which classically includes tears of the ACL, MCL, and medial meniscus.
- Mechanism: Typically caused by a high-energy valgus and external rotation force on a weight-bearing knee. Common in sports (e.g., football, soccer, skiing) and motor vehicle accidents.

Clinical Presentation

- A significant traumatic event with a sensation of the knee "popping" or "giving out".
- Symptoms:
  - Immediate, severe pain and rapid swelling (hemarthrosis).
  - A profound feeling of instability, inability to bear weight.
- Physical exam:
  - Positive Lachman test & pivot shift test: indicative of ACL insufficiency.
  - Pain and laxity on valgus stress testing.
  - Medial joint line tenderness: often present, suggesting possible medial meniscal involvement.

Imaging Findings

- Radiography
  - May be normal or show a joint effusion.
  - In high-grade MCL tears, there may be avulsion fractures at the MCL's femoral or tibial attachment.
  - Assess for associated fractures (e.g., tibial plateau, Segond fracture).
- MRI
  - MRI is essential for confirming the diagnosis, grading the tears, and identifying all associated injuries.
  - ACL complete tear: Full-thickness fibre discontinuity with a visible gap. The ligament appears wavy or retracted.
  - T2/PDFS: Fluid signal intensity filling the gap and surrounding the torn ends.
  - MCL Grade III tear: Complete disruption of all fibres (superficial and deep) from the femur or tibia. There is a visible gap with interposed fluid.
  - Grade II: partial tear with high signal intensity involving >50% of the fibre thickness but with some intact fibres remaining.
  - Surrounding edema and haemorrhage are prominent.
  - Associated injuries: medial meniscus tear: very common (~60% of cases).
  - Lateral compartment "kissing" bone bruises: classic pattern on the lateral femoral condyle and posterolateral tibial plateau from the subluxation event.
  - Other ligaments: Evaluate the posterolateral corner (PLC) and PCL.

Management

- Management is complex and must address both ligaments, often in a staged manner.
- Acute phase management (first 1–3 Weeks):
  - Protection: Hinged knee brace locked in extension to protect the MCL and allow it to heal in a reduced position.
  - Weight-bearing: Non-weight-bearing or toe-touch weight-bearing with crutches.
- Definitive management:
  - The treatment strategy is primarily determined by the grade of the MCL injury.
  - MCL repair/reconstruction + ACL reconstruction in a single surgery. This is common for proximal MCL avulsions or when the MCL is incarcerated in the joint.

- Rehabilitation:
  - Post-operative/healing phase: focus on restoring range of motion (avoiding valgus stress), reducing swelling, and quadriceps activation.
  - Strengthening & proprioception: gradual progression to dynamic stabilization exercises.
  - Return to sport: typically takes 9–12 months of dedicated rehabilitation.

Suggested Reading

Cristiani R, van de Bunt F, Kvist J, Stålman A. High prevalence of associated injuries in anterior cruciate ligament tears: a detailed magnetic resonance imaging analysis of 254 patients. Skeletal Radiol. 2024;53(11):2417–27.

Wright ML, Coladonato C, Ciccotti MG, Tjoumakaris FP, Freedman KB. Combined anterior cruciate ligament and medial collateral ligament reconstruction shows high rates of return to activity and low rates of recurrent valgus instability: an updated systematic review. Arthrosc Sports Med Rehabil. 2023;5(3):e867–79.

Case 28

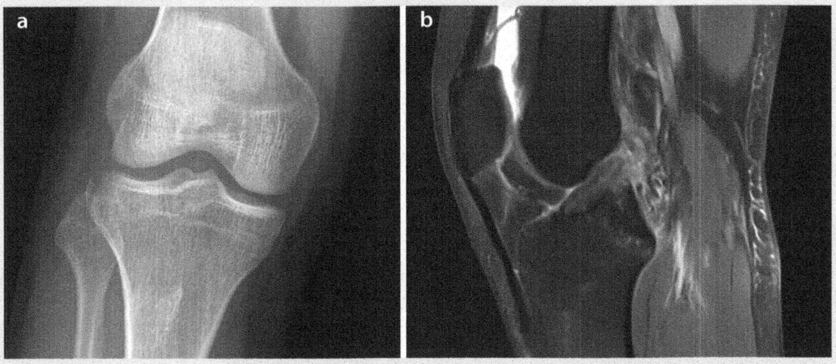

■ A 32-year-old male presented with a twisting knee injury followed by swelling of the knee joint and painful limitation of movements

S. Saran et al., *101 Knee Imaging Case Series*, 101 MSK Imaging 1,
https://doi.org/10.1007/978-3-032-21567-3_28

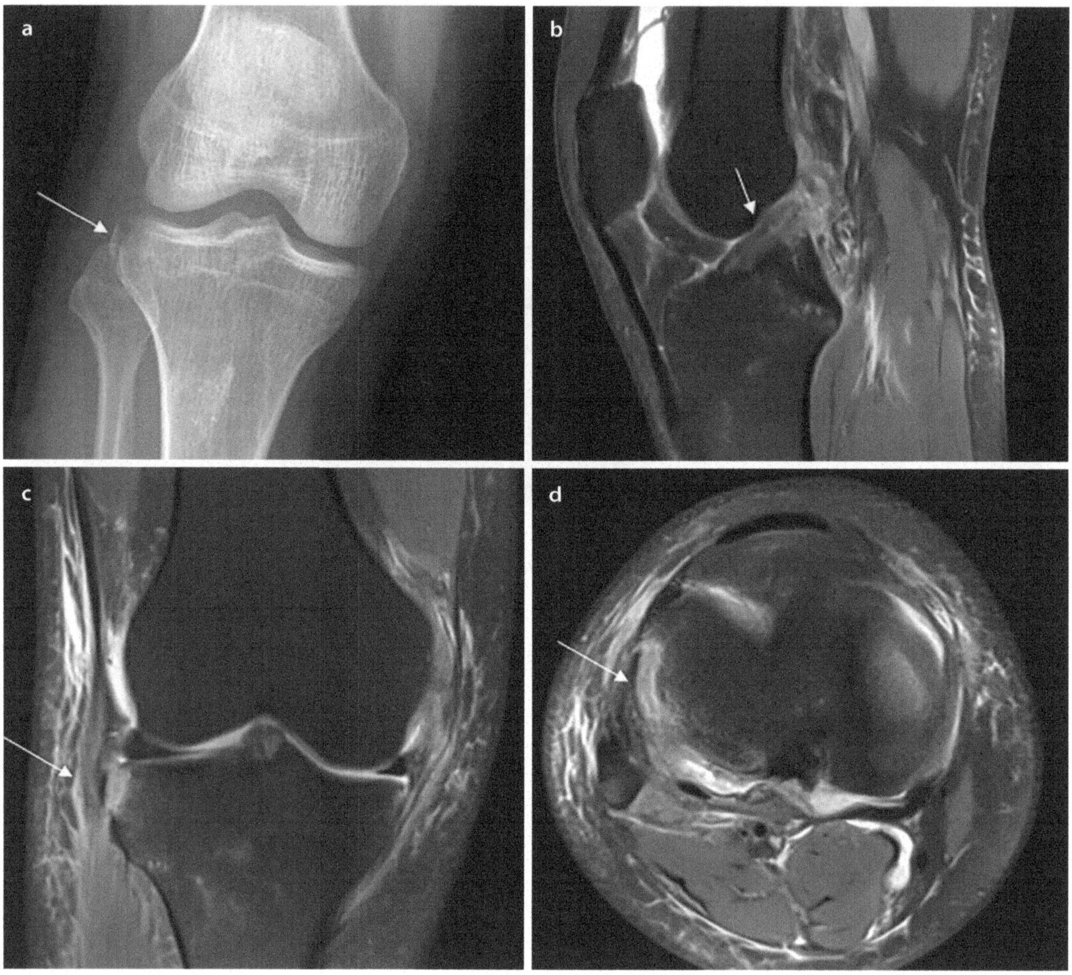

■ Radiograph **a** shows a curvilinear bone fragment lying parallel to the lateral aspect of the tibial plateau (arrow). MRI knee, PDFS weighted sagittal **a**, coronal **b**, and axial **c**, sequences showing a complete ACL tear (arrow in **b**) with a curvilinear bone fragment avulsed from the underlying lateral aspect of the tibial plateau (arrows in **c** and **d**). Imaging findings are suggestive of a complete ACL tear with Segond's fracture. The torn ligament is the Anterolateral ligament

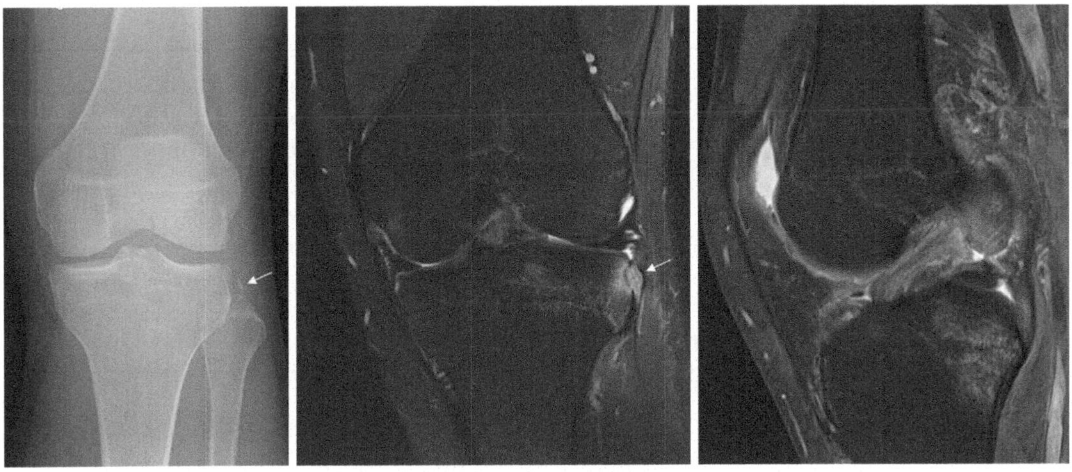

Companion case: Another case of complete ACL tear with Segond's fracture (arrows)

Segond's Fracture - Definition and Pathophysiology

- A Segond fracture is an avulsion fracture of the lateral aspect of the proximal tibia, just below the knee joint. It is not a primary injury but rather a highly significant secondary sign of profound internal knee derangement.
- Avulsed structure: The fracture fragment is avulsed by the Anterolateral ligament and the middle third of the lateral capsular ligament.

Clinical Significance: The "Tell-Tale" Sign

- The paramount importance of a Segond fracture lies in its near-pathognomonic association with soft tissue injuries inside the knee. It is a marker of severe trauma.
- ACL Tear: found in 75–100% of cases. The same forces that cause the Segond fracture almost always rupture the ACL.
- Meniscal tears: associated with lateral meniscal tears (66–75% of cases) and medial meniscal tears.
- Other ligament injuries: possible injury to the medial collateral ligament (MCL) or posterior cruciate ligament (PCL).

Clinical Presentation

- Significant acute knee trauma (e.g., sports injury, fall, car accident) with a twisting mechanism.
- Immediate pain, swelling (hemarthrosis), and a feeling of the knee "giving way".
- Signs: clinical signs of ACL deficiency (e.g., positive Lachman test) and lateral joint line tenderness.

Imaging Findings

- Radiography
  - A small, elliptical, curvilinear bone fragment avulsed from the lateral tibial plateau.
  - Typically, 2–4 mm below the cortex and posterior to Gerdy's tubercle (ITB insertion).
  - Best seen on the anteroposterior and internal rotation views of the knee.
  - If seen, it mandates MRI.
- MRI
  - Confirms the avulsion and associated bone marrow oedema.
  - ACL tear: identifies the complete rupture.
  - Meniscal and other ligament injuries.
  - Bone bruise pattern: often shows classic "kissing contusions" on the lateral femoral condyle and lateral tibial plateau.

Management

Treatment is never directed at the Segond fracture itself but at the associated ligamentous and meniscal injuries.

- Acute phase:
  - RICE Protocol (Rest, Ice, Compression, Elevation)
  - Hinged knee brace and crutches for protection.
- Definitive management:
  - ACL reconstruction: The cornerstone of treatment. This is almost always required to restore knee stability.
  - Meniscal repair vs. meniscectomy: depending on the type and location of the meniscal tear.
  - The Segond fragment: The small bony fragment is typically left alone. It often heals uneventfully once the knee is stabilised. It is rarely fixed surgically unless it is very large and displaced.

Prognosis

The prognosis is determined by the success of the ACL reconstruction and the treatment of any associated meniscal or ligament injuries. The presence of a Segond fracture indicates a high-energy injury, but outcomes are generally excellent with appropriate surgical and rehabilitative management.

Suggested Reading

Gottsegen CJ, Eyer BA, White EA, et al. Avulsion fractures of the knee: imaging findings and clinical significance. Radiographics. 2008;28(6):1755–70. https://doi.org/10.1148/rg.286085503.

Roberts CC, Towers JD, Spangehl MJ, et al. Advanced MR imaging of the cruciate ligaments. Radiol Clin North Am. 2007;45(6):1003–16., vi–vii. https://doi.org/10.1016/j.rcl.2007.08.007.

Case 29

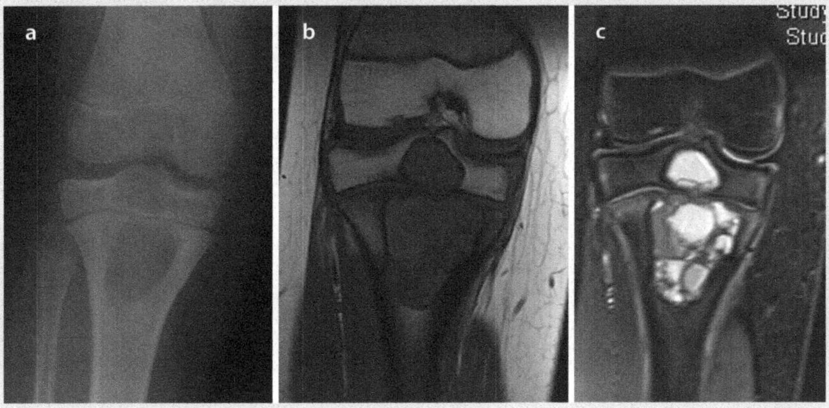

■ A 11-year-old male presented with pain in the right knee joint

S. Saran et al., *101 Knee Imaging Case Series*, 101 MSK Imaging 1,
https://doi.org/10.1007/978-3-032-21567-3_29

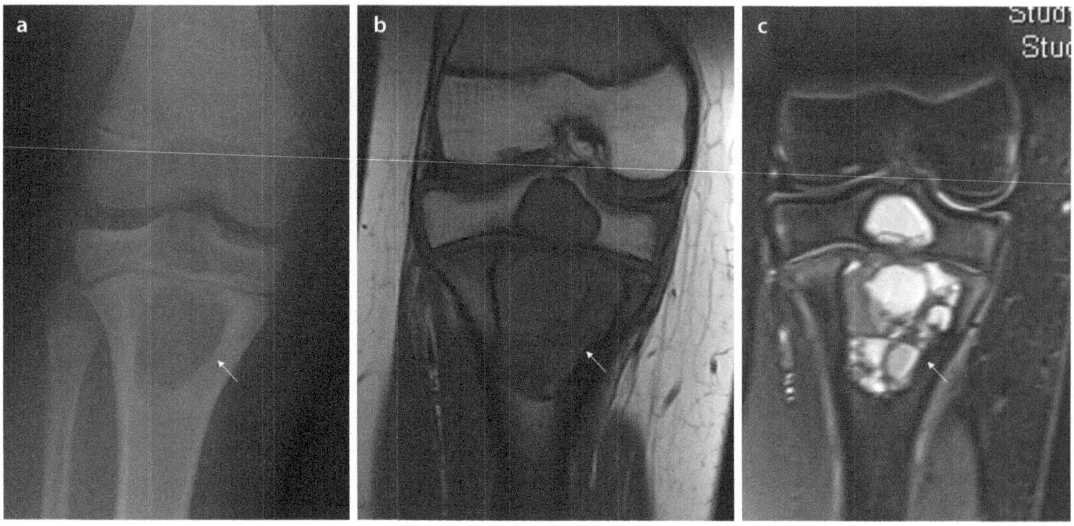

Radiograph **a** shows the presence of an expansile osteolytic lesion (arrow) in the proximal tibial metaphysis with extension into the epiphysis. MRI coronal; T1 **b** and STIR **c** shows the lesion as a multiloculated cystic lesion with varying signal intensities (arrows). The lesion was diagnosed as an aneurysmal bone cyst on histopathology

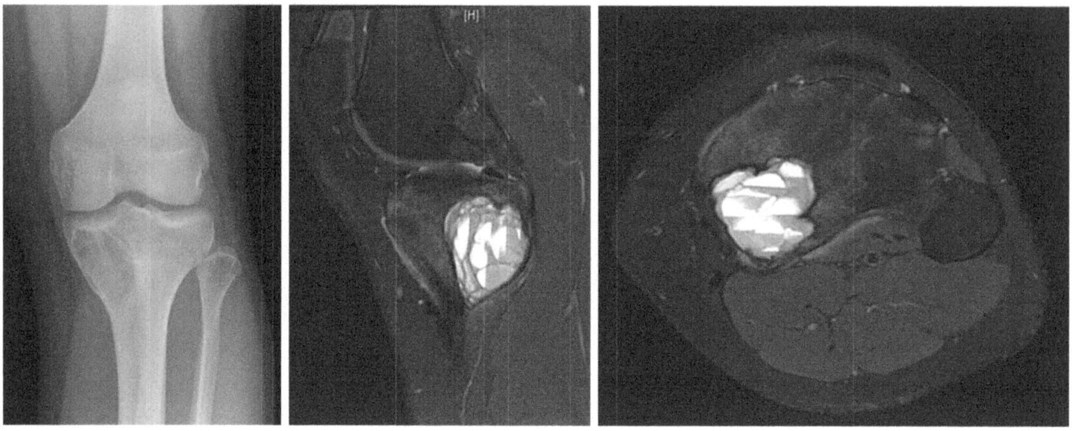

Companion case: another case of ABC in the proximal tibia with multiple fluid-fluid levels

Aneurysmal Bone Cyst

Definition and Pathophysiology

- An aneurysmal bone cyst (ABC) is a benign, locally destructive, expansile, osteolytic lesion of bone characterised by blood-filled spaces separated by connective tissue septae containing osteoclast-type giant cells and reactive bone. It can be primary (~70%) or secondary to an underlying bone

lesion (e.g., chondroblastoma, giant cell tumour, osteoblastoma).
- Pathogenesis: The primary form is driven by a specific genetic alteration—a translocation involving the USP6 gene on chromosome 17. This leads to increased matrix metalloproteinase activity, causing the characteristic expansile and destructive growth.
- It is a "blow-out" or "ballooned" lytic lesion filled with blood-filled cavities, giving it a characteristic multiloculated, "soap-bubble" appearance on imaging.

Clinical Presentation

- Demographics: Most common in children and adolescents (over 80% occur in patients under 20 years).
- Location: The proximal tibia is a very common site, along with the distal femur.
- Symptoms:
  - Pain and swelling: the most common symptoms, often present for weeks to months.
  - Palpable mass: a firm, sometimes tender expansion of the bone.
  - Pathologic fracture: can occur due to cortical thinning.
  - Limited range of motion: if located near the knee joint.

Imaging Findings

- Radiography
  - An eccentric, expansile, lytic ("blow-out") lesion.
  - Margin: typically has a well-defined, sclerotic rim.
  - Cortex: markedly thinned and expanded ("eggshell thinning"), but usually intact unless fractured.
  - Internal pattern: often shows a "soap-bubble" or multiloculated appearance due to internal septations.
  - No matrix mineralisation: the lesion is purely lytic.
- MRI
  - MRI is the best modality for confirming the diagnosis and defining the full extent, including any soft tissue component.
  - T1-Weighted: The lesion is heterogeneous with predominantly low to intermediate signal intensity. The septations are seen as low-signal lines.
  - T2-weighted fat-saturated/ STIR: The lesion is multiloculated with multiple fluid-fluid levels of varying signal intensity (due to blood products of different ages).
  - T1-weighted post-contrast: The septations and solid components (if present) enhance vividly, while the fluid-filled cavities do not.

Differential Diagnosis

- Simple bone cyst (unicameral bone cyst): Typically central, less expansile, and does not show fluid-fluid levels or enhancement. The "fallen fragment sign" is classic for a fracture in a simple bone cyst.
- Giant cell tumour of bone: occurs in skeletally mature patients. It is purely lytic, extends to the subchondral bone, and lacks a sclerotic rim and prominent fluid-fluid levels.
- Chondromyxoid fibroma: an eccentric, expansile lytic lesion with a sclerotic rim that can look very similar, but it typically lacks the prominent fluid-fluid levels of an ABC.
- Telangiectatic osteosarcoma: The most important mimic. It can appear identical with expansile growth and fluid-fluid levels. Key differentiators are its more aggressive, permeative margins, and the solid, enhancing tissue is typically more nodular and mass-like.

Management

- Minimally invasive interventions
  - Percutaneous sclerotherapy: an option for selected lesions. Under imaging guidance, a sclerosing agent is injected into the cyst to induce fibrosis and ossification. This avoids a large open surgery but has a variable success rate.
  - Embolisation: may be used pre-operatively for very vascular lesions or as a primary treatment in surgically challenging locations (e.g., the spine).
- Surgical intervention
  - Procedure: intralesional curettage and adjuvant therapy.

Suggested Reading

Restrepo R, Zahrah D, Pelaez L, Temple HT, Murakami JW. Update on aneurysmal bone cyst: pathophysiology, histology, imaging and treatment. Pediatr Radiol. 2022;52(9):1601–14.

Zishan US, Pressney I, Khoo M, Saifuddin A. The differentiation between aneurysmal bone cyst and telangiectatic osteosarcoma: a clinical, radiographic and MRI study. Skeletal Radiol. 2020;49(9):1375–86.

Case 30

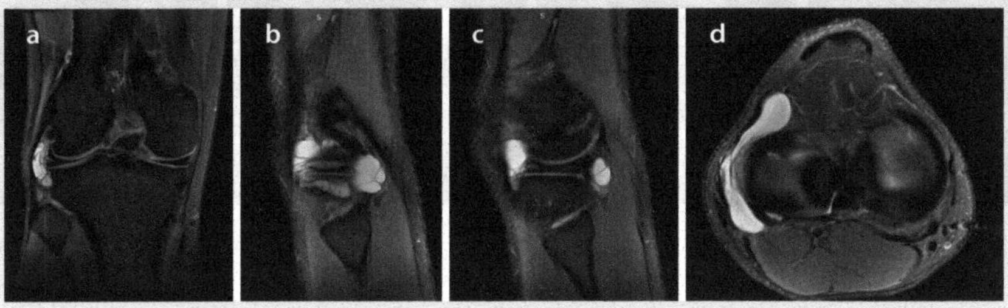

A 26-year-old male presented with pain and swelling along the medial joint line in the knee joint

S. Saran et al., *101 Knee Imaging Case Series*, 101 MSK Imaging 1,
https://doi.org/10.1007/978-3-032-21567-3_30

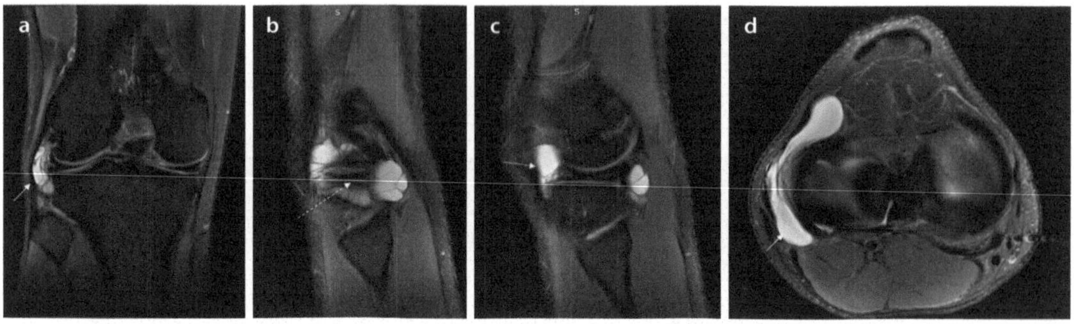

■ MRI knee, PDFS weighted coronal **a**, sagittal **b** and **c**, and axial **d**, sequences showing a well-defined multi-loculated cystic lesion (arrows) adjacent to the lateral meniscus with a horizontal tear (dashed arrow) in the body of the lateral meniscus. Imaging findings are of a horizontal lateral meniscal tear with a parameniscal cyst

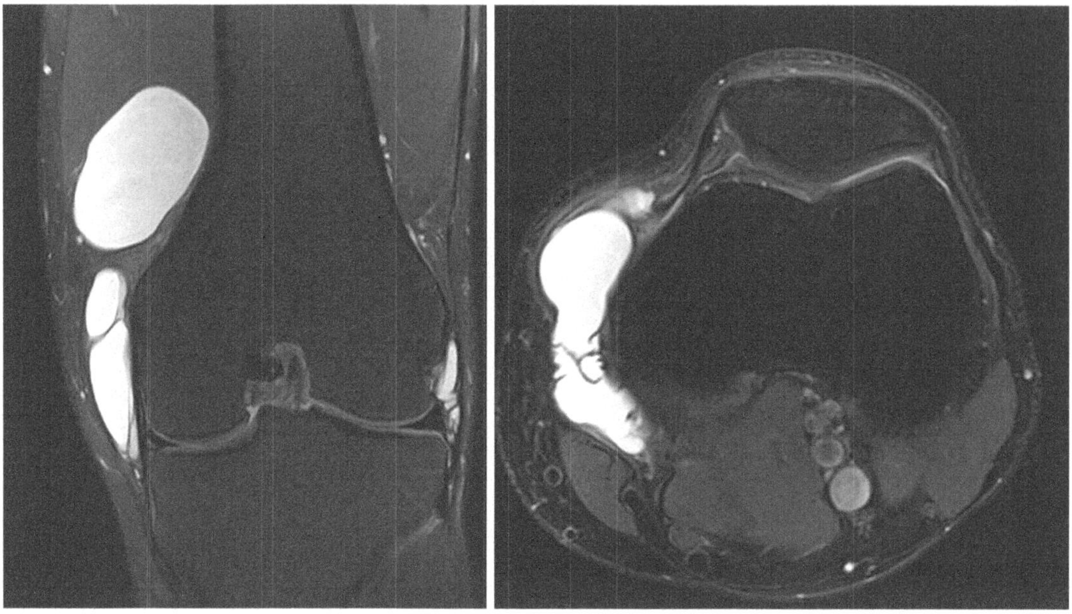

■ Companion case: A complex cystic lesion along the medial joint line with no obvious visible communication with the meniscus

Parameniscal Cyst – Definition and Pathophysiology

- A parameniscal cyst is a fluid-filled sac that forms adjacent to a torn meniscus. It is not a standalone condition but a direct consequence of a meniscal tear.
- Synovial fluid extrudes from the joint space through a horizontal cleavage tear (most common) or a complex tear in the meniscus. The fluid becomes trapped outside the joint, forming a cystic cavity.

- "Check-valve" mechanism: The tear acts as a one-way valve, allowing fluid to pump out of the joint during movement but preventing its return, leading to cyst enlargement.

Clinical Presentation

- Palpable mass: a firm, tender lump near the joint line.
- Pain: localised pain over the cyst, often worsened with activity.
- Clicking, locking, or catching if the underlying meniscal tear is unstable.

Imaging Findings

- MRI
  - A well-defined, fluid-intensity mass (hyperintense on T2-weighted and PDFS images) located adjacent to the meniscus, often in the pericapsular soft tissues.
  - The "Tail Sign": A crucial diagnostic feature. A linear fluid signal is seen tracking from the cyst back to the underlying meniscal tear, confirming the connection.
  - Meniscal tear: Evidence of the causative tear, almost always a horizontal cleavage tear or complex degeneration.
- Ultrasound
  - Shows a well-defined anechoic cystic structure with posterior acoustic enhancement.
  - Can be used to guide diagnostic or therapeutic aspiration/injection.

Management

Treatment is directed at the underlying meniscal tear, not just the cyst itself. Addressing the tear eliminates the fluid leak that causes the cyst.

- Conservative management
  - Activity modification: Avoid activities that aggravate symptoms.
  - NSAIDs: for pain and inflammation.
  - Image-guided aspiration: Ultrasound-guided drainage of the cyst can provide temporary relief, but recurrence is very high if the meniscal tear is not addressed.
- Surgical management
  - Indication: Persistent pain or mechanical symptoms despite conservative care.
  - Procedure: Arthroscopic surgery.

- Partial meniscectomy: The primary treatment. Debriding the unstable torn meniscal tissue and removing the "one-way valve" allows the cyst to decompress and resolve spontaneously.
- Cyst decompression: Occasionally, the cyst is directly decompressed or excised arthroscopically or open if it is very large, but this is often unnecessary after the tear is addressed.
- Outcome: Excellent. Resection of the torn meniscal tissue eliminates the fluid pathway, leading to cyst resolution and symptom relief.

Suggested Reading

De Smet AA, Graf BK, del Rio AM. Association of parameniscal cysts with underlying meniscal tears as identified on MRI and arthroscopy. AJR Am J Roentgenol. 2011;196(2):W180–6. https://doi.org/10.2214/AJR.10.4754.

Stensby JD, Pringle LC, Crim J. MRI of the meniscus. Clin Sports Med. 2021;40(4):641–55. https://doi.org/10.1016/j.csm.2021.05.004.

Case 31

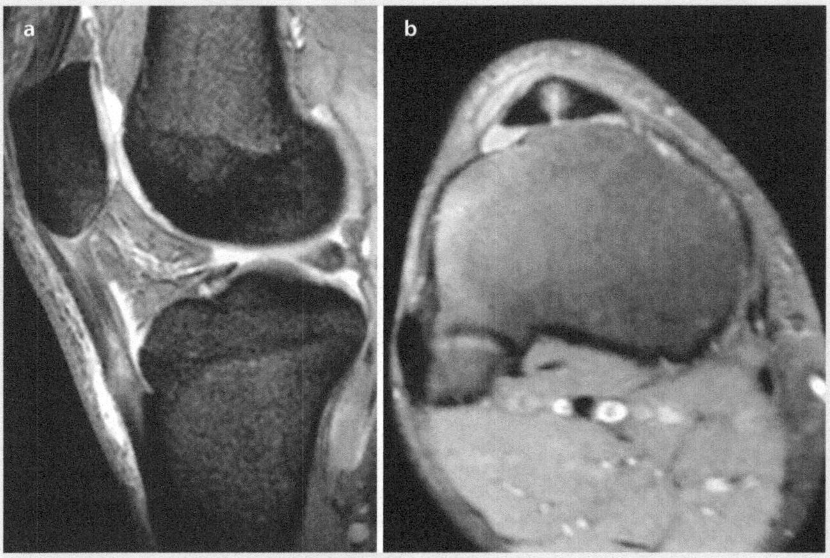

A 23-year-old male presented with knee pain predominantly in the extensor aspect

S. Saran et al., *101 Knee Imaging Case Series*, 101 MSK Imaging 1,
https://doi.org/10.1007/978-3-032-21567-3_31

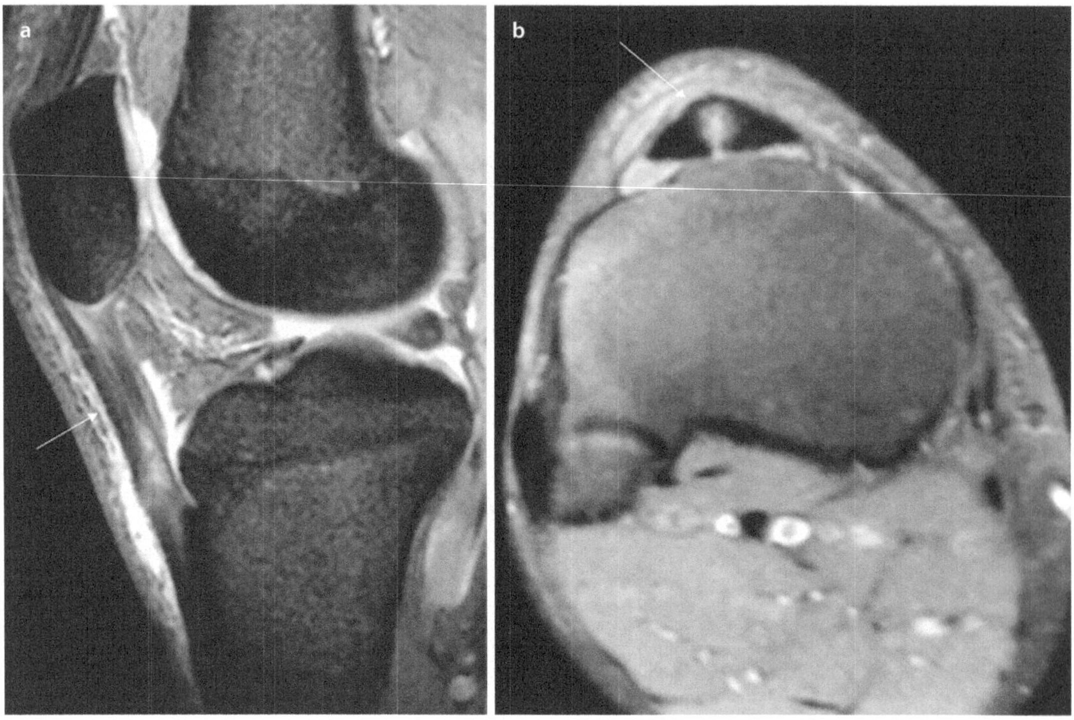

◘ MRI **a** and **b** shows diffuse thickening of the patellar tendon (arrows) with increased signal intensity on PDFS weighted sagittal **a** and axial **b** sequences, suggestive of patellar tendinosis/tendinopathy

Patellar Tendinosis/Tendinopathy ("Jumper's Knee")

Definition & Pathophysiology

- Patellar tendinosis is a degenerative condition of the patellar tendon, characterised by collagen breakdown, fibre disorganisation, and failed healing response at the tendon's origin on the inferior pole of the patella or sometimes the entire patellar tendon.
- Mechanism: Caused by repetitive mechanical overload (microtrauma) from activities involving forceful quadriceps contraction, such as jumping, landing, and cutting. This leads to microscopic tears and a degenerative cascade without adequate repair.

Clinical Presentation

- Demographics: Common in athletes involved in basketball, volleyball, soccer, and track & field ("Jumper's Knee").

- Symptoms: pain exacerbated by loading the extensor mechanism, point tenderness at the patellar tendon origin and stiffness, especially after periods of inactivity.

Imaging Findings

- Ultrasound
  - Shows a hypoechoic and thickened patellar tendon, particularly involving the deep posterior fibres. There may be focal defects, calcifications, or neovascularity.
  - Doppler may show hyperaemia (neovascularisation) within the tendon, indicating active repair/angiofibroblastic response.
- MRI
  - T1-Weighted & PD-Weighted: The patellar tendon appears thickened with focal or diffuse intermediate signal intensity replacing the normal low-signal tendon fibres.
  - T2-weighted/STIR: Shows increased signal intensity within the thickened tendon, representing mucoid degeneration, oedema, and tearing.
  - There may be reactive oedema in the inferior pole of the patella and Hoffa's fat pad oedema adjacent to the abnormal tendon segment.
  - Partial tearing in severe cases can be seen.

Differential Diagnosis

- Patellar tendon tear (partial or complete): presents with acute pain and functional loss; MRI shows a discrete, fluid-signal defect.
- Sinding-Larsen-Johansson syndrome: traction apophysitis at the inferior patellar pole in skeletally immature patients.
- Hoffa's fat pad impingement: pain is located deeper, adjacent to the tendon, and worsens with hyperextension.
- Infrapatellar bursitis: inflammation of the superficial or deep infrapatellar bursa.

Management

- Conservative management (first-line):
  - Activity modification and physical therapy form the cornerstone of treatment.
  - Extracorporeal shockwave therapy (ESWT): Can stimulate healing in refractory cases.

- Image-guided intervention (corticosteroid injection):
  - Use is controversial. Provides short-term pain relief but may impair long-term tendon healing and carries a risk of tendon rupture. Generally avoided.
- Ultrasound-guided percutaneous tenotomy (needling): A needle is used to repeatedly fenestrate the degenerative tendon to stimulate a healing response.
- Platelet-Rich Plasma (PRP) Injection: An emerging treatment where concentrated growth factors from the patient's own blood are injected into the degenerative focus to promote biologic healing. Often used after failed physical therapy.
- Surgical Intervention (for refractory cases):
  - Indication: Persistent, debilitating symptoms after 6–12 months of failed comprehensive non-operative management.
  - Procedure: Arthroscopic or open debridement.
  - A prolonged, structured rehabilitation program is essential post-operatively.

Suggested Reading

Everhart JS, Cole D, Sojka JH, Higgins JD, Magnussen RA, Schmitt LC, Flanigan DC. Treatment options for patellar tendinopathy: a systematic review. Arthroscopy. 2017;33(4):861–72.

Sugrañes J, Jackson GR, Mameri ES, Schundler S, Obioha OA, Pascual TA, Chahla J. Current concepts in patellar tendinopathy: an overview of imaging, pathogenesis, and nonoperative and operative management. JBJS Rev. 2023;11(8).

Case 32

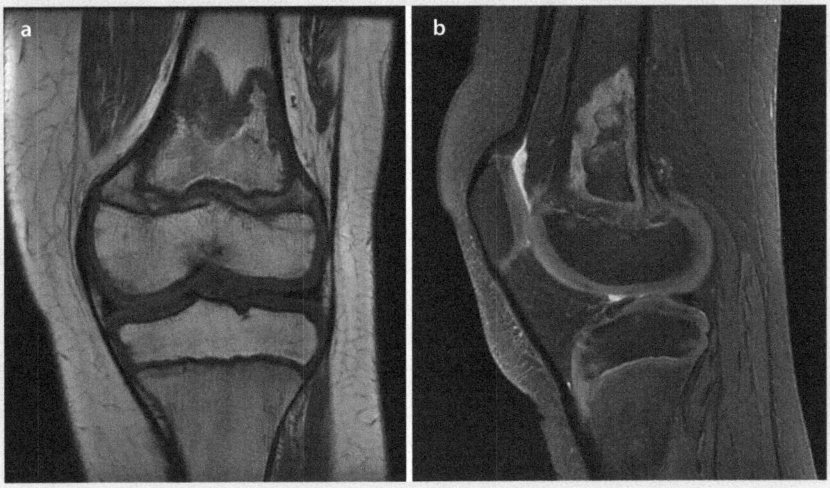

A 9-year-old male patient presented with pain around the knee joint

S. Saran et al., *101 Knee Imaging Case Series*, 101 MSK Imaging 1,
https://doi.org/10.1007/978-3-032-21567-3_32

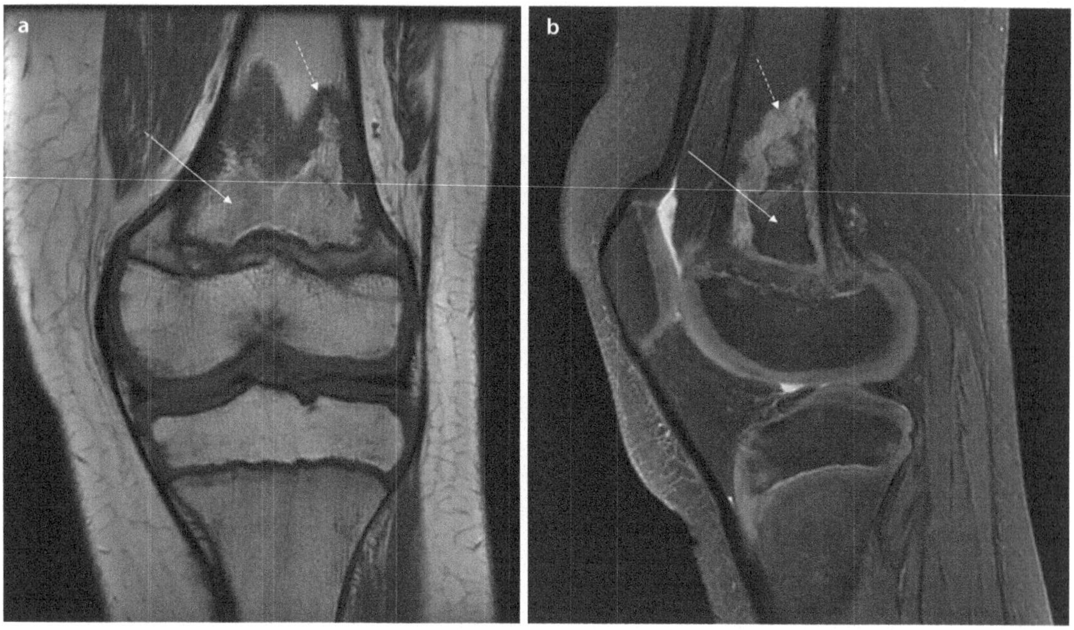

■ MRI knee, T1 weighted coronal **a** and PDFS sagittal **b**, sequences showing a geographic area of low signal intensity on T1 and high signal intensity on PDFS in the distal femur (dashed arrow) with a well-defined, serpentine border and central fatty marrow signal (arrow). Findings are consistent with bone infarct or osteonecrosis

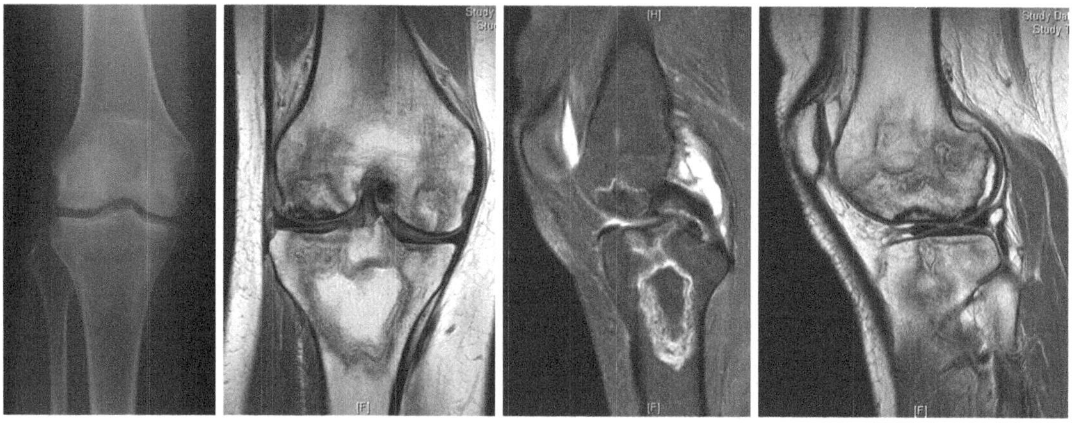

■ Companion case: Another case of multiple bone infarcts affecting the distal femur and proximal tibia, also involving the subchondral region

Bone Infarcts

Definition & Pathophysiology

- A bone infarct, also known as aseptic or avascular osteonecrosis (AVN), is the death of bony and marrow components due to a disruption of its blood supply. In the distal femur, it typically occurs in the metaphysis or epiphysis.
- Mechanism: Interruption of the blood flow leads to ischemia → death of osteocytes and bone marrow → structural weakening. The body attempts to repair the area with a process called "creeping substitution", where new bone forms on dead trabeculae. This repair process is slow and can be incomplete, leaving the area mechanically weak and prone to collapse, especially if it occurs in a weight-bearing area like the femoral condyles.

Common Causes & Risk Factors

- Corticosteroid use (most common association)
- Alcohol abuse
- Trauma (fractures disrupting blood supply)
- Sickle cell disease (vaso-occlusive crisis)
- Decompression sickness
- Connective tissue diseases (e.g., SLE)
- Radiotherapy
- Idiopathic

Clinical Presentation

- Early stages: often asymptomatic and discovered incidentally on imaging.
- Symptomatic stages:
  - Pain: deep, aching, or throbbing pain in the knee (if distal femur is involved), which is insidious in onset and worsens with weight-bearing.
  - Limited range of motion: if the articular surface is involved or collapses.
  - Sudden worsening: if subchondral collapse occurs, it can lead to acute severe pain and joint dysfunction.

Imaging Findings: Imaging Evolution Mirrors the Pathological Process

- Radiography
  - Early stages: normal.
  - Intermediate stages:
    - Mottled lucency: Areas of decreased density due to bone resorption.
    - Sclerosis: A surrounding rim of sclerosis as the body attempts to wall off the infarct.
  - Late stages:
    - "Serpiginous" or "map-like" pattern: A classic appearance of a well-defined, serpentine, sclerotic rim surrounding a lucent area.
    - Subchondral collapse: If the infarct is subarticular, a crescent sign (a subchondral lucent line) may appear, indicating fracture and impending collapse.
    - Secondary osteoarthritis: From collapse of the articular surface.
- MRI
  - MRI is the most sensitive and specific modality, detecting changes long before X-rays.
  - Classic "double line" sign: Pathognomonic on T2-weighted images.
  - An outer low-signal rim (sclerotic bone).
  - An inner high-signal rim (granulation tissue at the repair interface).
  - T1-weighted: A geographic area of low signal intensity with a well-defined, serpentine border and central fatty marrow.
  - Bone marrow oedema on fluid-sensitive sequences (STIR, T2 FS) in acute or symptomatic phases.
- Bone scan: Can show increased uptake ("hot spot") in the reparative phase, but is less specific than MRI.

Differential Diagnosis

- Enchondroma and low-grade chondrosarcoma: A cartilaginous tumour that can be lucent on X-ray but has a different MRI appearance (lobulated, T2 hyperintense, no serpentine border). The central marrow signal seen in an infarct is not seen in an enchondroma and low-grade chondrosarcoma.

Management

- Treatment depends on the size, location, and stage of the infarct, and whether the articular surface has collapsed.
- Asymptomatic infarct: Observation and risk factor modification (e.g., reduce steroid dose, manage lipid levels).

- Symptomatic infarct without collapse.
  - Goal: To prevent collapse and preserve the joint.
  - Core decompression: A surgical procedure where a core of bone is removed from the involved area. This decreases intraosseous pressure and stimulates neovascularisation and healing. It can be combined with bone grafting (vascularized or non-vascularized) or biologic adjuvants (e.g., BMP).
  - Protected weight-bearing: Not proven to prevent collapse, but is often used.
- Symptomatic infarct with articular collapse.
  - Joint-preserving procedures: For younger patients, options include:
    - Osteotomy: To realign the limb and shift weight away from the collapsed area.
    - Bone grafting: Structural grafts to support the collapsed articular surface.
  - Joint arthroplasty (replacement):
    - Unicompartmental knee arthroplasty (UKA): If only one femoral condyle is affected.
    - Total knee arthroplasty (TKA): For extensive involvement or advanced secondary osteoarthritis. This is the most common definitive treatment for end-stage disease.

Suggested Reading

Gulghane A, Gomase K, Taksande V, Sood A. Avascular necrosis of lateral femoral condyle in a middle-aged woman from Central India. Radiol Case Rep. 2025;20(6):2870–3.

Hedayati R, Soltanabadi M. Incidental osteonecrosis in the distal left femur in a case of beta-thalassemia with COVID-19: role of [99mTc]Tc-MDP whole-body bone scan. Nucl Med Rev Cent East Eur. 2023;26:46–8.

van Houten P, de Rooy J, van der Geest I, Netea-Maier R, van de Ven A. Spontaneous bone infarction of the distal femur in a patient with Cushing's disease: a case report. Bone Rep. 2021;14:100756.

Case 33

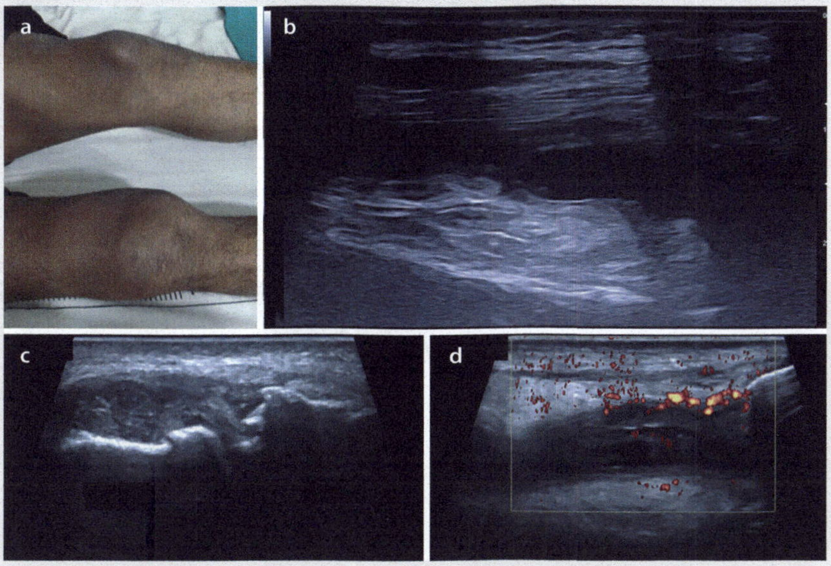

A 16-year-old male presented with pain and swelling in the right knee joint

S. Saran et al., *101 Knee Imaging Case Series*, 101 MSK Imaging 1,
https://doi.org/10.1007/978-3-032-21567-3_33

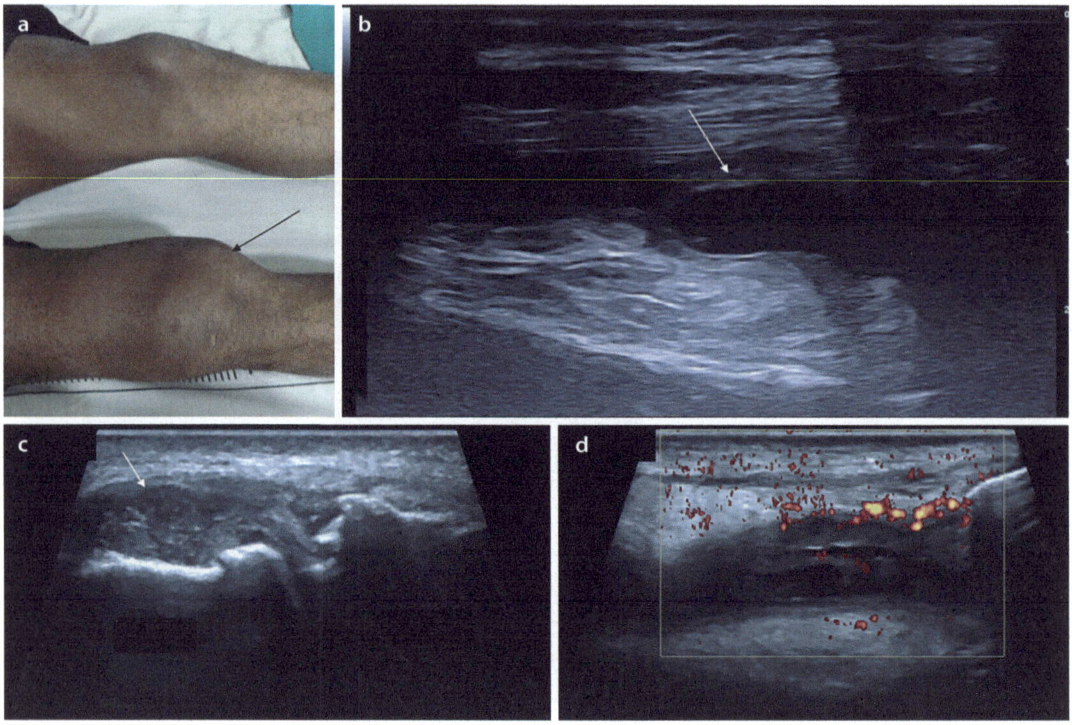

◘ Clinical picture **a** depicts swelling in the right knee joint (arrow). Ultrasound **b–d** shows the presence of joint effusion and synovial thickening (arrows) with the presence of increased Doppler activity, suggesting active inflammation. Ultrasound findings and clinical profile favoured the diagnosis of juvenile idiopathic arthritis

Juvenile Idiopathic Arthritis

Definition & Pathophysiology

- Juvenile Idiopathic Arthritis (JIA) is the most common chronic rheumatic disease in children, defined as arthritis of unknown cause that begins before the 16th birthday and persists for at least 6 weeks. It is an umbrella term for a heterogeneous group of conditions characterised by chronic joint inflammation. The knee is the most commonly affected joint.
- JIA is considered an autoimmune disorder. The exact trigger is unknown, but it is believed to involve a combination of genetic predisposition and environmental factors.
- The primary site of pathology is the synovial membrane lining the joint. It becomes infiltrated by inflammatory cells (lymphocytes, plasma cells), leading to synovial hyperplasia, pannus formation and joint effusion with cartilage and bone damage.

- Chronic inflammation near growth plates (physes) can stimulate or inhibit bone growth, leading to leg length discrepancies, bony overgrowth (epiphyseal enlargement), or angular deformities.

Clinical Features

- Demographics: onset before 16 years of age, with peak onset between 1 and 3 years and 8–12 years.
- Subtypes: several subtypes exist (e.g., oligoarticular, polyarticular, systemic-onset), each with different presentations and prognoses.
- Symptoms:
  - Joint swelling, warmth, and morning stiffness or stiffness after inactivity.
  - Pain: often less pronounced than in adults; a child may be pain-free but show a limp or refusal to walk.
  - Limp: a common presenting sign.
  - Limited range of motion.
  - Muscle atrophy & weakness.

Imaging Findings

- Radiography
  - Soft tissue swelling, periarticular osteoporosis, and growth disturbances like epiphyseal hypertrophy or premature growth plate closure.
  - Later stages may show joint space narrowing, bone erosions, and joint damage.
- Ultrasound
  - Synovitis (synovial thickening and joint effusion), increased blood flow (detected by Doppler), and damage to cartilage and bone.
  - Over time, this can lead to thinning and eventual loss of cartilage, and in later stages, bone erosions.
- MRI
  - Synovial hyperplasia, joint effusion and bone marrow oedema (ill-defined T2 hyperintensity in the epiphyses and metaphyses) indicating active inflammation.
  - Chronic damage, bone erosions and growth abnormalities.
  - Enlarged femoral or tibial condyles compared to the contralateral side.
  - Premature physeal closure can lead to leg length discrepancy.
  - Baker's cyst: a common secondary finding.

Management

- The goal of management is to control inflammation, preserve joint function, prevent long-term damage, and promote normal growth and development.
- Multidisciplinary Team: Involves pediatric rheumatologists, physiotherapists, and occupational therapists.
- First-line: non-steroidal anti-inflammatory drugs (NSAIDs) for pain and inflammation.
- Second-line/disease-modifying antirheumatic drugs (DMARDs): Methotrexate is the cornerstone to suppress the underlying disease process.
- Biologic agents: TNF-alpha inhibitors (e.g., Etanercept, Adalimumab) and other biologics are used for patients unresponsive to DMARDs.
- Intra-articular corticosteroid injections: highly effective for rapidly reducing inflammation in a specific joint like the knee, often providing months of relief.

Suggested Reading

Hemke R, Herregods N, Jaremko JL, Maas M. Imaging of juvenile idiopathic arthritis. Radiol Clin North Am. 2024;62(5):889–902.

Tsujioka Y, Nishimura G, Sugimoto H, Nozaki T, Kono T, Jinzaki M. Imaging findings of juvenile idiopathic arthritis and autoinflammatory diseases in children. Jpn J Radiol. 2023;41(11):1186–207.

Moderately Difficult Cases

Contents

Case 34

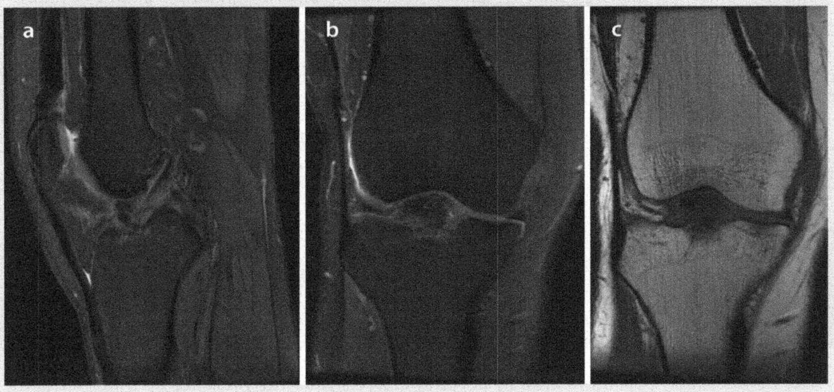

A 20-year-old male presented with pain and instability following a twisting knee injury

S. Saran et al., *101 Knee Imaging Case Series*, 101 MSK Imaging 1,
https://doi.org/10.1007/978-3-032-21567-3_34

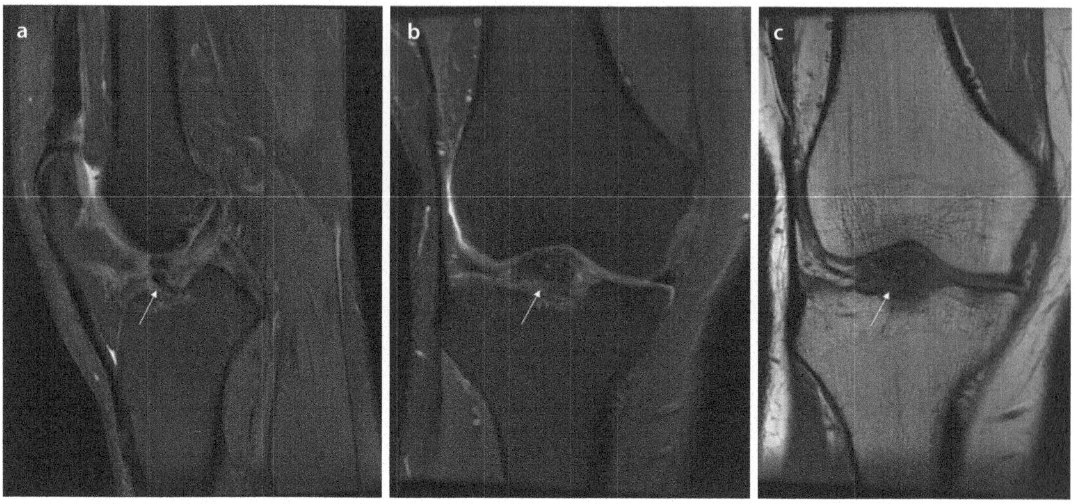

■ MRI knee, PDFS sag **a**, coronal **b** and T1 coronal **c**. **a–c** shows the presence of a bony fragment (arrows) in the intercondylar region at the tibial attachment site of the anterior cruciate ligament, suggesting an avulsion fracture

Avulsion Fracture at the Tibial Attachment Site of the Anterior Cruciate Ligament (ACL)

Definition & Pathophysiology

- An avulsion fracture at the tibial attachment of the ACL is a bony injury where the ACL, under extreme tension, pulls a fragment of its tibial insertion point away from the main bone.
- This is distinct from a mid-substance ligament tear and is more common in skeletally immature patients (children and adolescents) because the physes (growth plates) are the weakest link in the musculoskeletal chain.
- Mechanism: Typically caused by the same forces that cause an ACL tear, a sudden deceleration, hyperextension, or a forceful pivot with the foot planted.
- The strength of the ligament exceeds the strength of the immature bone, resulting in a bony avulsion rather than a ligamentous rupture.

Clinical Presentation

- Acute knee pain and swelling following a traumatic event.
- Inability to bear weight.
- A feeling of instability or "giving way".
- Positive Lachman test & anterior drawer test.

Imaging Findings

- Radiography
  - Lateral view: Shows a bony fragment avulsed from the anterior aspect of the tibial spine (the intercondylar eminence).
- CT
  - Excellent for pre-operative planning in complex or comminuted fractures (Type III/IV).
  - Precisely defines the size, rotation, and degree of displacement of the fragment.
- MRI
  - While the fracture is visible, MRI's primary role is to evaluate the entire ligament and other structures.
  - ACL Ligament: The ligament fibres appear continuous but are seen attached to the avulsed bone fragment.

Classification (Meyers & McKeever)

- Type I: Non-displaced or minimally displaced fragment.
- Type II: Hinged fragment, elevated anteriorly but with posterior cortex contact ("beak" fracture).
- Type III: Completely displaced fragment, often rotated.
- Type IV: Comminuted fracture.

Management

- The goal is to achieve anatomic reduction of the fragment to restore the normal tension of the ACL and prevent non-union, instability, and arthrofibrosis.
- Non-surgical management (for non-/minimally displaced fractures):
  - Indications: Meyers & McKeever Type I and some stable Type II fractures.
  - Immobilisation: long leg cast or brace with the knee in full extension (to relax the ACL and allow the fragment to settle) for 4–6 weeks.
  - Non-weight-bearing with crutches.
- Surgical intervention (open reduction and internal fixation—ORIF):
  - Indications: displaced fractures (Type III and IV) and non-union after conservative treatment.
  - Procedure: arthroscopic or open reduction.

Prognosis & Complications

- Excellent prognosis with anatomic reduction, as the native ACL is preserved.
- Arthrofibrosis: A common complication, especially with prolonged immobilisation. Early, controlled motion is key to prevention.

Suggested Reading

Kosco ED, Montalbano AN, Scarano K, Sohn D. Tibial eminence fracture and pediatric ACL avulsion diagnosis and treatment: a case report. J Orthop Case Rep. 2024;14(4):90–4.

White EA, Patel DB, Matcuk GR, Forrester DM, Lundquist RB, Hatch GF 3rd, Vangsness CT, Gottsegen CJ. Cruciate ligament avulsion fractures: anatomy, biomechanics, injury patterns, and approach to management. Emerg Radiol. 2013;20(5):429–40.

Case 35

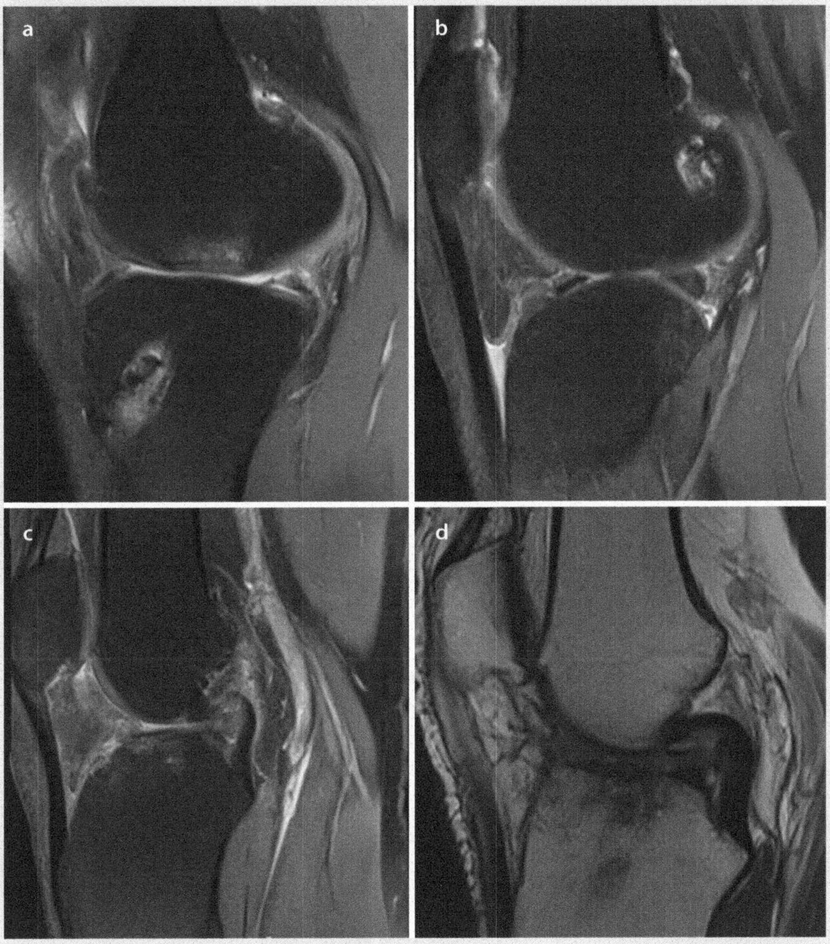

■ A 27-year-old male with post-ACL reconstruction presented with pain and instability for 2 months

S. Saran et al., *101 Knee Imaging Case Series*, 101 MSK Imaging 1,
https://doi.org/10.1007/978-3-032-21567-3_35

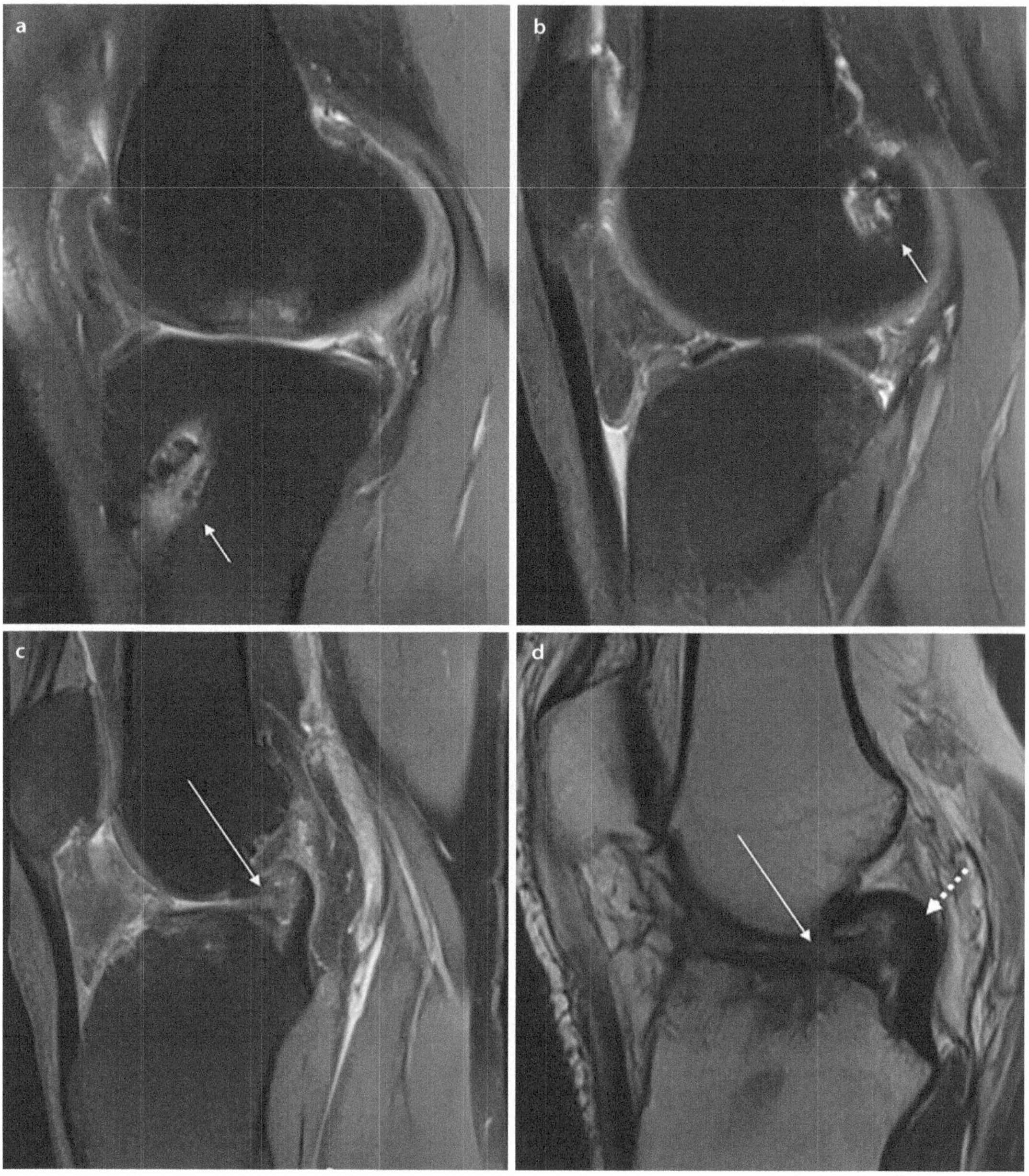

◘ MRI knee, PDFS weighted sagittal **a**–**c**, and T2 weighted sagittal **d** sequences showing tibial and femoral tunnel (short arrows) with non-visualisation of ACL graft in the intercondylar region (long arrows). Additionally, buckling of PCL (dashed arrow) is also noted, signifying anterior tibial translation. The constellation of findings is suggestive of a tear of ACL graft

Tear of the ACL Graft

Definition & Pathophysiology

- A torn ACL graft represents the failure of the surgically reconstructed ligament. This can be a devastating complication, often requiring revision surgery. Graft failure is not a single event but typically the result of a combination of factors.
- Mechanism of re-rupture: A new significant force (e.g., pivoting, cutting, or hyperextension) that exceeds the graft's strength, similar to the initial injury.
- Technical errors: The most common cause of early failure.
  - Non-anatomic tunnel placement: malpositioned femoral or tibial tunnels leading to graft impingement and progressive failure.
  - Inadequate graft fixation: weak initial fixation leading to graft slippage or laxity.
  - Biologic failure: failure of the graft to "ligamentise" (incorporate and develop a viable blood supply).
  - Rehabilitation errors: overly aggressive rehab or premature return to sport.

Clinical Presentation

- The presentation often mirrors that of a primary ACL tear. History is often a distinct re-injury event with a "pop" sensation, followed by swelling and pain. In some cases, failure is insidious, with a gradual return of instability.
- Giving way/instability: the most telling symptom, especially during pivoting activities.
- Pain and swelling: acute onset after a traumatic event.
- Loss of confidence in the knee.

Physical Exam

- Positive Lachman test & pivot shift test: Indicating restored anterior and rotational laxity.
- Effusion.

Imaging Findings

- MRI is essential for confirming the tear and identifying the cause of failure.

- Direct signs of graft tear:
  - Discontinuity: complete disruption of the graft fibres.
  - Abnormal signal & morphology: The graft appears indistinct, thickened, or attenuated with diffuse high signal on T2/PD-weighted images (indicating mucoid degeneration or tearing).
- Indirect signs & evaluation of cause:
  - Tunnel position: critical to assess for malposition (e.g., vertical femoral tunnel, anterior tibial tunnel).
  - Tunnel widening ("lytic tibia"): bone resorption around the tunnels, often a sign of chronic instability or biologic reaction.
- Secondary signs: bone bruising pattern (e.g., on the lateral femoral condyle and posterior tibia) from the subluxation event, and meniscal tears. Anterior tibial translation and buckling of PCL.

Management

Management is highly individualised, depending on the patient's age, activity level, and the cause of failure.

- Decision-making: conservative vs. surgical
  - Conservative management: may be considered for lower-demand patients with minimal functional instability. Involves physical therapy for strengthening and activity modification.
  - Surgical revision ACL reconstruction: this is the standard for active patients who wish to return to sports or have significant instability.
- Revision ACL reconstruction (a complex procedure): a revision is significantly more complex than a primary reconstruction and requires meticulous pre-operative planning.
  - Existing hardware: may need to be removed.
  - Tunnel widening & bone loss: Compromised bone stock is a major challenge.
  - Stage 1: remove old graft and hardware; bone graft the widened tunnels.
  - Stage 2: perform the new ACL reconstruction (after 4–6 months of healing) once the bone stock has been restored.
  - Graft choice: allograft (donor tissue) is often preferred in revisions to avoid harvesting from the already compromised knee, but autografts from the contralateral leg or quadriceps tendon are also common.
  - Technique: the surgeon must use new, correctly placed anatomic tunnels, which may require specialised fixation devices.

Prognosis & Outcomes

- Outcomes after revision ACL reconstruction are generally good but inferior to primary reconstructions.
- Return to sport rates are lower.
- Risk of re-failure is higher than with primary surgery.
- Higher risk of post-traumatic osteoarthritis.

Suggested Reading

Bencardino JT, Beltran J, Feldman MI, Rose DJ. MR imaging of complications of anterior cruciate ligament graft reconstruction. Radiographics. 2009;29(7):2115–26.

Somanathan A, Tandon A, Yang LW. Review of magnetic resonance imaging features of complications after anterior cruciate ligament reconstruction. Singapore Med J. 2019;60(2):63–8.

Case 36

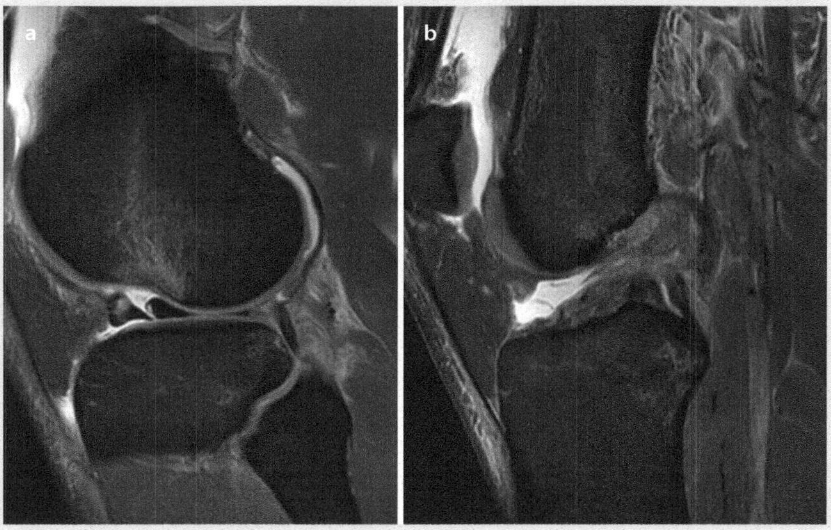

A 24-year-old football player presented with a twisting knee injury

S. Saran et al., *101 Knee Imaging Case Series*, 101 MSK Imaging 1,
https://doi.org/10.1007/978-3-032-21567-3_36

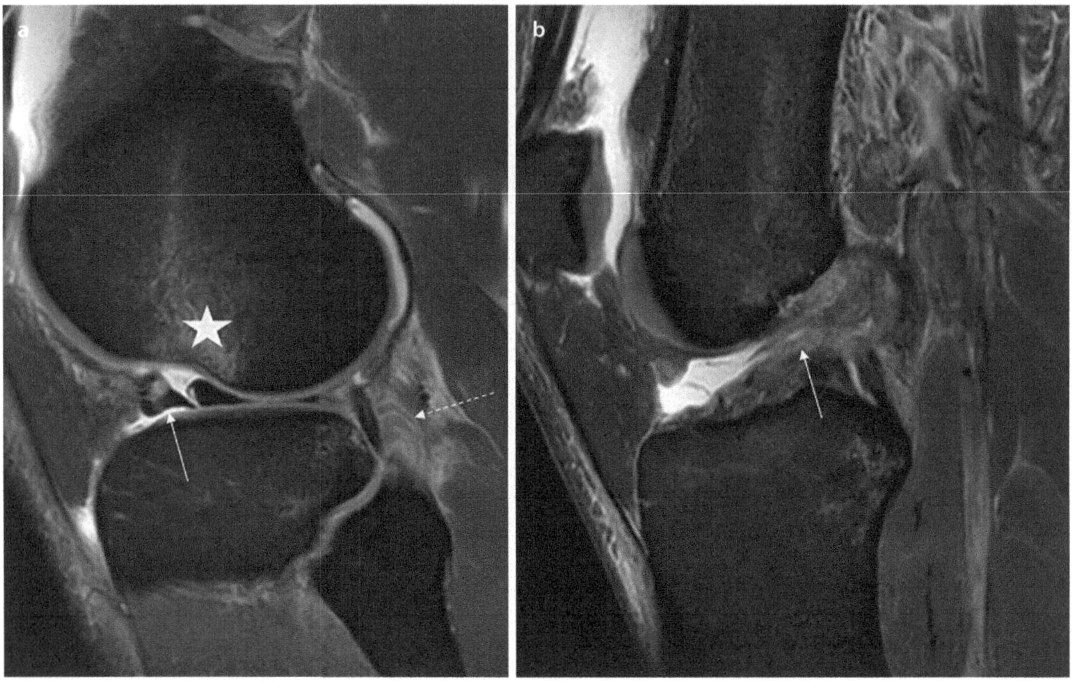

■ MRI knee, PDFS weighted sagittal **a** and **b** sequences showing anterior flipping of the posterior horn of the lateral meniscus, giving double anterior horn or double delta signs (arrow in **a**). Full-thickness ACL tear is seen (arrow in **b**) with the deep sulcus sign and underlying marrow oedema in the lateral femoral condyle (star). Posterolateral corner injury is also seen (dashed arrow)

Flipped Meniscus

Definition & Pathophysiology

- A "flipped meniscus" is a specific, displaced pattern of a bucket-handle tear (BHT). In this variant, the separated inner fragment (the "handle") is not just displaced into the intercondylar notch but is completely flipped or rotated 180 degrees on its axis, often lying anterior to the remaining meniscal rim.
- Mechanism: The same as a standard BHT—a high-energy twisting injury on a flexed knee. The forces involved are significant enough to not only detach the fragment but also cause it to flip over.
- Consequence: This flipped fragment can cause mechanical blocking of knee extension and is often associated with more severe symptoms than a standard displaced tear.

Clinical Presentation

- Mechanical locking: inability to fully extend the knee is a cardinal sign.
- Pain localised to the lateral joint line.
- Catching or clicking sensation during movement.
- Loss of motion: significant loss of terminal flexion and extension.
- Effusion: rapid swelling due to hemarthrosis.

MRI Findings

- MRI is crucial for identifying the flipped fragment and planning surgery. The classic signs of a standard BHT may be absent or altered.
- "double anterior horn" sign: this is the most characteristic finding. On sagittal MRI images, two structures resembling the anterior horn of the lateral meniscus are seen adjacent to each other. One is the true anterior horn, and the other is the flipped posterior horn fragment.
- Absent/truncated posterior horn: the native posterior horn appears small, truncated, or "missing" because a large portion of it has flipped anteriorly.
- Altered "bowtie" sign on sagittal images.

Management

- Treatment is always surgical due to the mechanical block and symptoms. The goal is to preserve meniscal tissue whenever possible.
- Arthroscopic surgery:
  - Meniscal repair: this is the preferred option if the tissue is of good quality and the tear is in the vascular zone (especially in younger patients). Sutures or fixation devices are used to secure the fragment back to the meniscal rim.
  - Partial meniscectomy (debridement): if the tissue is degenerated, frayed, or the tear is in the avascular zone, the unstable flipped fragment is trimmed and removed, leaving a stable, balanced meniscal rim.

Prognosis & Complications

- Repair: Carries an excellent prognosis for long-term joint health if healing is achieved, though it requires a longer, protected rehabilitation.
- Meniscectomy: Provides good short-term relief but increases the long-term risk of lateral compartment osteoarthritis due to the loss of load-bearing meniscal tissue.
- The "flipped" pattern often indicates a more complex tear, making a successful repair more challenging but highly desirable.

Suggested Reading

Ahn JH, Yim SJ, Seo YS, Ko TS, Lee JH. The double flipped meniscus sign: unusual MRI findings in bucket-handle tear of the lateral meniscus. Knee. 2014;21(1):129–32.

Pakdemirli E, Cesur T, Bozkurt İ. MRI in the diagnosis of bucket handle tears: what is the current situation? Cureus. 2023;15(8):e43324.

Shah A, Iyengar KP, Gavvala SN, Shah A, Beale D, Botchu R. The pelican sign: case series demonstrating a unique description of an anteriorly flipped bucket-handle meniscal tear of the knee. Indian J Radiol Imaging. 2022;33(2):157–61.

Case 37

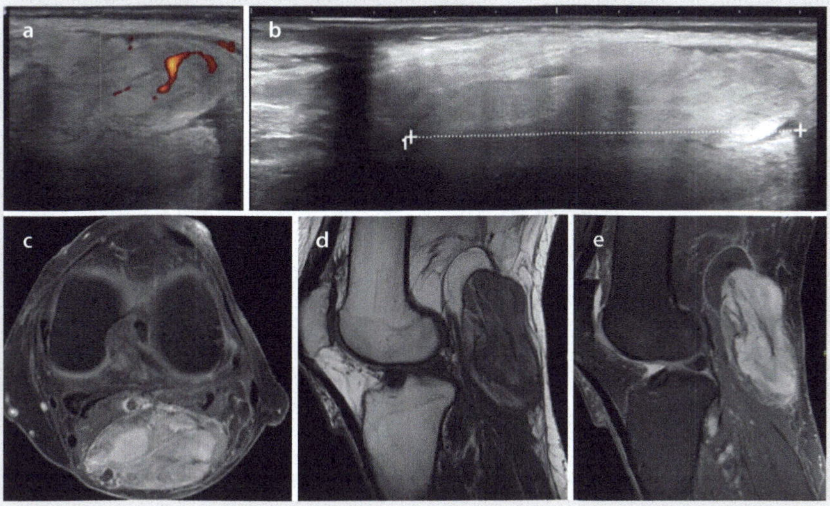

A 45-year-old male presented with firm swelling in the popliteal region for 2 years with a recent increase in size

S. Saran et al., *101 Knee Imaging Case Series*, 101 MSK Imaging 1,
https://doi.org/10.1007/978-3-032-21567-3_37

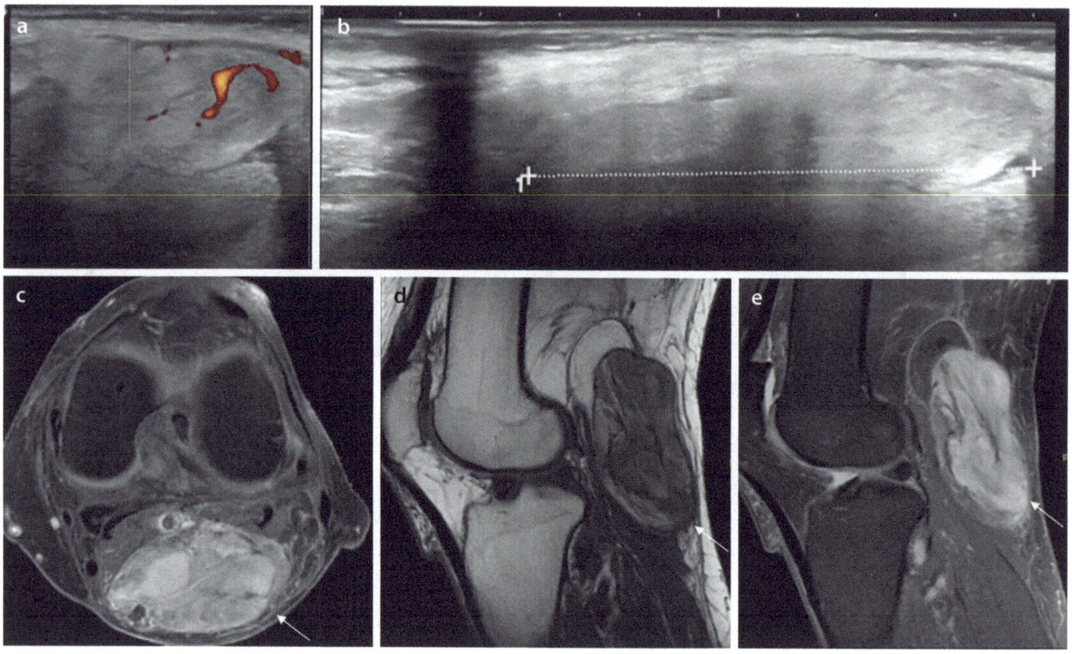

▣ Ultrasound **a** and **b** examination of the popliteal region revealed a well-defined hyperechoic mass lesion with internal Doppler activity. MRI **c**–**e** shows the lesion (arrows) as heterogeneously hyperintense on PDFS weighted axial **c** and sagittal **e** sequences and hypointense on T1 weighted sequences **d**. There is a presence of a fat signal intensity area in the cranial aspect and sarcomatous component in the caudal aspect. Imaging findings favour the diagnosis of Atypical lipomatous tumour

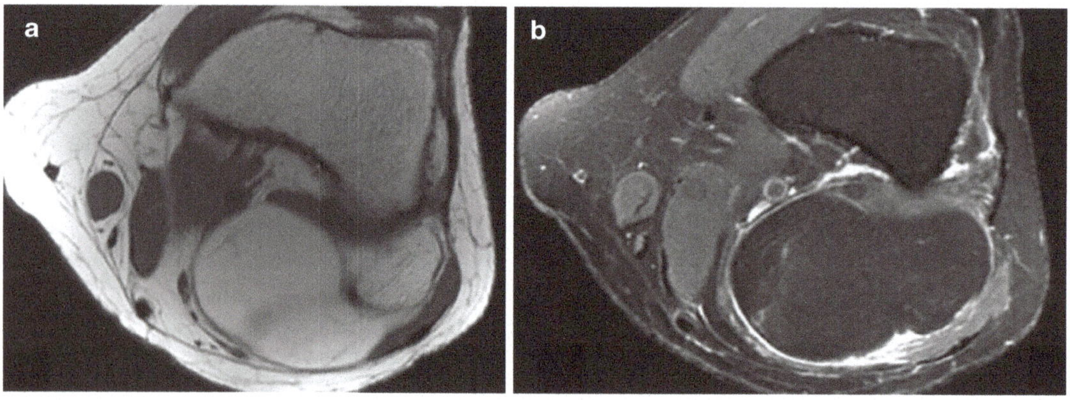

▣ Companion case: A case of typical lipoma in the popliteal region with thin internal septa and no obvious soft tissue component

Atypical Lipomatous Tumour (ALT)/ Well-Differentiated Liposarcoma (WDLS)

Definition & Pathophysiology

- Atypical lipomatous tumour (ALT) and well-differentiated liposarcoma (WDLS) are two names for the same entity, representing a locally aggressive, intermediate-grade malignant adipocytic tumour with virtually no potential for distant metastasis, but a significant risk of local recurrence. The terminology used depends on the anatomical location, which dictates the potential for complete surgical resection and thus the clinical risk.
- It is characterised by the proliferation of mature adipocytes with significant variation in cell size and the presence of scattered, hyperchromatic, atypical stromal cells. The hallmark genetic finding is supernumerary ring and giant chromosomes containing amplification of the 12q14–15 region, which includes the MDM2 gene.

Terminology

- Atypical lipomatous tumour (ALT): The preferred term for tumours in anatomically expendable or readily resectable locations (e.g., limbs, subcutaneous tissue). This name emphasises its excellent prognosis when widely excised.
- Well-differentiated liposarcoma (WDLS): The traditional term used for tumours in sites where complete surgical resection is often difficult or impossible (e.g., retroperitoneum, mediastinum, spermatic cord). In these locations, the inability to achieve wide margins leads to high rates of local recurrence and significant morbidity/mortality, justifying the more ominous "sarcoma" designation.

Clinical Presentation

- Demographics: typically presents in adults, 50–70 years old.
- Location: deep intramuscular location in the thigh or popliteal fossa.
  - Symptoms: a slow-growing, painless, deep-seated mass that has often been present for years.

Imaging Findings

- Imaging is highly characteristic and often allows for a presumptive diagnosis.
- Ultrasound:
  - Multilobulated, well-defined hyperechoic mass with areas of hypoechogenicity and internal vascularity.
- MRI:
  - MRI shows a mass that is predominantly fatty but with non-adipose components.
  - The presence of thick, nodular, non-fatty septa (>2 mm) and/or non-lipomatous masses/nodules that show enhancement is the hallmark imaging finding.

Differential Diagnosis

- Lipoma: A benign fatty tumour. It typically has thin, uniform septa (<2 mm) that do not enhance significantly and no non-fatty nodules.
- Dedifferentiated liposarcoma: A more aggressive sarcoma that develops within a pre-existing ALT/WDLS. It appears as a distinct, non-lipomatous, solid, enhancing mass abruptly arising from the fatty tumour.
- Myxoid liposarcoma: Appears as a cystic, non-fatty mass on MRI and is often misdiagnosed as a cyst or hematoma; it typically contains very little macroscopic fat.

Diagnostic Confirmation

- MDM2 Immunohistochemistry or FISH: The definitive diagnostic test. Overexpression or amplification of the MDM2 gene is seen in >95% of ALT/WDLS and is negative in benign lipomas.

Management

- The cornerstone of treatment is wide local excision.
- Role of radiation therapy: may be used pre-operatively or post-operatively for large, deep limb tumours to reduce the local recurrence risk, especially if margins are close or positive.
- Surveillance: follow-up with imaging is required due to the persistent risk of late local recurrence and the potential for dedifferentiation (which occurs in ~5–10% of cases, more commonly in the retroperitoneum).

Suggested Reading

Gupta P, Potti TA, Wuertzer SD, Lenchik L, Pacholke DA. Spectrum of fat-containing soft-tissue masses at MR imaging: the common, the uncommon, the characteristic, and the sometimes confusing. Radiographics. 2016;36(3):753–66.

Kallen ME, Hornick JL. The 2020 WHO classification: what's new in soft tissue tumor pathology? Am J Surg Pathol. 2021;45(1):e1–e23.

Case 38

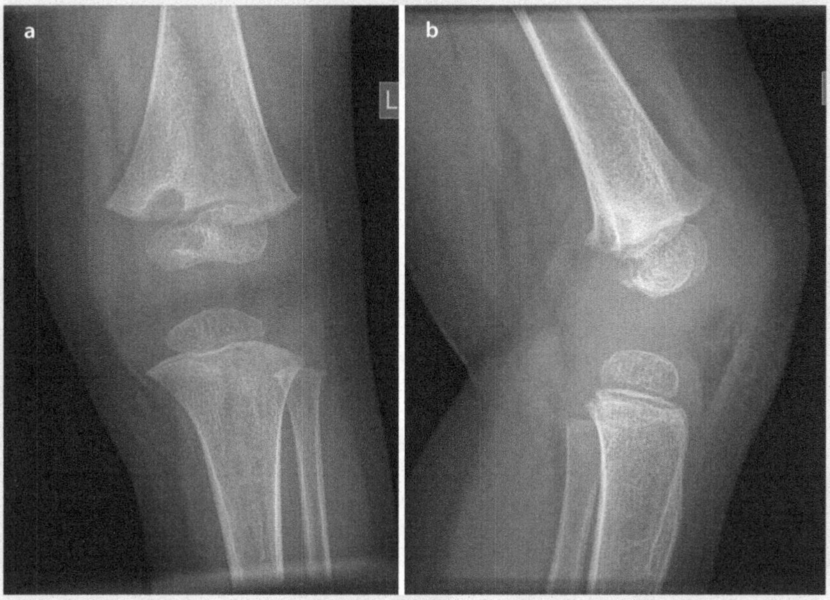

■ A 9-year-old male presented with a 6-week history of intermittent, dull, aching pain in his left knee. The pain has been gradually worsening over the past 2 weeks

S. Saran et al., *101 Knee Imaging Case Series*, 101 MSK Imaging 1,
https://doi.org/10.1007/978-3-032-21567-3_38

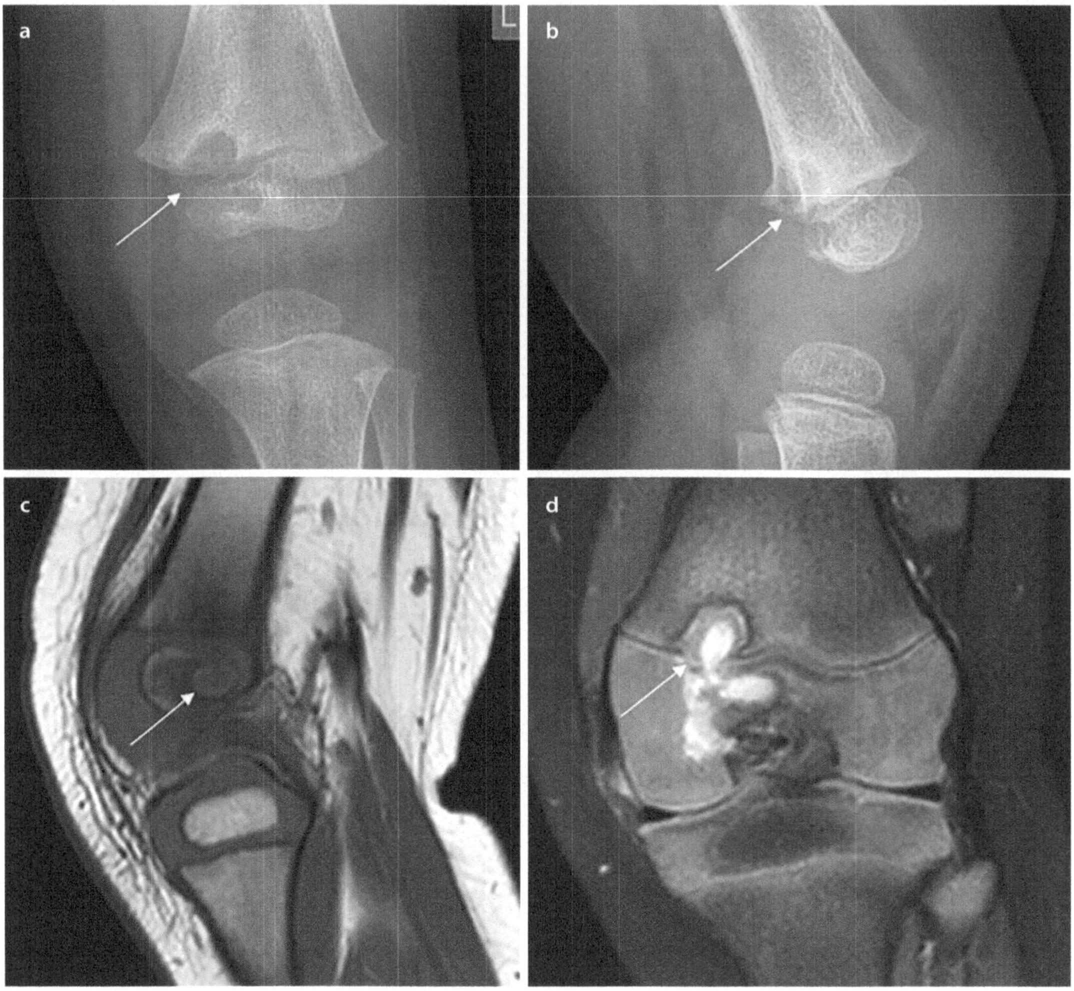

■ Radiographs **a** and **b** show an osteolytic area (arrows) in the distal femoral metaphysis and epiphysis. MRI knee, sagittal T1 **c** and coronal STIR **d** shows the lesion as a well-defined osteolytic area (arrow) with an internal rim of hyperintensity on T1-weighted sequence **c**, suggestive of the penumbra sign. The lesion appears as a hyperintense area with an isointense rim and adjacent marrow oedema on the PDFS sequence **d**. The constellation of clinical findings, along with imaging, is suggestive of Brodie's abscess

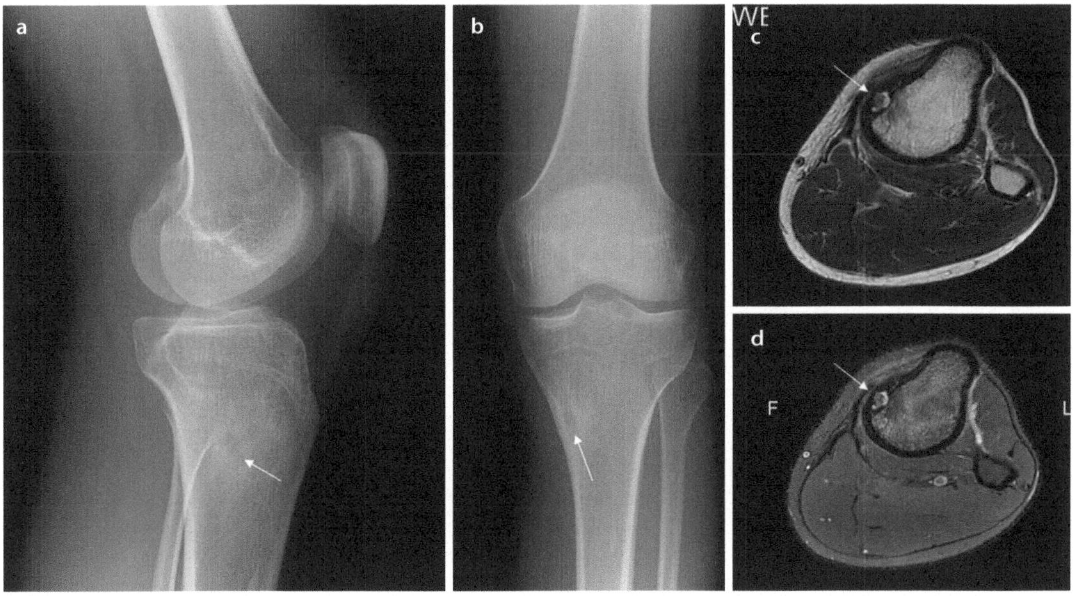

Cortical abscess (Brodie's abscess) in the proximal tibia (arrows) in another patient

Brodie's Abscess

Definition & Pathophysiology

- A Brodie's abscess is a localised, subacute-to-chronic bone abscess characterised by a walled-off collection of pus within the bone. It represents an indolent form of osteomyelitis where the body successfully contains the infection but fails to eradicate it completely.
- Pathogenesis: It typically follows hematogenous spread of bacteria or, less commonly, a minor trauma that introduces bacteria. The patient's immune system walls off the infection, creating a well-defined abscess cavity.
- Staphylococcus aureus is the most common cause.
- Location: The metaphysis of long bones is the classic site, with the distal femur and proximal tibia being most commonly affected. In adults, it can also occur in the epiphysis.

Clinical Presentation

- Most common in children and adolescents, but can occur at any age.
- Symptoms:
  - "The Great Mimicker": Presentation is often insidious and nonspecific.

- Dull, aching pain: the most common symptom, often worse at night and of long duration (weeks to months).
- Localised tenderness.
- Minimal systemic symptoms: the patient is usually afebrile and does not appear systemically ill, which distinguishes it from acute osteomyelitis.
- Mild swelling: there may be slight swelling over the affected area.

Imaging Findings

- Radiography
  - A well-defined, lytic lesion in the metaphysis of the long bone.
  - Surrounding sclerosis: there is often a large area of reactive bone sclerosis around the abscess, indicating the chronic nature of the infection.
  - Serpiginous tract: a faint, winding, linear lucency (the "cloquet canal") may be seen extending from the abscess cavity towards the growth plate (physis). This represents a sinus tract.
- MRI
  - T1-Weighted: The central abscess cavity is hypointense and is surrounded by a well-defined, hyperintense rim suggestive of granulation tissue. This is known as the "penumbra sign".
  - T2-Weighted/PDFS: The central abscess cavity is hyperintense due to its fluid/pus content. There is extensive, confluent hyperintense bone marrow oedema surrounding the lesion.
  - T1-Weighted post-contrast: Shows a characteristic "double-line" or "target" sign.

Differential Diagnosis

- Osteoid Osteoma: Also causes night pain, relieved by NSAIDs. The central nidus may enhance, but it lacks the fluid-filled cavity and "penumbra sign" on T1.
- Eosinophilic Granuloma (Langerhans Cell Histiocytosis).
- Chondroblastoma: An epiphyseal lesion in a young patient, often with chondroid matrix calcification.
- Giant cell tumour of bone: Occurs in skeletally mature patients and is subchondral, abutting the articular surface. It lacks a sclerotic rim.

Management

The goal is to eradicate the infection, which typically requires surgical intervention combined with antibiotics.

- Surgical intervention
  - Curettage: The abscess cavity is surgically opened, and all purulent material, necrotic tissue, and granulation tissue are thoroughly removed using a curette.
  - Tissue is sent for culture and sensitivity to guide antibiotic therapy. This is both diagnostic and therapeutic.
- Antibiotic therapy
  - Empirical therapy: Started intravenously to cover for S. aureus and other common pathogens (e.g., Cefazolin, Clindamycin).
  - Culture-directed therapy: Once culture results are available, therapy is narrowed to the specific organism.
  - Duration: Typically, 2–6 weeks of IV antibiotics, followed by a course of oral antibiotics for a total duration of 3–6 months.

Suggested Reading

Afshar A, Mohammadi A. The "Penumbra Sign" on magnetic resonance images of Brodie's abscess: a case report. Iran J Radiol. 2011;8(4):245–8.

Kamio S, Arai M, Matsumoto S, Saito M, Asano N, Nakayama R. Radiological changes in the formation of Brodie's abscess by sequential magnetic resonance imaging: a case report. Radiol Case Rep. 2021;16(10):2993–7.

Case 39

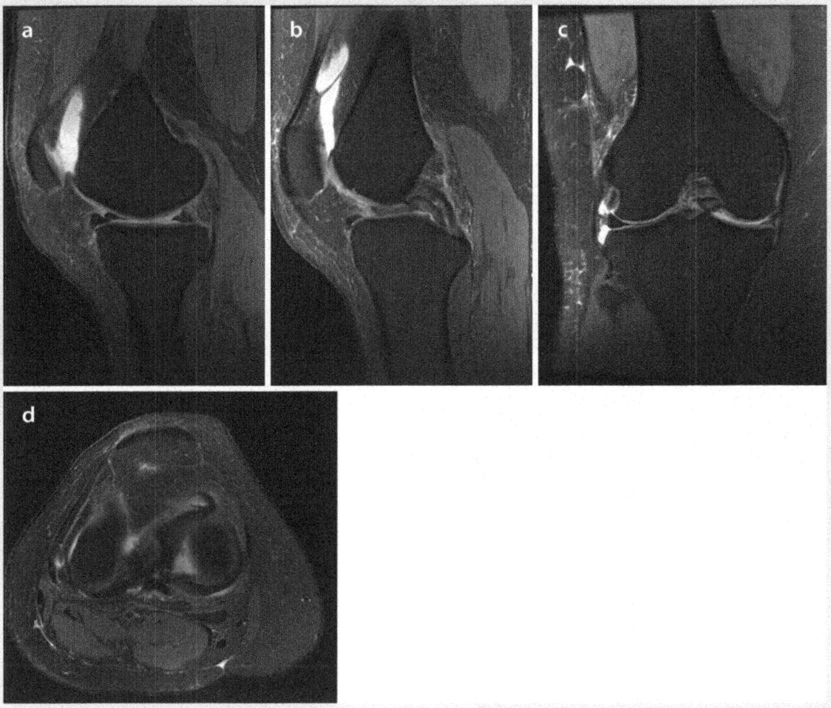

A 28-year-old male presented with pain and locking sensation 2 months after a twisting injury to the knee joint

S. Saran et al., *101 Knee Imaging Case Series*, 101 MSK Imaging 1,
https://doi.org/10.1007/978-3-032-21567-3_39

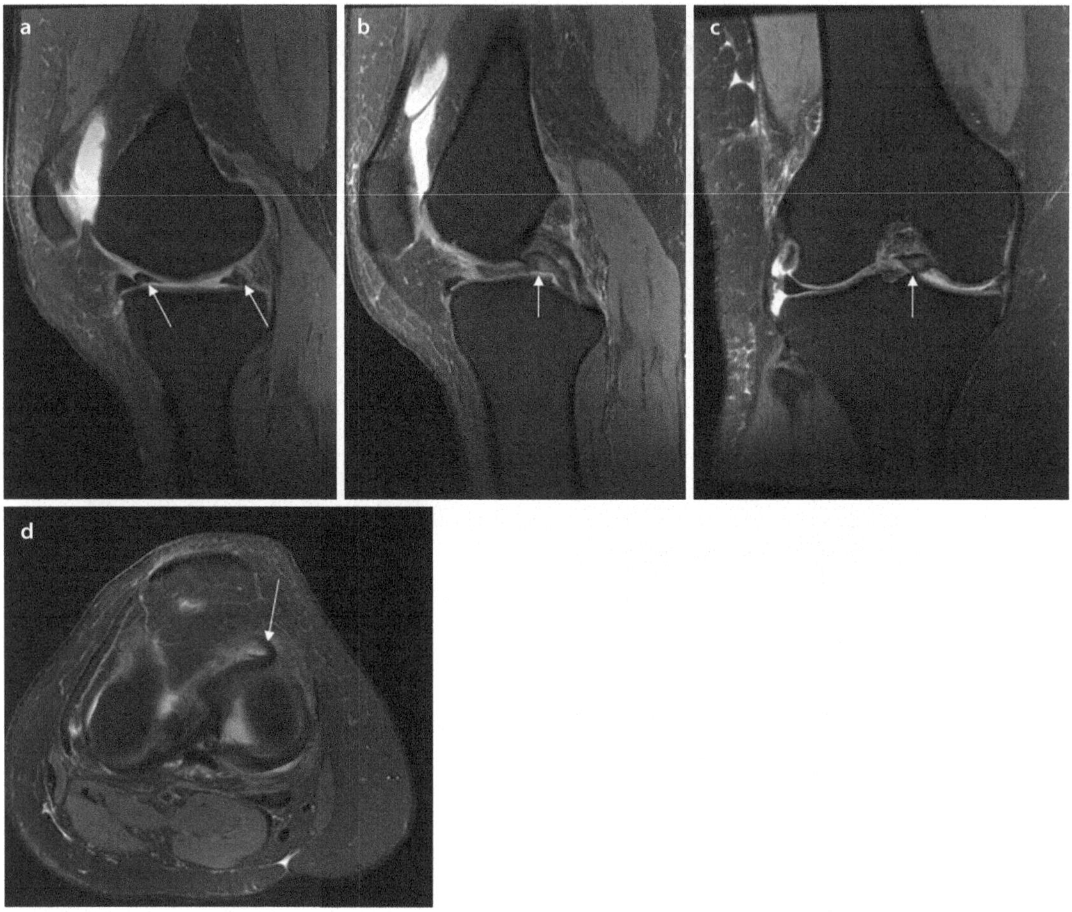

▪ MRI knee, PDFS weighted sagittal **a**, **b**, coronal **c**, and axial **d**, sequences showing vertical longitudinal tear involving both horns and body of the medial meniscus (arrows in **a**) with displaced inner fragment in the intercondylar groove (arrow in **c**) giving double PCL sign (arrow in **b**). Axial slice shows the inner displaced fragment (arrow in **d**) forming the handle of the bucket. Absence of ACL in mid-sagittal slice **b** suggests a complete ACL tear. Final diagnosis is bucket handle medial meniscal tear with complete ACL tear

Bucket Handle Meniscal Tear

Definition

A bucket-handle tear (BHT) is a specific, severe type of longitudinal vertical tear most commonly seen in the medial meniscus. The inner fragment of the tear becomes displaced, often into the intercondylar notch, resembling the handle of a bucket, while the outer rim remains, resembling the bucket itself.

▪▪ Pathophysiology and Mechanism

Typically, a high-energy twisting injury on a flexed knee, often seen in sports or trauma. It can also occur in conjunction with an ACL tear. The displaced fragment can cause mechanical locking of the knee, preventing full extension.

Clinical Presentation

History of a significant traumatic event followed by
- Mechanical locking: inability to fully extend the knee is a classic sign. The knee may "catch" at a certain angle.
- Catching or clicking: sensation during movement.
- Pain: localized to the medial joint line.

Physical Exam Findings

- Joint line tenderness: maximal over the medial joint line.
- Positive McMurray test: A "clunk" or painful click may be felt when the knee is rotated from a flexed to an extended position.
- Loss of extension: The patient may walk with a slightly flexed knee.

MRI Findings

- "Double PCL Sign" (Pathognomonic): On sagittal MRI images, the displaced meniscal fragment lies inferior and parallel to the Posterior Cruciate Ligament (PCL), making it appear as if there are two PCLs.
- "Double Delta Sign" (or "Double Anterior Horn Sign"): On coronal images, the flipped fragment and the native anterior horn of the meniscus are seen side-by-side, forming two triangular structures.
- "Absent Bowtie Sign": On sagittal images, a normal meniscus appears as two consecutive "bowties". In a BHT, the body of the meniscus (the bowtie) is absent because it has flipped into the notch.
- Fragment in the Intercondylar Notch: The displaced handle is visibly seen within the notch on multiple sequences.

Management

Treatment is almost always surgical due to the mechanical nature of the symptoms. The goal is to preserve as much healthy meniscal tissue as possible to prevent future osteoarthritis.
- Arthroscopic meniscal repair: ideal for young patients, acute tears (< 6 weeks), tears in the vascular "red-red" or "red-white" zone, and tears associated with ACL tears.

- Arthroscopic partial meniscectomy (debridement): indicated for irreparable tears (chronic, complex, degenerative tissue), tears in the avascular "white-white" zone, or patients who cannot comply with the strict rehab protocol of a repair.

Prognosis & Complications

- Repair: Good to excellent outcomes if healing is achieved. The main risk is re-tear.
- Meniscectomy: Good short-term pain relief, but increased risk of medial compartment osteoarthritis over 10–20 years due to altered knee biomechanics.
- Untreated: Persistent locking can lead to arthrofibrosis and accelerated cartilage wear.

Suggested Reading

Mihoubi F, Tordjman M, Khaled W, Guerini H, Thevenin F, Campagna R, Pluot E, Drapé JL, Feydy A. Overview of meniscal injuries. Semin Musculoskelet Radiol. 2025;29(3):403–16.

Tsakiri V, Kyriakidis T, Papadopoulos P, Davitis V, Chalidis B, Papadopoulos P, Gigis I. Meniscal bucket-handle tears and return to sports in young adults: a systematic review and meta-analysis. Cureus. 2025;17(3):e81329.

Case 40

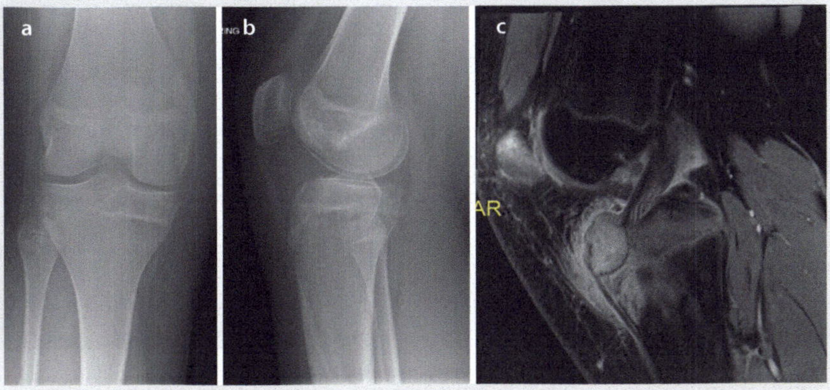

■ A 12-year-old boy presented with chief complaints of pain and swelling in the knee joint

S. Saran et al., *101 Knee Imaging Case Series*, 101 MSK Imaging 1,
https://doi.org/10.1007/978-3-032-21567-3_40

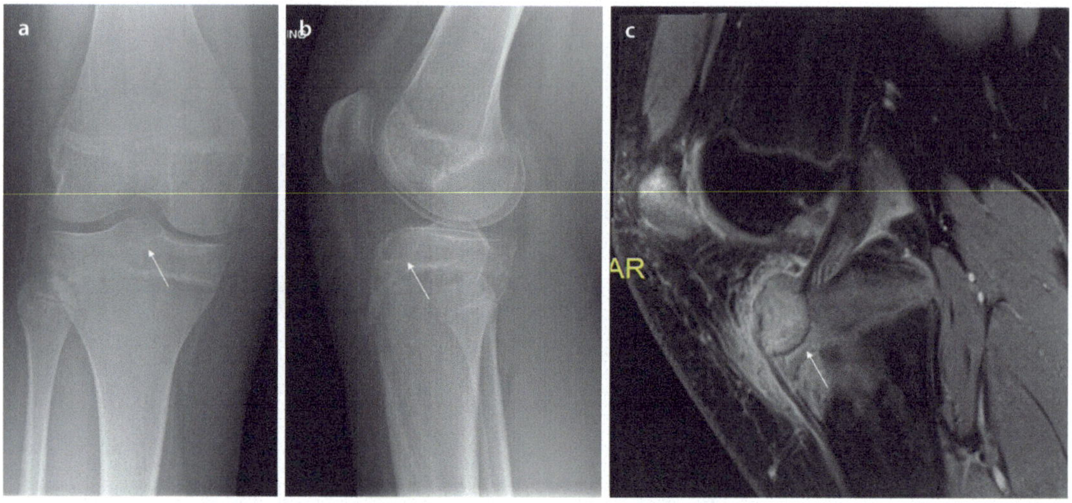

■ Radiographs Anteroposterior **a** lateral **b** of the knee joint show a well-defined osteolytic lesion in the proximal tibial epiphysis with a narrow zone of transition and a thin sclerotic rim (arrows). MRI PDFS weighted sagittal sequence **c** shows the lesion (arrow) to be hyperintense in signal intensity with intense adjacent marrow oedema. The diagnosis was chondroblastoma

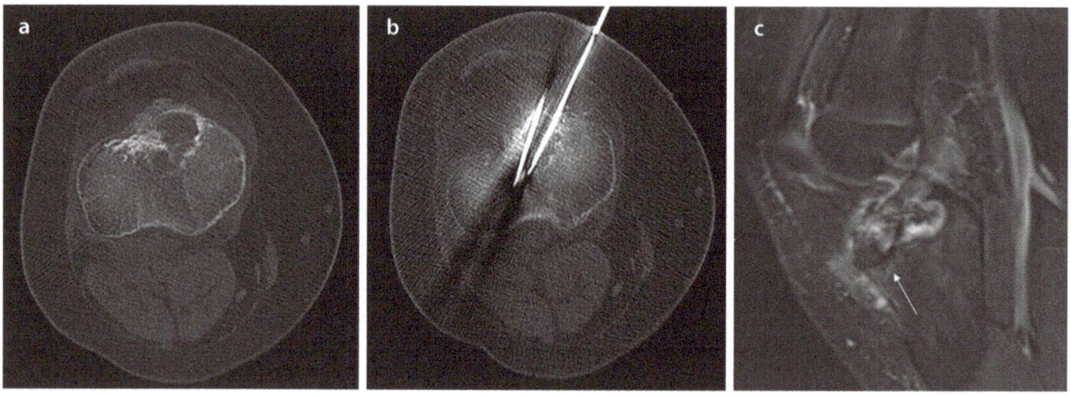

■ CT-guided biopsy and radio-frequency ablation **a** and **b** were performed. Follow-up MRI **c** shows a good response, characterised by sclerosis of the lesion and decreased adjacent marrow oedema (arrow)

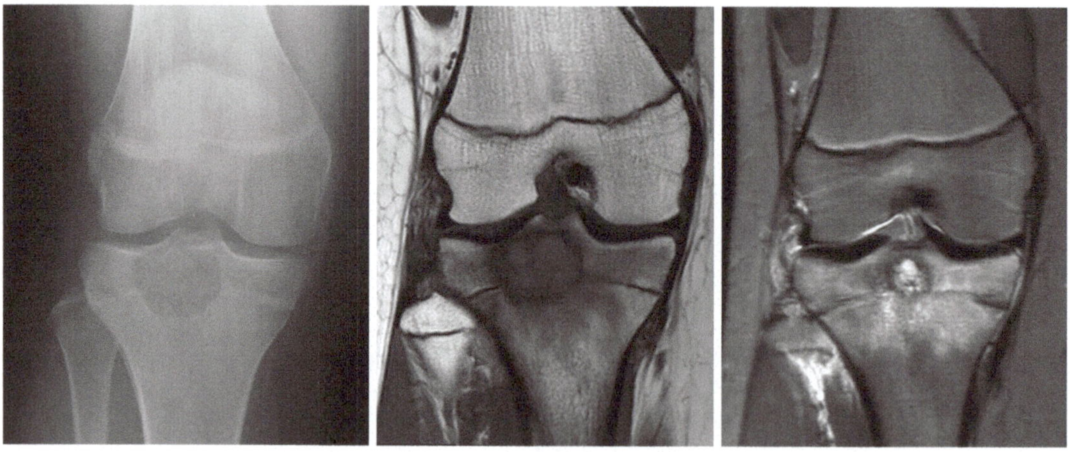

■ Companion case: Chondroblastoma in the proximal tibia

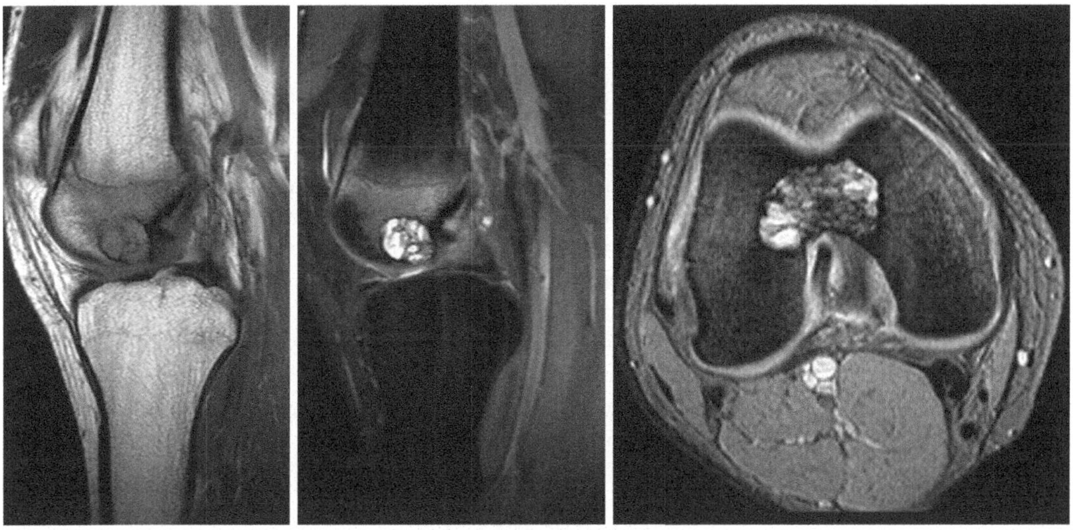

Companion case: Chondroblastoma in the distal femur epiphysis

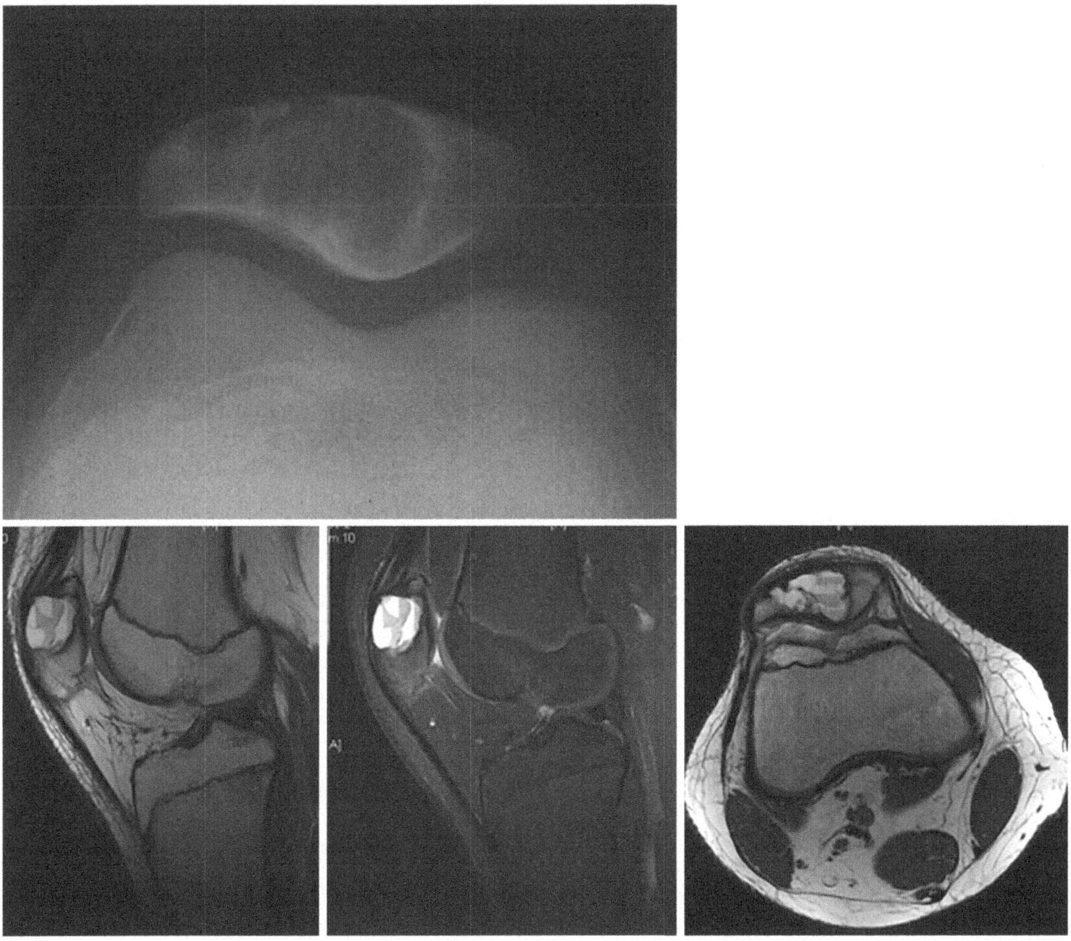

Companion case: Chondroblastoma in the patella with secondary aneurysmal bone cyst transformation

Chondroblastoma

Definition & Pathophysiology

- Chondroblastoma is a rare, benign, cartilaginous bone tumour that arises from epiphyseal cartilage. Despite being benign, it can be locally aggressive.
- It is one of the few primary bone tumours that almost exclusively arise in the epiphysis or apophysis of a long bone before skeletal maturity.
- Location: Most common in the distal femur, proximal tibia, and proximal humerus.
- Secondary aneurysmal bone cyst transformation can develop in Chondroblastoma.

Clinical Presentation

- Age: primarily affects children and young adults (10–25 years old), with open growth plates.
- Pain: the most common symptom, often localised to the joint. It can be dull and persistent or more severe.
- Joint effusion & swelling: due to the lesion's proximity to the joint.
- Decreased range of motion: pain and swelling can limit joint movement.
- Limp: if in the lower extremity.

Imaging Findings

- Radiography
  - Location: Eccentric or central lytic lesion in the epiphysis or apophysis of the long bone. It may cross the open physis.
  - Margin: Well-defined, geographic with a thin sclerotic rim.
  - Matrix: May show "chondroid" matrix calcification (punctate or "popcorn-like").
- MRI
  - T1-weighted: Low to intermediate signal intensity.
  - T2-weighted/PD FS/STIR: A heterogeneous high signal is classic. The solid components are often low to intermediate signal, while areas of secondary aneurysmal bone cyst change are very bright.
  - Perilesional oedema: Prominent, extensive bone marrow oedema surrounding the lesion is a hallmark finding. There is also often soft tissue and joint effusion.
  - Post-contrast (T1+C): Shows solid, heterogeneous enhancement.

Key Pathologic Feature

"Chicken-Wire" Calcification: A histological hallmark where calcification surrounds individual chondroblasts, creating a lace-like pattern.

Differential Diagnosis: For an epiphyseal lesion in a young person, consider

- Giant cell tumour of bone: occurs in skeletally mature patients (20–40 yrs) after physeal closure. It is purely lytic and lacks a sclerotic rim and matrix calcification.
- Subchondral cyst (ganglion): typically smaller, associated with osteoarthritis or trauma.
- Clear cell chondrosarcoma: a rare low-grade malignant tumour that mimics chondroblastoma but occurs in an older age group.
- Brodie's abscess: a subacute osteomyelitis that can occur in the metaphysis or epiphysis, often with a serpiginous tract.

Management

- CT-guided Radiofrequency or cryoablation
  - Both methods offer a less invasive alternative to surgery, but potential risks include damage to nearby cartilage or bone, especially in weight-bearing areas or near joints, necessitating careful, individualised case evaluation.
- Surgical intervention: reserved for cases not responding to minimally invasive treatment
  - Intralesional curettage: the standard treatment.
  - Adjuvant therapy: to reduce the risk of local recurrence, the cavity is often treated with a high-speed burr (to extend the margin), cryotherapy (liquid nitrogen), or phenol.
  - Bone grafting/bone cement: the resulting defect is filled with bone graft (allograft or autograft) or polymethylmethacrylate (PMMA) cement.

Prognosis

- Recurrence rate is reported in 10–20% of cases, typically within 2 years, emphasising the need for meticulous management.
- Malignant transformation is exceedingly rare.
- The primary risks are local recurrence and, in growing children, potential damage to the physis (growth plate) during surgery, which could result in limb-length discrepancy or angular deformity.

Suggested Reading

Karbhari A, Vijan A, Janu AK, Gulia A, Kulkarni S, Shetty N, Gala K, Panjwani P. Retrospective study of multimodality imaging features of chondroblastoma. Indian J Orthop. 2024;58(9):1303–9.

Salmon V, Gondim Teixeira PA, Blum A. Bone lesions of the tibia: multimodal iconographic review and diagnostic algorithms, part 2: metaphyseal and epiphyseal lesions. Eur J Radiol Open. 2025;14:100654.

Case 41

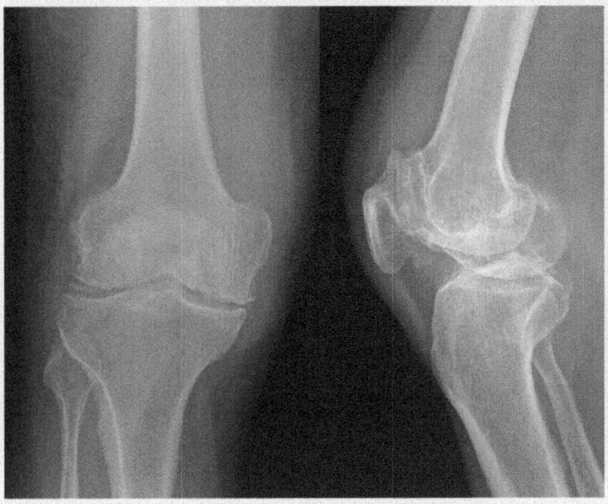

A 48-year-old male presented with chronic pain in the knee joint

S. Saran et al., *101 Knee Imaging Case Series*, 101 MSK Imaging 1,
https://doi.org/10.1007/978-3-032-21567-3_41

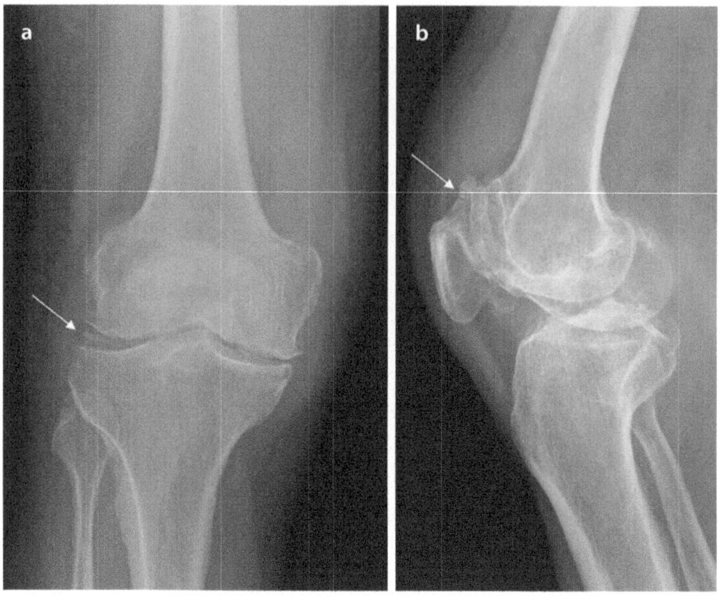

■ Radiograph (AP **a** and lateral **b**) shows the presence of calcification in the lateral meniscus region (arrow in **a**) with degenerative changes, more severely involving the patellofemoral joint (arrow in **b**). Radiographic findings suggest the possibility of Calcium pyrophosphate dihydrate deposition (CPPD) disease

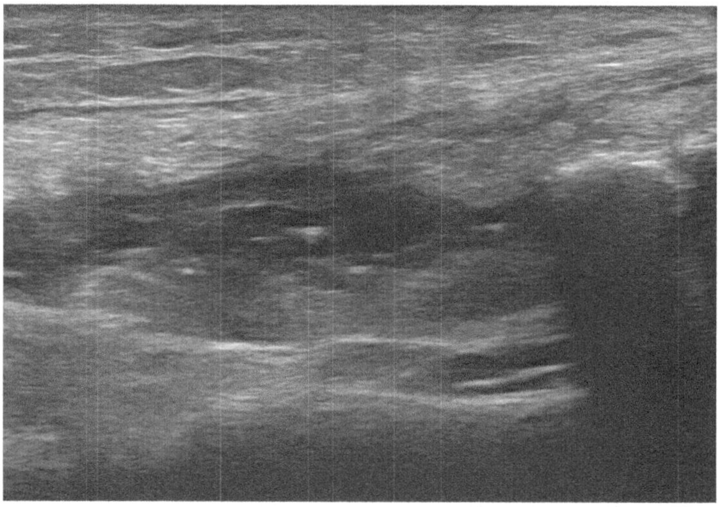

■ Ultrasound of the supra-patellar region in the same patient shows the presence of floating crystals in the joint recess

Calcium Pyrophosphate Dihydrate Crystal Deposition (CPPD) Disease

Definition & Pathophysiology

- Calcium Pyrophosphate Dihydrate Crystal Deposition (CPPD) Disease is a metabolic arthropathy characterised by the deposition of calcium pyrophosphate dihydrate crystals in articular and periarticular tissues, most notably hyaline cartilage and fibrocartilage (menisci). The term "Pseudogout" refers to the acute, gout-like inflammatory attacks caused by these crystals.
- The underlying cause is often idiopathic but is associated with disordered pyrophosphate metabolism in cartilage. This leads to crystal formation, which can shed into the joint space, triggering an intense acute neutrophilic inflammatory response.
- The disease has a wide spectrum of clinical presentations, from asymptomatic to acutely inflammatory to chronically degenerative.

Clinical Presentation

- Asymptomatic CPPD (Most Common): Incidental finding on imaging; no symptoms.
- Acute Pseudogout: Presents as a monoarticular, acute-onset arthritis mimicking gout or septic arthritis. The knee is the most commonly affected joint. Features include:
  - Severe pain, swelling, warmth, and erythema.
  - Can be triggered by surgery, trauma, or illness.
- Chronic Pyrophosphate Arthropathy: A progressive, degenerative arthritis that can mimic severe osteoarthritis but with distinctive features.

Imaging Findings

Imaging, particularly radiography, plays a crucial diagnostic role.

- Radiography
  - Unusual distribution (affects joints not typically involved in primary osteoarthritis, like the patellofemoral and radiocarpal joints).
  - Patellofemoral joint predominance: often shows disproportionately severe joint space narrowing and sclerosis compared to the tibiofemoral compartments.
  - Fibrocartilage: linear calcification in the medial and lateral menisci.

  - Hyaline cartilage: thin, linear calcification parallel to the subchondral bone of the femoral condyles and tibial plateau.
  - Degenerative changes with subchondral cysts (often numerous and large) and osteophytes.
- CT
  - More sensitive for detecting chondrocalcinosis and characterising the extent of osseous changes.
- MRI
  - Chondrocalcinosis: Appears as punctate or linear areas of low signal intensity on all sequences within the menisci and articular cartilage.
  - Synovitis: shows thickened, enhancing synovium.
  - Complications: can identify associated meniscal tears, ligamentous injury, or bone marrow oedema patterns.
  - Note: MRI is less specific than radiography for diagnosing CPPD; the crystals can be inconspicuous.

Differential Diagnosis

- Gout (uric acid crystal deposition): calcifications are typically not seen in cartilage (no chondrocalcinosis) but are seen on the surface. Erosions are characterised by "overhanging edges".
- Primary osteoarthritis: Typically has a different distribution (e.g., medial tibiofemoral compartment predominance) and lacks chondrocalcinosis.
- Septic arthritis: A medical emergency that can be indistinguishable from acute pseudogout clinically; joint aspiration is mandatory for diagnosis.

Diagnostic Gold Standard

- Joint aspiration with synovial fluid analysis: The definitive diagnosis is made by identifying positively birefringent, rhomboid-shaped crystals under polarised light microscopy.

Management

- Acute pseudogout attack
  - Joint aspiration: therapeutic and diagnostic; reduces intra-articular pressure and inflammation.
  - NSAIDs: First-line for pain and inflammation.
  - Colchicine: effective for acute attacks and prophylaxis.
  - Intra-articular corticosteroids: highly effective if infection has been ruled out.

- Chronic pyrophosphate arthropathy
  - Analgesics (e.g., acetaminophen).
  - Physical therapy for quadriceps strengthening and range of motion.
  - Assistive devices (e.g., cane, unloader brace).
  - Total Knee Arthroplasty (TKA): The definitive treatment for end-stage, debilitating arthropathy.

Suggested Reading

Cowley S, McCarthy G. Diagnosis and treatment of Calcium Pyrophosphate Deposition (CPPD) disease: a review. Open Access Rheumatol. 2023;15:33–41.

Reijnierse M, Schwabl C, Klauser A. Imaging of crystal disorders: calcium pyrophosphate dihydrate crystal deposition disease, calcium hydroxyapatite crystal deposition disease and gout pathophysiology, imaging, and diagnosis. Radiol Clin North Am. 2022;60(4):641–56.

Case 42

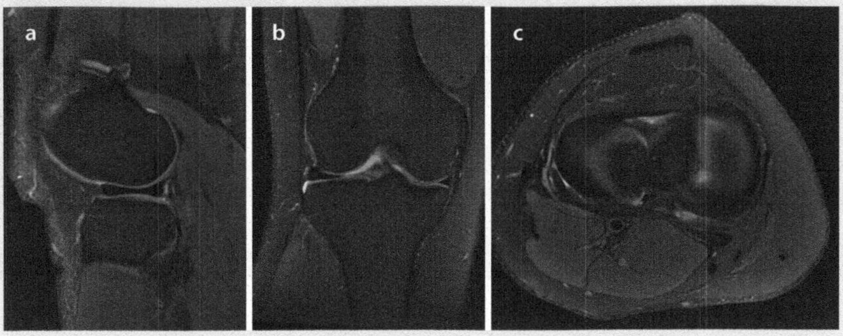

■ A 42-year-old male with pain and locking sensation in the knee joint

S. Saran et al., *101 Knee Imaging Case Series*, 101 MSK Imaging 1,
https://doi.org/10.1007/978-3-032-21567-3_42

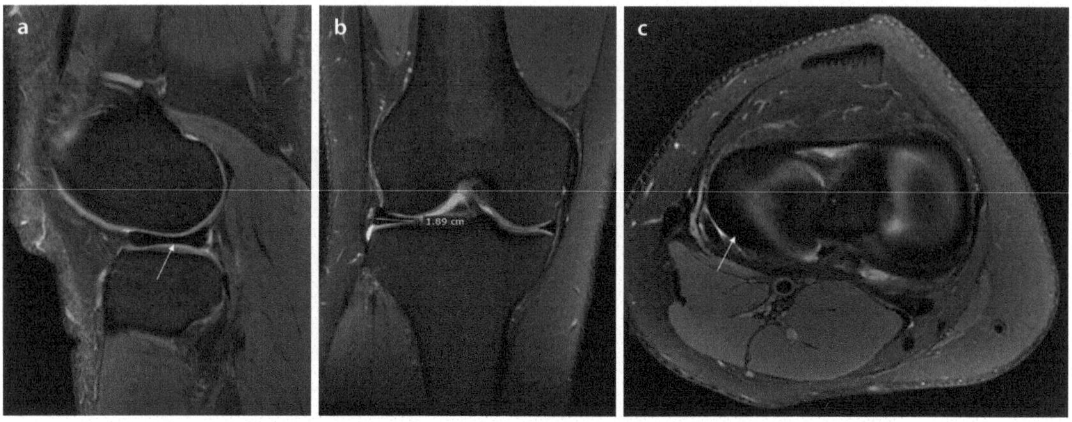

◘ MRI knee, PDFS weighted sagittal **a**, coronal **b**, and axial **c**, sequences showing a thicker and disk-shaped lateral meniscus (arrows) with a width of 18.9 mm. An incomplete discoid lateral meniscus

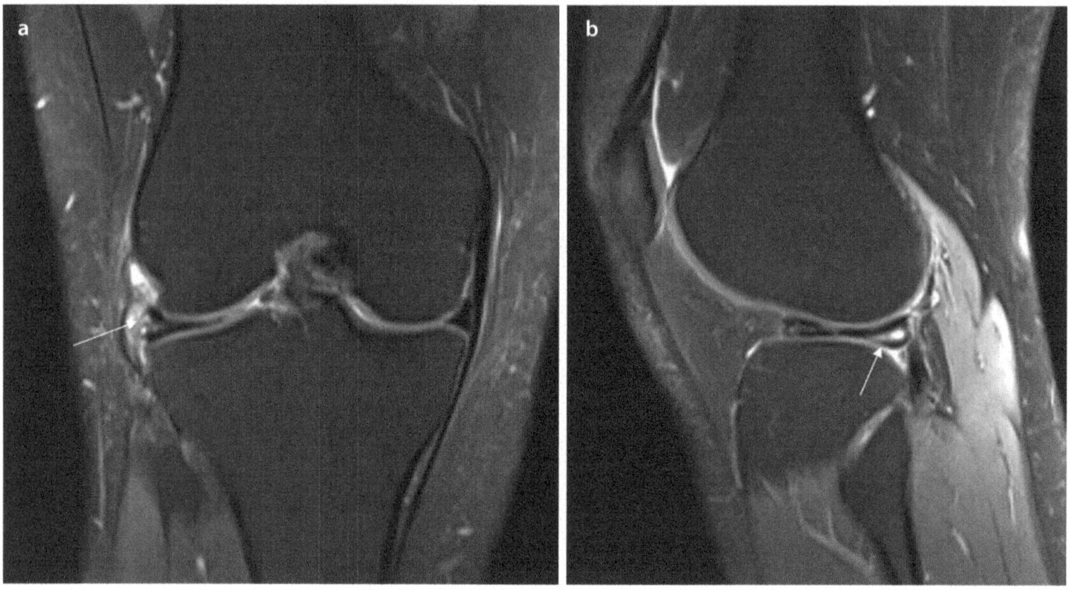

◘ Companion case: MRI knee, PDFS weighted coronal **a** and sagittal **b** sequences showing a discoid lateral meniscus with degenerative horizontal tear (arrow) and associated para-meniscal cyst

Discoid Lateral Meniscus – Definition & Pathophysiology

- A congenital variant of the lateral meniscus where the meniscus is thicker and disk-shaped (instead of the normal crescent shape), leading to altered biomechanics and increased risk of tears, instability, and degeneration.
- Prevalence: ~3–5% of the population (more common in Asians).
- Aetiology: Failure of normal meniscal embryological remodelling.

Classification (Watanabe System)

- Complete discoid—Covers the entire tibial plateau.
- Incomplete discoid—Wider than normal but doesn't fully cover the plateau.
- Wrisberg-ligament type—Lacks posterior meniscotibial attachments → hyper-mobile, prone to snapping.

Clinical Presentation

- Asymptomatic (incidental finding on MRI).
- Symptomatic cases: pain (lateral joint line); snapping/clicking (especially with knee motion—"snapping knee syndrome"); locking or giving way (if torn or unstable); and swelling (if secondary cystic degeneration).

MRI Findings

- Coronal view: "Continuous Bowtie sign" (meniscal Bowtie on ≥3 consecutive 4–5 mm slices); thickened meniscus (>15 mm).
- Sagittal view:
  - "Block-like" appearance (loss of normal triangular shape).
  - Tear (if present): Increased T2/PD signal (intrasubstance or peripheral tear).
  - Parameniscal cyst (if horizontal cleavage tear).

Management

- Asymptomatic: no treatment (observation).
- Symptomatic (no tear): physical therapy (quad strengthening, proprioception) and NSAIDs for pain/inflammation.
- Symptomatic with tear or instability: arthroscopic surgery.

Prognosis & Complications

- Good outcomes after repair.
- Risk of early osteoarthritis if a significant portion of the meniscus is removed.

Suggested Reading

Arora G, Parvir K, Jolly A, Kantroo AA, Patel JH, Chaliawala Y. Surgical management of symptomatic discoid meniscus: a case report and review of outcomes. J Orthop Case Rep. 2025;15(7):152–6.

Qin C, Zhang Y, Tian Z, Shang Y, Li P. Prevalence and correlation analysis of lateral discoid meniscus with degeneration or injury of the meniscus and articular cartilage in the entire tibiofemoral joint. BMC Musculoskelet Disord. 2025;26(1):740.

Watanabe M, Takeda S, Ikeuchi H. Atlas of arthroscopy. Tokyo: Igaku-Shoin; 1979. p. 156.

Case 43

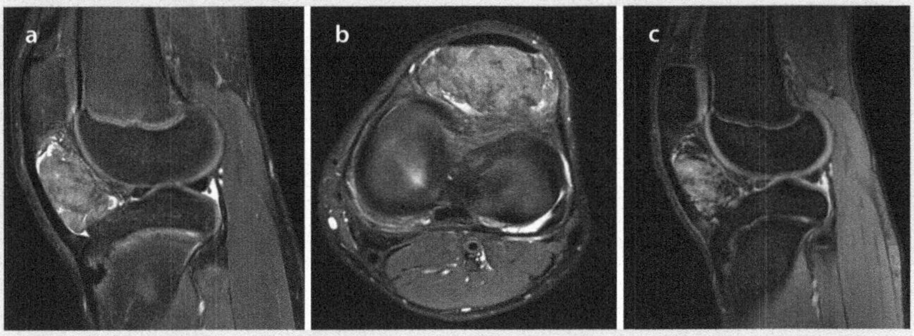

■ A 38-year-old man presented with a 3-year history of pain in the right knee joint

S. Saran et al., *101 Knee Imaging Case Series*, 101 MSK Imaging 1,
https://doi.org/10.1007/978-3-032-21567-3_43

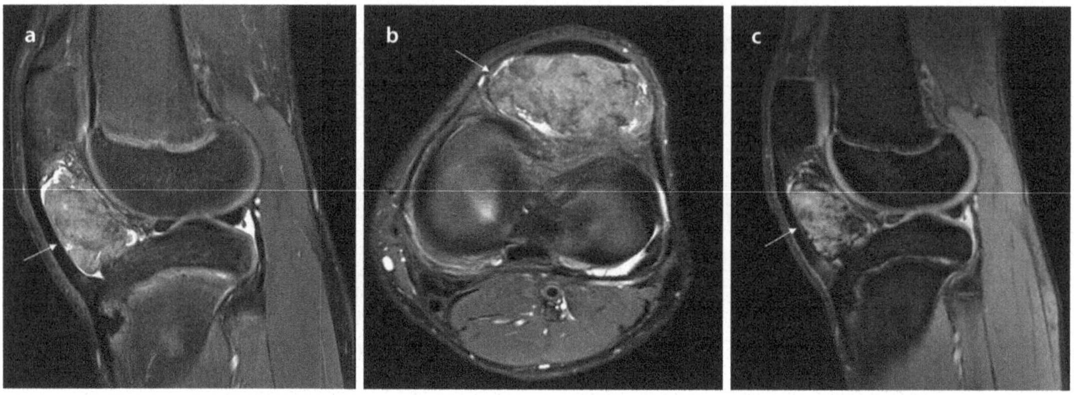

MRI knee **a**–**c** shows the presence of a large well-defined lesion in the infrapatellar fat pad (arrows) showing hyperintense signals on PDFS **a** and **b** weighted sequences with hypointense internal areas. The lesion demonstrates areas of "blooming" on gradient echo sequence **c**, suggesting hemosiderin deposition. MRI findings favour the diagnosis of focal pigmented villonodular synovitis of the knee

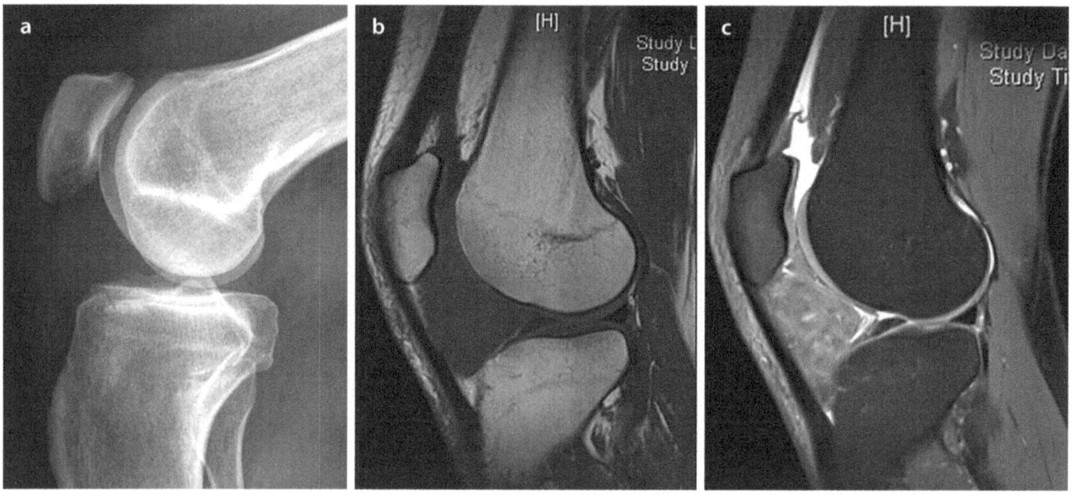

Companion case: Another case of focal pigmented villonodular synovitis of the knee in the infrapatellar fat pad

Focal Pigmented Villonodular Synovitis (PVNS)

Definition & Pathophysiology

- Focal pigmented villonodular synovitis (PVNS), also known as localised nodular synovitis, is a benign, proliferative disorder of the synovial lining of joints, bursae, and tendon sheaths. The "focal" form presents as a single, pedunculated or sessile nodule, in contrast to the diffuse form, which involves the entire synovium.

- It is characterised by a fibrous stroma, lipid-laden macrophages, multinucleated giant cells, and heavy hemosiderin deposition from recurrent microhemorrhages.
- The localised form is less aggressive than the diffuse type, typically causing mechanical symptoms due to the nodule itself rather than joint-wide destruction.
- Important: The 2020 WHO Soft Tissue and Bone Tumors Classification (fifth edition) has updated the nomenclature for this condition, replacing "pigmented villonodular synovitis" with the preferred term "tenosynovial giant cell tumor". Despite this change, the outdated terminology persists in common usage.

Clinical Presentation

- Demographics: Most common in adults aged 30–50 years.
- Symptoms:
  - Mechanical symptoms: intermittent pain, locking, catching, or giving way as the nodule becomes interposed between the joint surfaces.
  - Recurrent effusion.
  - Differentiator from diffuse PVNS: Symptoms are more intermittent and mechanical, rather than the constant pain, progressive stiffness, and diffuse swelling seen in the diffuse form.

Imaging Findings

- Radiography
  - Often normal.
  - May show a non-specific soft tissue density within the joint.
  - Unlike the diffuse form, bone erosions and cysts are rare.
- MRI
  - The MRI appearance is driven by the paramagnetic effects of hemosiderin, which cause magnetic susceptibility artifact.
  - T1-weighted: The nodule is typically isointense or slightly hypointense to muscle.
  - T2-weighted/PD/STIR: The lesion is predominantly hypointense due to the magnetic "blooming" effect of hemosiderin. This is a pathognomonic finding. Areas of inflammation or fluid may show mixed signals. The cellular component shows hyperintense signals.
  - Gradient-Echo (GRE): Shows the most dramatic "blooming artifact".
  - T1-weighted post-contrast: The nodule typically shows intense, homogeneous enhancement of the viable cellular tissue.

Differential Diagnosis

- Diffuse PVNS: Involves most or all of the synovium, leading to widespread thickening and innumerable nodules. Carries a higher recurrence rate.
- Synovial hemangioma: A vascular malformation that is hyperintense on T2-weighted images, unlike the dark T2 signal of PVNS.
- Synovial osteochondromatosis: Characterised by multiple intra-articular loose bodies that may be calcified. The synovium itself is not as thickened or hemosiderin-laden.

Management

- The treatment of choice is complete surgical excision, which is typically curative for the focal form.
- Surgical intervention (definitive treatment)
  - Procedure: arthroscopic excision.
  - Complete removal is critical to prevent recurrence. The focal form has an excellent prognosis with a low recurrence rate (<10%) after complete arthroscopic resection.

Suggested Reading

Bassetti E, Candreva R, Santucci E. Pigmented villonodular synovitis of the knee: a case report. J Ultrasound. 2011;14(3):167–9.

Sahin MS. Localized pigmented villonodular synovitis of the knee joint: a case report. J Orthop Case Rep. 2022;12(4):44–8.

Case 44

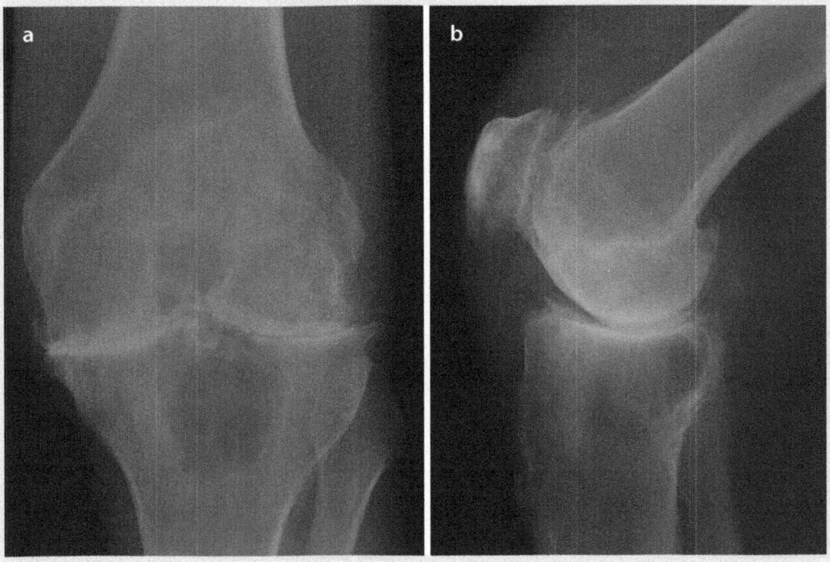

■ A 72-year-old woman presented with a long-standing history of bilateral knee pain with significantly worsened pain in the left knee over the past 6 months

S. Saran et al., *101 Knee Imaging Case Series*, 101 MSK Imaging 1,
https://doi.org/10.1007/978-3-032-21567-3_44

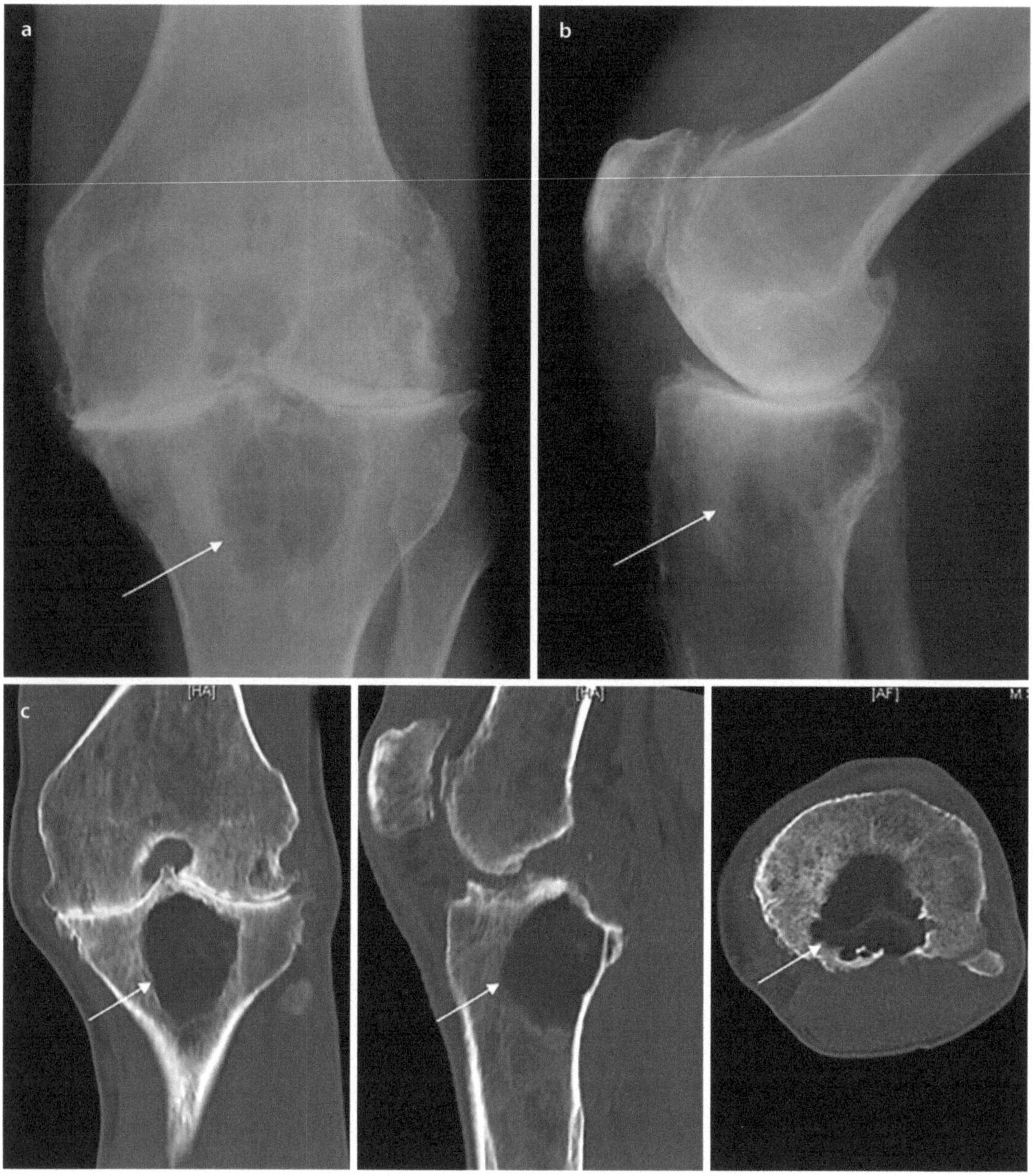

Radiographs AP **a**, Lateral **b** of the left knee show severe joint space narrowing with osteophytes and subchondral sclerosis. A large, well-defined, radiolucent cystic area (arrows) is present within the proximal tibia in the subchondral region. Radiographic findings are highly suggestive of a large geode (subchondral bone cyst) in the context of severe knee osteoarthritis. CT **c** confirms the presence of a geode (arrow) in the background of severe knee osteoarthritis

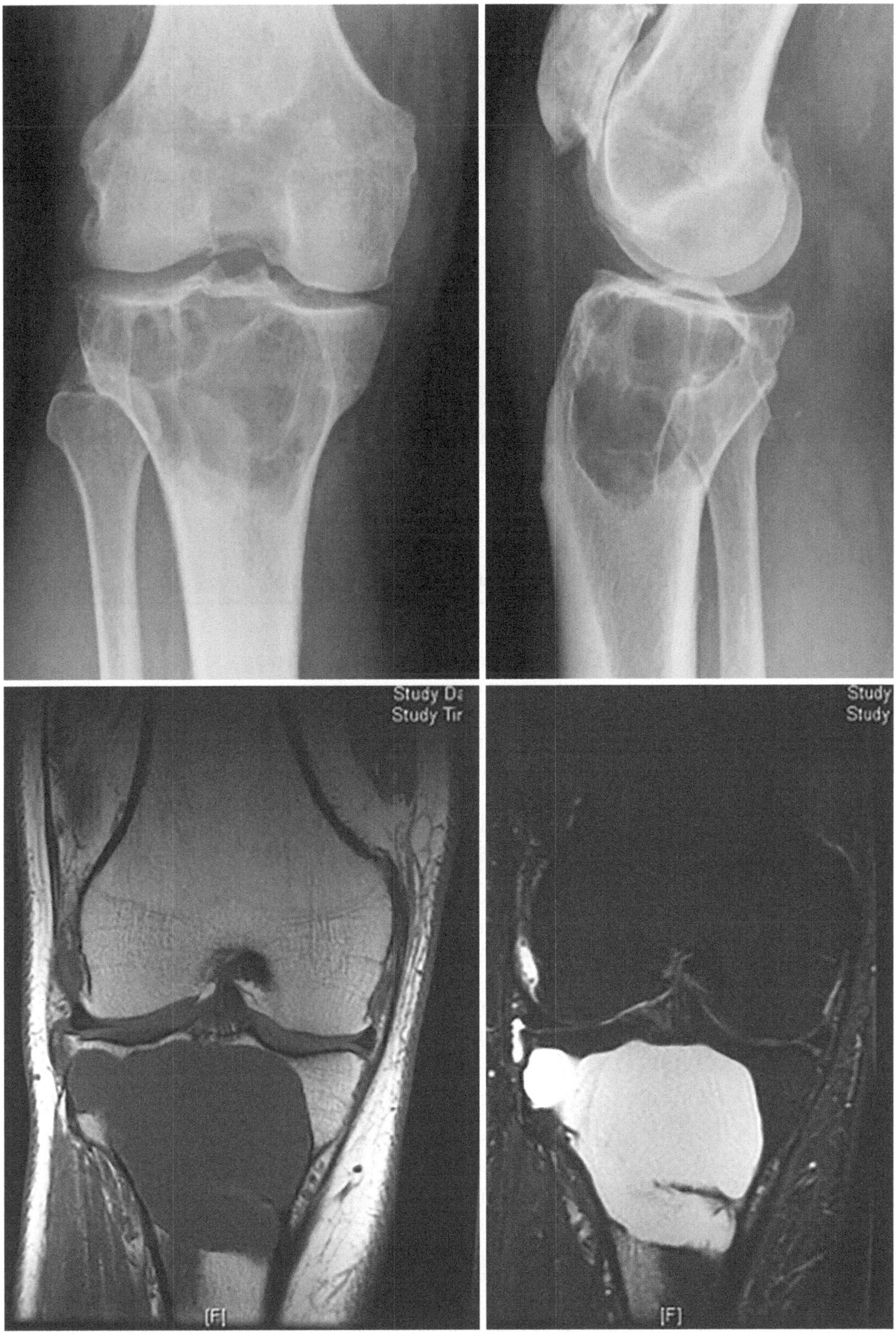

Companion case: Large Geode in proximal tibia in a case of degenerative knee arthritis

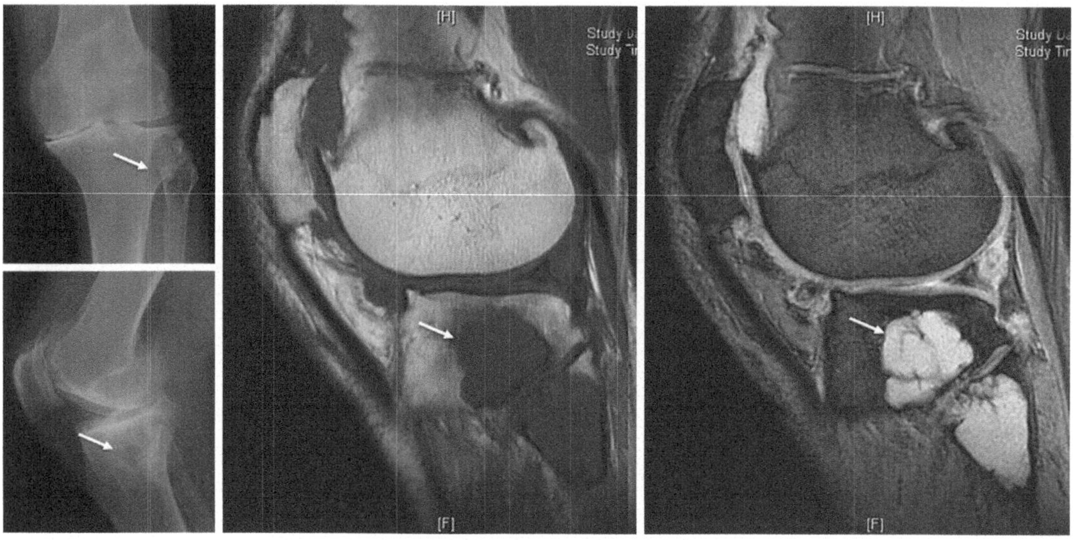

Companion case: Another case of Geode involving proximal tibio-fibular joint (arrows)

Geode (Subchondral Cyst)

Definition & Pathophysiology

- A geode (subchondral cyst) is a fluid-filled, cystic lesion found in the bone just beneath the articular cartilage.
- Pathogenesis: Two primary theories explain their formation in OA:
  - Synovial fluid intrusion (bone contusion theory): Repetitive high stress on the denuded, worn-out cartilage (eburnated bone) causes microfractures in the subchondral bone plate. Synovial fluid is then forced ("pumped") into the bone marrow, forming a cystic cavity.
  - Synovial tissue invasion: Synovial tissue from the joint extends into the bone through the damaged subchondral plate, forming a cyst lined with fibrous tissue and synovial cells.

Clinical Presentation

- The symptoms are those of severe, end-stage osteoarthritis.
- Persistent pain: deep, aching pain in the knee, present at rest and worsening with any weight-bearing activity.
- Stiffness: significant morning stiffness and stiffness after inactivity.
- Deformity: visible varus (bow-legged) or valgus (knock-kneed) deformity is typical.

- Loss of function: profound difficulty with walking, climbing stairs, and rising from a chair due to pain and mechanical instability.
- Crepitus: audible and palpable grinding during knee movement.

Imaging Findings

- Radiography
  - Large osteophytes with "bone-on-bone" joint space loss.
  - Subchondral sclerosis with gross deformity (varus/valgus angulation).
  - Geode appearance: a well-defined, rounded lucency in the subchondral bone of the proximal tibia or distal femur with a thin, sclerotic rim, indicating a chronic, walled-off process.
- MRI
  - MRI is excellent for confirming the cystic nature of the lesion and ruling out other pathologies.
  - T1-weighted: Geodes appear as sharply marginated, homogeneously low signal intensity lesions.
  - T2-weighted/STIR: They are homogeneously hyperintense, confirming their fluid content.
  - Post-contrast (T1+C): The cyst itself does not enhance, but the thin fibrous wall and the surrounding inflamed bone marrow may show mild enhancement.

Differential Diagnosis

In a joint with severe osteoarthritis, a geode is the most likely diagnosis. However, it's important to distinguish it from:
- Intraosseous ganglion: A similar cyst, but it is not associated with advanced osteoarthritis.
- Giant cell tumour of bone (GCT): In younger patients, a GCT is purely lytic, eccentric, and abuts the articular surface but lacks the sclerotic rim and surrounding degenerative changes.

Management

Management is directed at the underlying end-stage osteoarthritis, not the geode itself. The geode is a sign of the disease severity, and may not be the cause of the pain.
- Conservative management (palliative)
  - Analgesics for pain control.
  - Unloader braces.
  - Activity modification.
  - Walking aid.

  - Corticosteroid injections: For temporary relief of inflammatory pain and synovitis.
  - Visco supplementation (hyaluronic acid) Injections: May provide limited symptomatic relief in some patients.
- Surgical management (definitive treatment)
  - Total knee arthroplasty: The gold standard and definitive treatment.
  - During surgery, the geodes are routinely treated by curettage and packing with bone graft or bone cement to provide a solid foundation for the tibial implant.

Suggested Reading

Amirthalingam S, Kumar P, Harshavardhan JKG. A massive proximal tibia geode – can we afford to miss it? J Orthop Case Rep. 2023;13(7):116–20.

Resnick D, Niwayama G, Coutts RD. Subchondral cysts (geodes) in arthritic disorders: pathologic and radiographic appearance of the hip joint. AJR Am J Roentgenol. 1977;128(5):799–806.

Case 45

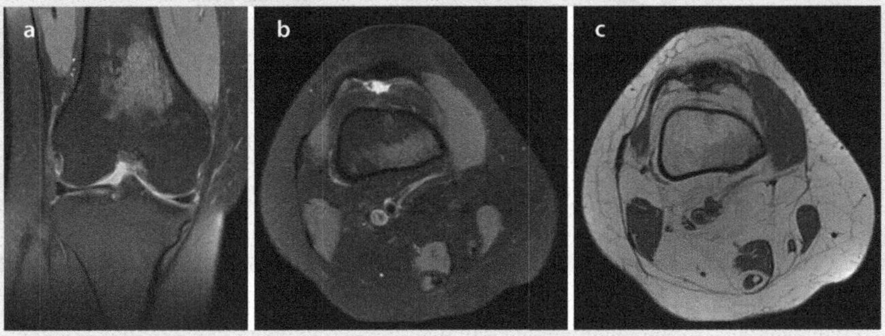

■ A 23-year-old female presented with pain in the knee joint. A MRI of the knee was performed

S. Saran et al., *101 Knee Imaging Case Series*, 101 MSK Imaging 1,
https://doi.org/10.1007/978-3-032-21567-3_45

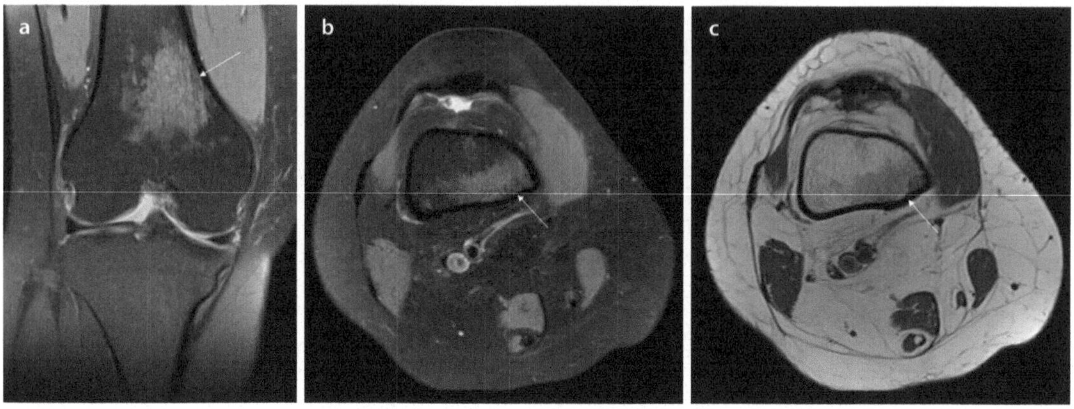

The MRI of the knee was reported as normal. A patchy area of altered signal intensity (arrows) is noted in the distal femoral metaphysis, showing high signal on PDFS sequences **a**, **b**. The area is hypo-intense on the T1 weighted sequence (arrow in **c**); however, the signal intensity is higher than that of the muscles. The MRI findings indicate the presence of hematopoietic marrow rest

Hematopoietic Marrow Rest

Definition & Pathophysiology

- A hematopoietic marrow rest refers to the persistence of red bone marrow in a location where it would typically be expected to have converted to yellow marrow with age. This is a normal physiological variant and not a pathological process.
- Normal marrow conversion: With ageing, the body undergoes a predictable conversion of red marrow to yellow marrow. This process occurs in a centripetal pattern—from the extremities toward the axial skeleton. In long bones, it progresses from the diaphysis to the metaphysis and finally to the epiphysis.
- Clinical significance: It is an incidental finding with absolutely no clinical symptoms or malignant potential. Its importance lies solely in not mistaking it for a pathological lesion such as a bone tumour, metastasis, or infection.

Clinical Presentation

- Asymptomatic: this is never the cause of a patient's pain or symptoms.
- Incidental finding: discovered purely by chance on an MRI scan performed for an unrelated reason, such as knee pain, trauma, or ligament injury.

Imaging Findings

- MRI is the primary modality where this finding is encountered and characterised. Its appearance is classic and follows the signal characteristics of normal red marrow.
- T1-weighted: The marrow rest appears as a geographic area of intermediate signal intensity (darker than subcutaneous fat but brighter than muscle). It blends imperceptibly with the surrounding fatty yellow marrow, which is bright.
- Fat-saturated T2-weighted / STIR: It shows intermediate to higher signal intensity. A key feature is its lack of mass effect and well-defined, often feathery, margins.
- Chemical shift imaging (in-phase/out-of-phase): This is a highly specific sequence. The lesion will show signal loss (drop-out) on the out-of-phase images because it contains both fat (from the marrow space) and water (from the hematopoietic cells). This "India ink" artifact at the interface confirms the presence of microscopic fat and is a hallmark of benign red marrow.
- Post-contrast (T1 + C): May show mild, diffuse enhancement due to the vascular nature of red marrow, but it is not a prominent or concerning feature.

Differential Diagnosis

- Bone metastasis: A malignant lesion is typically T1 hypointense (darker than muscle), brightly hyperintense on T2/STIR, demonstrates restricted diffusion (bright on high b-value DWI), and shows more intense, nodular enhancement. It may also cause a mass effect or bone destruction.
- Primary bone tumour (e.g., lymphoma, Ewing's sarcoma): These are aggressive lesions that are T1 hypointense, T2 hyperintense, and often have a large associated soft tissue mass.
- Osteomyelitis: presents with clinical signs of infection (fever, pain, elevated inflammatory markers). MRI shows confluent bone marrow oedema, cortical destruction, and periosteal reaction.

Management

- No treatment required: this is a "do-not-touch" lesion. No treatment, biopsy, or further imaging is indicated.
- Reassurance: the most important management step is to correctly identify the finding and reassure the patient and referring clinician that it is a normal variant of no clinical significance.

- Documentation: the radiologist should clearly describe it in the report as a "focus of persistent hematopoietic marrow, a normal physiological variant", to prevent unnecessary follow-up or concern.

Suggested Reading

Ahlawat S, Ghasemi A, Fayad LM. How I do it: MRI of the bone with marrow-specific sequences. Radiology. 2025;316(3):e242371.

Arslan G, Ozmen E, Soyturk M. MRI of residual red bone marrow in the distal femur of healthy subjects. Pol J Radiol. 2015;80:300–4.

Case 46

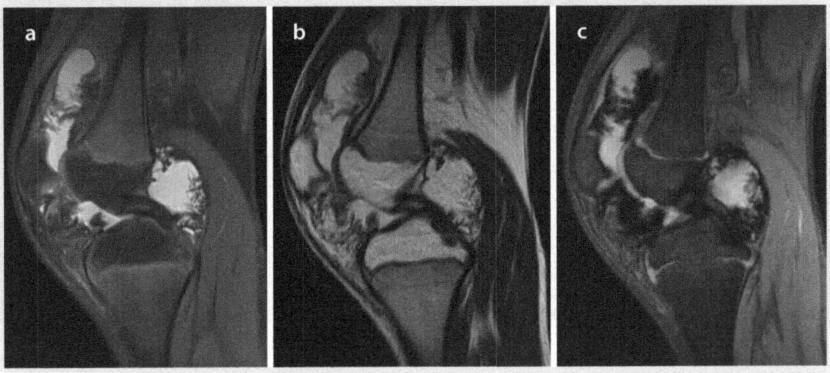

■ A 13-year-old child with a known genetic disorder presented with recurrent knee swelling and pain

S. Saran et al., *101 Knee Imaging Case Series*, 101 MSK Imaging 1,
https://doi.org/10.1007/978-3-032-21567-3_46

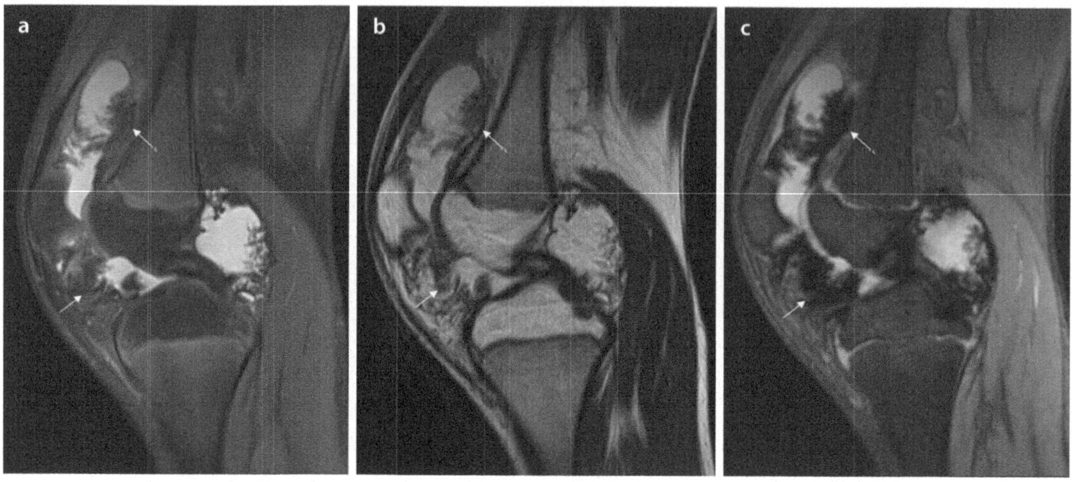

■ MRI of the knee shows the presence of diffuse proliferation of the synovium (arrows) with low signal on PDFS weighted sagittal **a**, T2-weighted sagittal **b** and blooming artifact on gradient echo **c** images. The patient is a known case of haemophilia, and recurrent haemarthrosis has led to siderotic synovitis

Hemosiderotic Synovitis in Haemophilia

Definition & Pathophysiology

- Hemosiderotic synovitis is a chronic, proliferative, and inflammatory synovial condition characterised by excessive iron deposition within the synovial membrane. In haemophilia, it is a direct consequence of recurrent haemorrhages.

Clinical Presentation

- Patient profile: individuals with severe haemophilia A or B.
- Symptoms:
  - Chronic joint pain and swelling.
  - Stiffness and progressive loss of range of motion.
  - Joint feels warm and boggy during acute bleeds.
- Physical exam:
  - Joint effusion.
  - Synovial hypertrophy: a thickened, rubbery, or firm synovium palpable around the joint.
  - Crepitus and joint contractures in advanced stages.
  - Muscle atrophy around the affected joint.

Imaging Findings

- Radiography
  - Early stages: may only show soft tissue swelling and effusion.
  - Late stages (haemophilic arthropathy):
    - Osteoporosis.
    - Joint space narrowing due to cartilage destruction.
    - Subchondral cysts and erosions.
    - Epiphyseal overgrowth and squaring of the patella.
    - Widening of the intercondylar notch.
- MRI
  - MRI is exquisitely sensitive for detecting hemosiderin.
  - T2-weighted/STIR: The hypertrophied synovium appears as thickened, frond-like, low-signal tissue lining the joint, outlined by effusion.
  - Hemosiderin deposition causes a profound “blooming artifact” on T2*-weighted Gradient-Echo (GRE) sequences, where it appears larger than its actual size.
  - Post-contrast (T1 + C): The inflamed, hypertrophied synovium shows intense, vivid enhancement.

Differential Diagnosis

- Pigmented villonodular synovitis (PVNS): The imaging appearance is identical, as it also features hemosiderin deposition. The key differentiator is the clinical history of a bleeding diathesis in individuals with haemophilia. PVNS is typically monoarticular and idiopathic.
- Rheumatoid arthritis: causes synovitis and erosions but does not show prominent hemosiderin deposition on MRI. It is typically polyarticular and symmetric.
- Synovial osteochondromatosis: characterised by multiple intra-articular calcified loose bodies, not low-signal synovium.

Management

Management is complex and requires a multidisciplinary approach (haematology, orthopaedics, physiotherapy).

- Medical management (primary prevention)
  - Factor replacement prophylaxis: The cornerstone of modern care. Regular intravenous infusion of the missing clotting factor to maintain a baseline level and prevent hemarthroses from occurring.
  - Non-factor therapies: Emicizumab (Hemlibra®), a bispecific monoclonal antibody, mimics the function of Factor VIII.

- Arthroscopic or open synovectomy
  - Surgical removal of the diseased synovium.
  - Indicated for persistent bleeding despite medical and radiation synovectomy.
- Surgical intervention (for end-stage arthropathy).

Suggested Reading

Gualtierotti R, Solimeno LP, Peyvandi F. Hemophilic arthropathy: current knowledge and future perspectives. J Thromb Haemost. 2021;19(9):2112–21.

Kessi EMCJ, Maslouhi K, Guelzim Y, Belkouchi L, Allali N, Chat L, El Haddad S. Severe hemophilic arthropathy of the knee: MRI has its place. Glob Pediatr Health. 2024;11:2333794X241280116.

Case 47

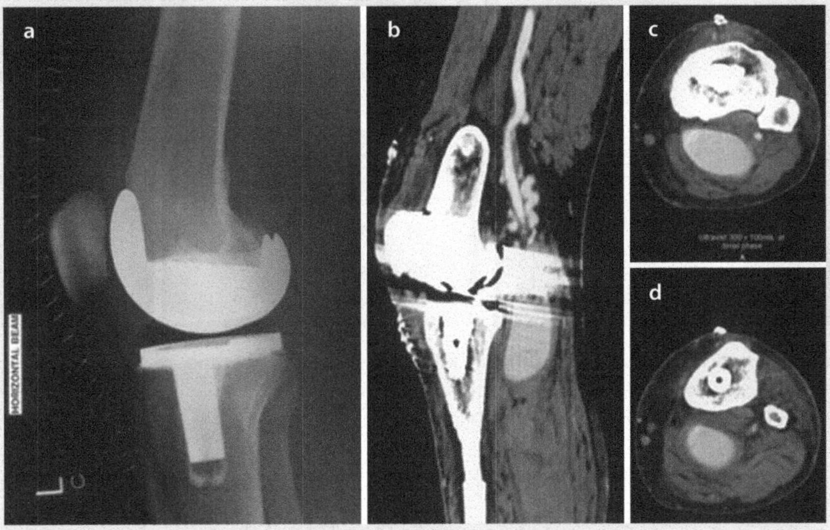

■ A 66-year-old female (post TKR) presented with pulsatile swelling in the popliteal region

S. Saran et al., *101 Knee Imaging Case Series*, 101 MSK Imaging 1,
https://doi.org/10.1007/978-3-032-21567-3_47

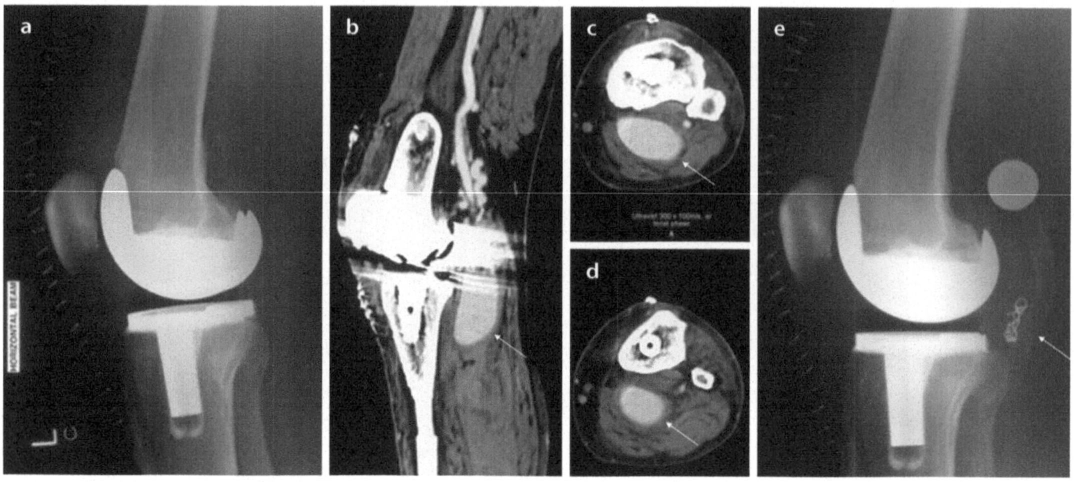

Lateral radiographs **a** shows the status post-TKR left knee. CT angiography **b**–**d** shows the presence of contrast-filled outpouching (arrows) arising from the popliteal artery, suggestive of iatrogenic popliteal artery aneurysm. Radiograph **e** shows status post endovascular repair of the aneurysm (arrow)

Iatrogenic Popliteal Artery Aneurysm

Definition & Pathophysiology

- An iatrogenic popliteal artery aneurysm is a false aneurysm (pseudoaneurysm) of the popliteal artery resulting from a breach in the arterial wall caused by a surgical procedure. Unlike a true aneurysm, it is not a dilation of all three vessel layers but a contained rupture where blood leaks through a defect in the artery and is contained by the surrounding adventitia, connective tissue, and haematoma.

Common Iatrogenic Causes

- Arthroscopic knee surgery: the most common cause. Injury can occur during posteromedial or posterolateral portal placement, posterior meniscal repair, or PCL reconstruction, where instruments are in close proximity to the popliteal artery.
- Total Knee Arthroplasty (TKA): From retractors, saws, or bone fragments.
- Manipulation under anaesthesia.
- Angiography or endovascular procedures (e.g., from catheterisation or balloon injury).

Clinical Presentation

- Timeline: Symptoms can present immediately postoperatively or in a delayed fashion (days to weeks).
- Symptoms & signs:
  - Pain, swelling, pulsatile mass with audible bruit.
  - Distal ischemia due to compression or thromboembolism.
  - Neurological deficit due to compression of the tibial nerve.

Imaging Findings

- Duplex ultrasound
  - B-mode: shows a cystic or complex mass adjacent to the popliteal artery.
  - Colour Doppler: Reveals the classic "yin-yang" sign—a swirling pattern of blood flow into the pseudoaneurysm sac during systole and out during diastole.
  - Spectral Doppler: Can identify the "to-and-fro" waveform in the neck of the pseudoaneurysm.
- CT Angiography (CTA)
  - Provides a comprehensive "roadmap" essential for deciding between endovascular and open repair:
    - The size and location of the pseudoaneurysm sac.
    - The diameter and length of the neck connecting it to the artery.
    - The relationship to surrounding structures (bone, veins, nerves).
    - The status of the distal runoff vessels.
- Conventional Angiography
  - Remains the diagnostic gold standard and allows for immediate endovascular intervention.

Differential Diagnosis

- True popliteal artery aneurysm: a dilation of all three arterial wall layers, typically bilateral and associated with atherosclerosis. It lacks a recent history of iatrogenic trauma.
- Baker's cyst: a non-pulsatile, fluid-filled synovial cyst from the knee joint. No internal flow on Doppler.
- Hematoma: a collection of blood without a communication to the artery; it will not show the characteristic "yin-yang" flow.
- Soft tissue tumour: a solid mass, not a vascular structure.

Management

- This is a vascular emergency. Treatment is required to prevent rupture, thrombosis, or distal embolisation. The choice of repair depends on the anatomy of the pseudoaneurysm and the patient's condition.
- Ultrasound-guided compression/thrombin injection:
  - Indication: first-line for simple pseudoaneurysms with a narrow, accessible neck.
  - Procedure: under ultrasound guidance, direct pressure is applied to the neck, or thrombin is injected into the sac to induce thrombosis.
  - Limitation: often not suitable if the neck is wide, the sac is multiloculated, or there is an active arteriovenous fistula.
- Endovascular Stent-Graft repair:
  - Indication: increasingly the preferred treatment, especially in stable patients with suitable anatomy.
  - Procedure: a covered stent (stent-graft) is deployed across the defect via a catheter, excluding the pseudoaneurysm from the circulation while maintaining arterial flow.
- Open surgical repair
  - Unstable patient, or failed endovascular therapy.
  - Complex anatomy not suitable for stenting.

Suggested Reading

Alammari N, Ananthan B, Alotaibi S, Asiri Y, Mohammed M, Almulla A. A rare presentation of pseudoaneurysm of the popliteal artery after total knee replacement: a case report and review of the literature. Cureus. 2024;16(7):e65772.

Nazari I, Zargar MA, Nazari A, Alavi SMA. Iatrogenic popliteal artery pseudoaneurysm: a case report. Int J Surg Case Rep. 2024;122:109988.

Case 48

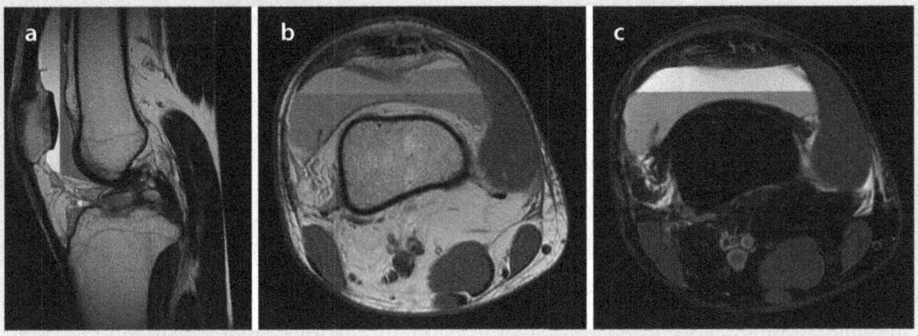

■ A 20-year-old male presented with a twisting knee injury followed by instability and a rapid onset of knee swelling

S. Saran et al., *101 Knee Imaging Case Series*, 101 MSK Imaging 1,
https://doi.org/10.1007/978-3-032-21567-3_48

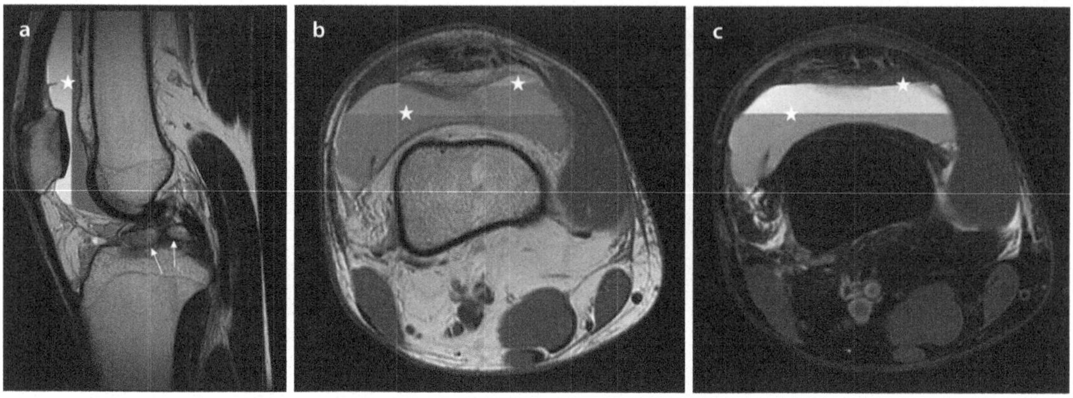

■ MRI knee **a**–**c** (T2 sagittal **a**, PD axial **b** and PDFS **c** axial sequences) shows the presence of avulsion fracture at the tibial attachment of the anterior cruciate ligament (arrows) with Lipohemarthrosis (stars) showing layering of marrow fat over fluid and blood

Lipohemarthrosis

Definition & Pathophysiology

- Lipohemarthrosis is the presence of fat and blood within a joint space. It is a specific and important diagnostic sign, indicating an intra-articular fracture that has extended into the marrow-containing bone, allowing marrow fat to escape into the joint alongside blood.
- The condition requires a fracture line that communicates with the joint capsule. Common site of fractures in the knee include tibial plateau fractures, condylar femoral fractures, and patellar fractures.
- The presence of fat in the joint fluid is virtually pathognomonic for an intra-articular fracture. It is not a disease in itself, but a sign of a significant underlying injury.

Clinical Features

- History of acute trauma (e.g., fall, motor vehicle accident).
- Knee pain, swelling, and significant joint effusion.
- Inability to bear weight.

Imaging Findings

- Cross-table lateral knee X-ray
  - Fat-fluid level: a horizontal line is visible within the suprapatellar bursa. The lucent fat layer floats on top of the denser sanguinous fluid layer.

  - Requirement: The X-ray beam must be horizontal (parallel to the floor) while the patient lies supine to allow the layers to separate by gravity.
  - Its identification on imaging is a critical clue to an occult intra-articular fracture that may not be clearly visible on initial X-rays.
- CT
  - Clearly demonstrates the fat-fluid level with high sensitivity.
  - Exquisitely defines the associated intra-articular fracture.
- MRI
  - Layer-specific signal intensities:
    - Superior layer (fat): hyperintense on T1 and T2; suppresses on fat-saturated sequences.
    - Inferior layer (blood): signal varies with the age of the bleed. Acute blood may be intermediate, while subacute blood is hyperintense on both T1 and T2. It does not suppress on fat-sat sequences.
    - Sometimes three layers are seen with fat as the most superficial one, followed by serous fluid and dependent sanguinous fluid.
  - MRI is also excellent for identifying the fracture, bone marrow oedema, and associated soft tissue injuries (menisci, ligaments).

Management

- Management is directed entirely at the underlying fracture, not the Lipohemarthrosis itself.
- Immobilisation of the knee with a splint or brace.
- Definitive fracture care:
  - Non-operative: for non-displaced or minimally displaced stable fractures. Involves casting or functional bracing with non-weight-bearing.
  - Surgical intervention: For displaced, unstable, or depressed intra-articular fractures (e.g., tibial plateau fractures). Open Reduction and Internal Fixation (ORIF) is performed to restore joint congruity and stability.

Suggested Reading

Porrino J, Shreve C, Marten E, Lee H, Haims A. Lipohemarthrosis in the detection of intraarticular fractures: looking beyond the tibial plateau. PM R. 2024;16(9):1041–8.

Schick C, Mack MG, Marzi I, Vogl TG. Lipohemarthrosis of the knee: MRI as an alternative to the puncture of the knee joint. Eur Radiol. 2003;13(5):1185–7.

Case 49

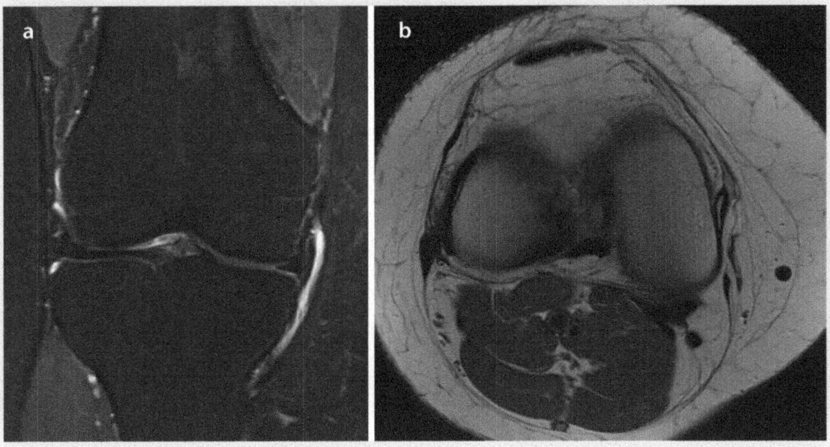

■ A 30-year-old female with pain in the knee joint along the medial joint line without any history of trauma

S. Saran et al., *101 Knee Imaging Case Series*, 101 MSK Imaging 1,
https://doi.org/10.1007/978-3-032-21567-3_49

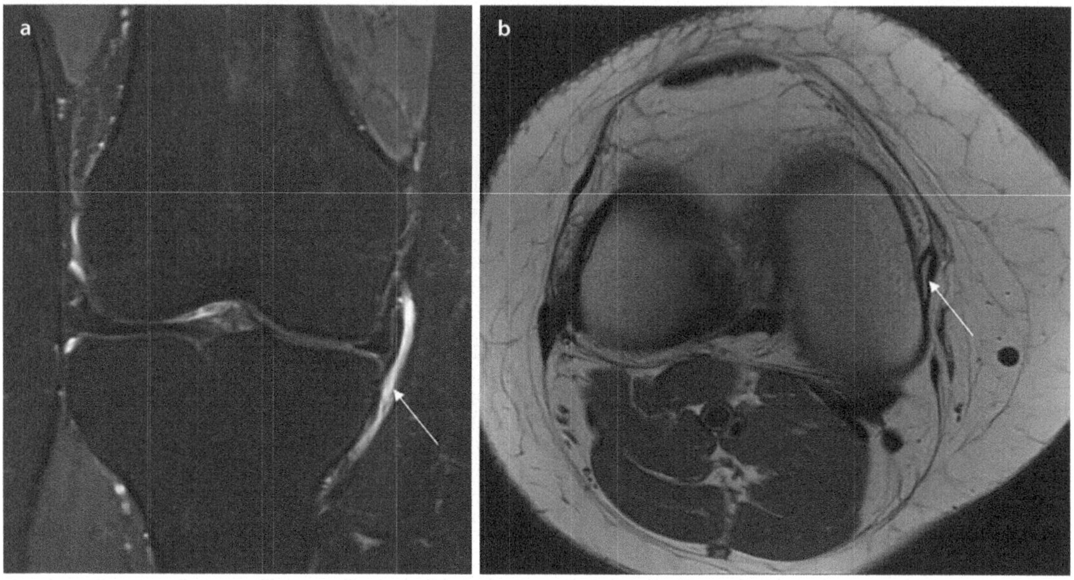

■ MRI knee, PDFS weighted coronal **a**, and T2 weighted axial **b**, sequences showing a well-defined vertical hyperintense area (arrows) between the superficial and deep components of the Medial collateral ligament (MCL). In the absence of a history of trauma, this represents MCL bursitis

MCL Bursitis

Definition & Pathophysiology

- MCL bursitis is the inflammation and fluid distension of the unique bursa located between the superficial and deep layers of the medial collateral ligament.
- The MCL bursa, also known as Voshell's bursa, is a distinct, vertically oriented compartment within the ligament complex itself.
- Function: It functions as a gliding plane, reducing friction between the superficial and deep layers of the MCL during knee motion, particularly during flexion and valgus stress.
- Cause of inflammation: Results from repetitive shear stress or a direct valgus force that causes pinching and irritation of this bursa. It is often associated with: chronic mechanical stress (e.g., in athletes); degenerative joint disease (osteoarthritis); trauma or direct impact to the medial knee; concurrent knee pathologies (e.g., meniscal tears, especially of the medial meniscus).

Clinical Presentation

- Pain: Localised, point tenderness over the medial joint line, typically superior to the pes anserinus.
- Swelling: A subtle, soft swelling may be palpable along the course of the MCL.
- Unlike a complete MCL tear, there is no joint laxity or instability on valgus stress testing; the pain is localised to the bursa itself.

MRI Findings

- MRI is the gold standard for confirming this diagnosis and distinguishing it from other causes of medial knee pain.
- A characteristic finding of a well-defined, fluid-signal intensity collection (hyperintense on T2/PD-weighted images) neatly interposed between the superficial and deep fibres of the MCL.
- Location: Confined to the middle third of the knee, along the joint line.
- Morphology: Typically appears as a vertical, curvilinear, or comma-shaped fluid collection.
- No underlying ligament disruption: The MCL fibres themselves appear intact, distinguishing them from a partial tear, which would show ligamentous oedema and disruption.

Management

- Conservative
  - Activity modification: Avoid activities that provoke symptoms (pivoting, cutting).
  - NSAIDs: To reduce pain and inflammation.
  - Physical therapy: Focus on strengthening the dynamic stabilisers of the knee (quadriceps, hip abductors) and improving flexibility to reduce stress on the MCL complex.
- Image-guided interventions
  - Corticosteroid injection: Ultrasound-guided injection of a corticosteroid and local anaesthetic directly into the bursa is highly effective for both diagnostic confirmation and therapeutic relief. This is often the definitive treatment if conservative measures fail.

Suggested Reading

Chatra P. Bursae around the knee joints. Indian J Radiol Imaging. 2012;22(1):27–30. https://doi.org/10.4103/0971-3026.95400.

Perdikakis E, Skiadas V. MRI characteristics of cysts and "cyst-like" lesions in and around the knee: what the radiologist needs to know. Insights Imaging. 2013;4(3):257–72. https://doi.org/10.1007/s13244-013-0240-1.

Case 50

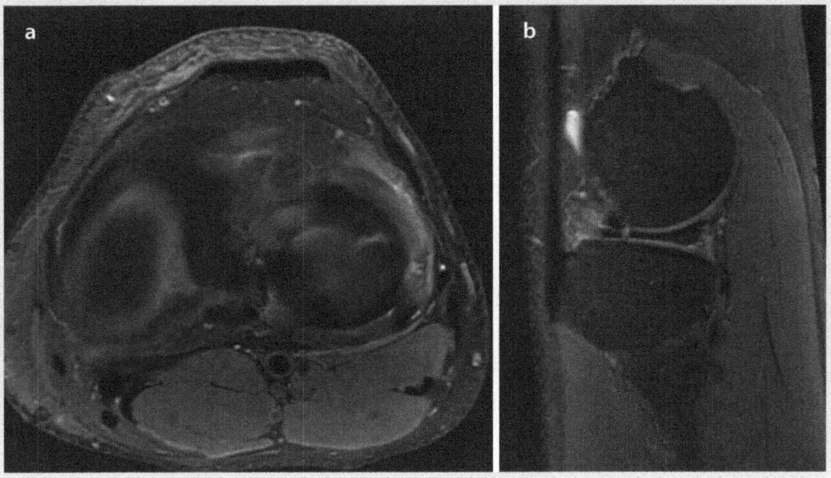

A 35-year-old male presented with pain in the knee joint

S. Saran et al., *101 Knee Imaging Case Series*, 101 MSK Imaging 1,
https://doi.org/10.1007/978-3-032-21567-3_50

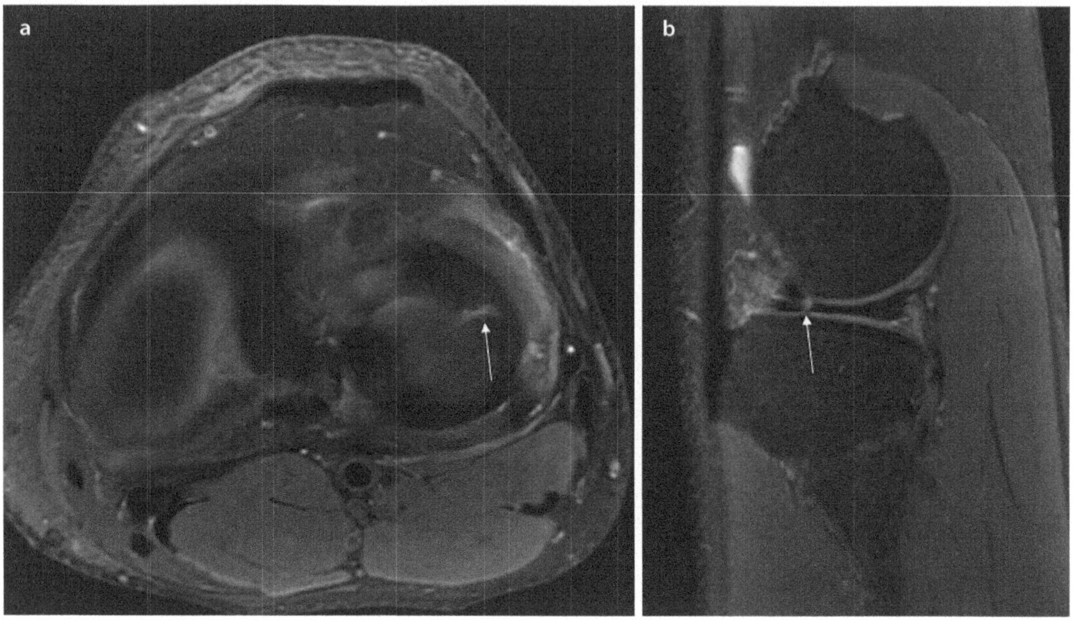

▪ MRI knee **a**. PDFS weighted axial image shows a fluid cleft involving the inner free edge of lateral meniscus at the junction of anterior horn and body (arrow). **b**. Corresponding cleft is also seen on PDFS weighted sagittal image (arrow in **b**). MRI findings are of radial tear

Radial Meniscal Tear

Definition & Pathophysiology

- A radial meniscal tear is a severe injury characterized by a tear that propagates perpendicular to the circumferential collagen fibers of the meniscus, from the free, inner edge toward the peripheral rim. This disrupts the meniscus's primary function of converting axial load into "hoop stresses".
- Mechanism: Typically caused by a sudden, high-load axial force combined with rotation, often during deep squatting, pivoting, or heavy lifting.
- Biomechanical Consequence: A full-thickness radial tear that reaches the peripheral capsule is biomechanically equivalent to a total meniscectomy. It completely disrupts the meniscus's ability to distribute load, leading to a dramatic increase in joint contact pressures and a high risk of rapid post-traumatic osteoarthritis.
- Root tear is a variety of radial tear.

Clinical Presentation

- Symptoms:
  - Acute, sharp pain at the time of injury, often localised to the joint line (medial or lateral).
  - Swelling develops hours after the injury.
  - Mechanical symptoms like clicking or catching, though locking is less common than with flap or bucket-handle tears.
  - A sensation of the knee "giving way".

Imaging Findings

- MRI appearance
  - The key is to identify a linear defect that extends perpendicularly from the free edge.
  - Sagittal images: the classic finding is the cleft sign. The tear appears as a vertical line of high signal intensity (on T2/PDFS) replacing the normal dark meniscus.
  - Coronal images: best for visualising the tear as it extends from the free edge toward the capsule. A truncated triangle is seen.
  - Axial images: can clearly show the tear as a linear defect radiating from the inner meniscal margin.

Classification by Location & Severity

- Partial radial tear: does not extend to the peripheral rim. The meniscus maintains some hoop-stress function.
- Complete radial tear (full-thickness): extends to the peripheral capsule, completely dividing the meniscus and abolishing its load-sharing function.
- Root tear: a specific, severe type of radial tear located at the meniscal attachment to the tibia (within 1 cm). This is biomechanically the most devastating.
- Oblique (parrot-beak) tear: a combination of radial and longitudinal components.

Management

- Treatment is dictated by the location, completeness, and stability of the tear, as well as the patient's age and activity level.
- Non-surgical management:
  - Indications: small (<5 mm), partial, non-displaced radial tears in the vascular "red-red" or "red-white" zone.

  - Physical therapy: focus on quadriceps and hip strengthening to improve dynamic knee stability.
- Surgical intervention (required for most symptomatic or complete tears).
  - The choice between repair and resection is critical and depends on the tear's characteristics.
  - Arthroscopic partial meniscectomy (debridement): Partial tears causing mechanical symptoms, or complete tears in the avascular "white-white" zone, or in older, low-demand patients.
  - Arthroscopic meniscal repair: Complete radial tears in the vascular zone (red-red or red-white) in young, active patients. This is the preferred treatment to preserve meniscal function.

Suggested Reading

Alaia EF, Samim M, Moore MR, Walter WR, Burke CJ, LaPorte ZL, Egol AJ, Golant A, Alaia MJ. The lateral meniscal oblique radial tear: MRI identification of a biomechanically important tear pattern associated with anterior cruciate ligament injury. AJR Am J Roentgenol. 2025.

Harper KW, Helms CA, Lambert HS 3rd, Higgins LD. Radial meniscal tears: significance, incidence, and MR appearance. AJR Am J Roentgenol. 2005;185(6):1429–34.

Lee SY, Jee WH, Kim JM. Radial tear of the medial meniscal root: reliability and accuracy of MRI for diagnosis. AJR Am J Roentgenol. 2008;191(1):81–5.

Case 51

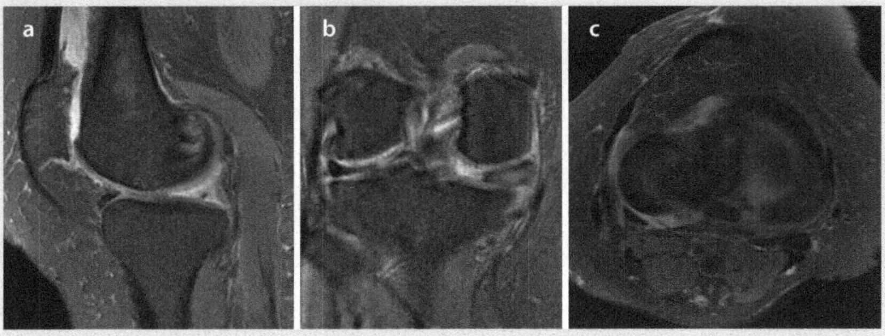

■ A 65-year-old female presented with chronic pain in the knee joint with decreased range of movement

S. Saran et al., *101 Knee Imaging Case Series*, 101 MSK Imaging 1,
https://doi.org/10.1007/978-3-032-21567-3_51

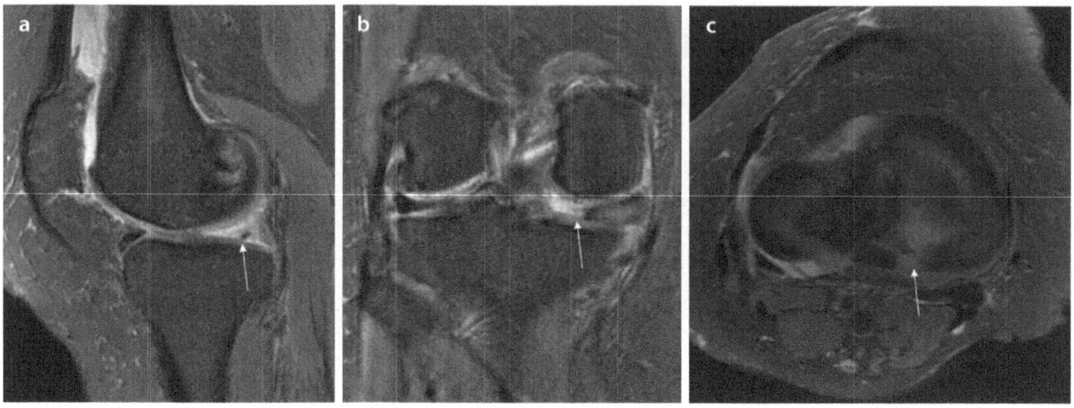

■ MRI knee PDFS weighted sequences **a**–**c** showing a "meniscal ghost sign" (absence of meniscal tissue) on the sagittal image (arrow in **a**), truncation sign on the coronal images (arrow in **b**) and absence of meniscal signals involving the posterior root of the medial meniscus on axial image (arrow in **c**) suggestive of posterior root tear of medial meniscus. Associated extrusion of the involved meniscus and degenerative osteoarthritis in the knee joint is also seen

Root Tear of the Meniscus

Definition & Pathophysiology

- A meniscal root tear is a specific, severe type of meniscal injury characterised by a complete radial tear located within 1 cm of the meniscal attachment site to the tibial plateau. This injury effectively detaches the meniscus from its bony anchor, destroying its ability to function as a load-sharing structure.
- The posterior root of the medial meniscus is most commonly affected.
- Biomechanical Consequence: A root tear is biomechanically equivalent to a total meniscectomy. It eliminates the "hoop stress" mechanism, which leads to:
  - Uncontrolled joint space narrowing.
  - Dramatically increased contact pressure on the articular cartilage.
  - Rapid progression to osteoarthritis.

Clinical Presentation

- Mechanism: Can be traumatic in younger patients (often a deep squat or twisting injury) or degenerative in older patients with minimal trauma.
- Symptoms:
  - Posterior knee pain: deep, aching pain, often localised to the medial or posteromedial joint line.

- Effusion: swelling after the injury.
- Mechanical symptoms: sensations of popping or clicking are common, but true locking is rare.

Imaging Findings

- MRI is the gold standard for diagnosis. The key is to scrutinise the meniscal roots on every knee MRI.
- Direct signs of a root tear on MRI:
  - The "Ghost Sign" (most specific sign): On sagittal MRI images, the meniscus is "ghosted" or missing.
  - Truncation sign: On coronal images, a vertical, linear defect is seen at the meniscal attachment site.
  - Extrusion of the meniscal body: The meniscus is pushed out of the joint. On a coronal image, meniscal extrusion >3 mm beyond the tibial margin is a key indirect sign of a root tear or other significant dysfunction.

Differential Diagnosis

- Radial tear in the meniscal body: located away from the root; has a different biomechanical impact.
- Complex degenerative meniscal tear: involves multiple planes but may not specifically detach the root.

Management

Management is highly time-sensitive. The goal is to restore the meniscal function and prevent rapid joint degeneration.

- Non-surgical management (rarely indicated)
  - Only for: low-demand, elderly patients with minimal symptoms and established, accepted osteoarthritis.
  - Treatment: NSAIDs, physical therapy for quadriceps strengthening, and activity modification.
- Surgical Intervention
  - Surgery is almost always recommended for complete root tears.
  - Procedure: arthroscopic meniscal root repair.

Suggested Reading

Ashir A, Chang EY. Common mistakes in meniscal injury. Semin Musculoskelet Radiol. 2025;29(5):757–66.

Beaufils P, Pujol N. Management of traumatic meniscal tear and degenerative meniscal lesions. Save the meniscus. Orthop Traumatol Surg Res. 2017;103(8S):S237–44.

Guimarães JB, Chemin RN, Araujo FF, Link TM, Silva FD, Bitar A, Nico MAC, Filho AGO. Meniscal root tears: an update focused on preoperative and postoperative MRI findings. AJR Am J Roentgenol. 2022;219(2):269–78.

Case 52

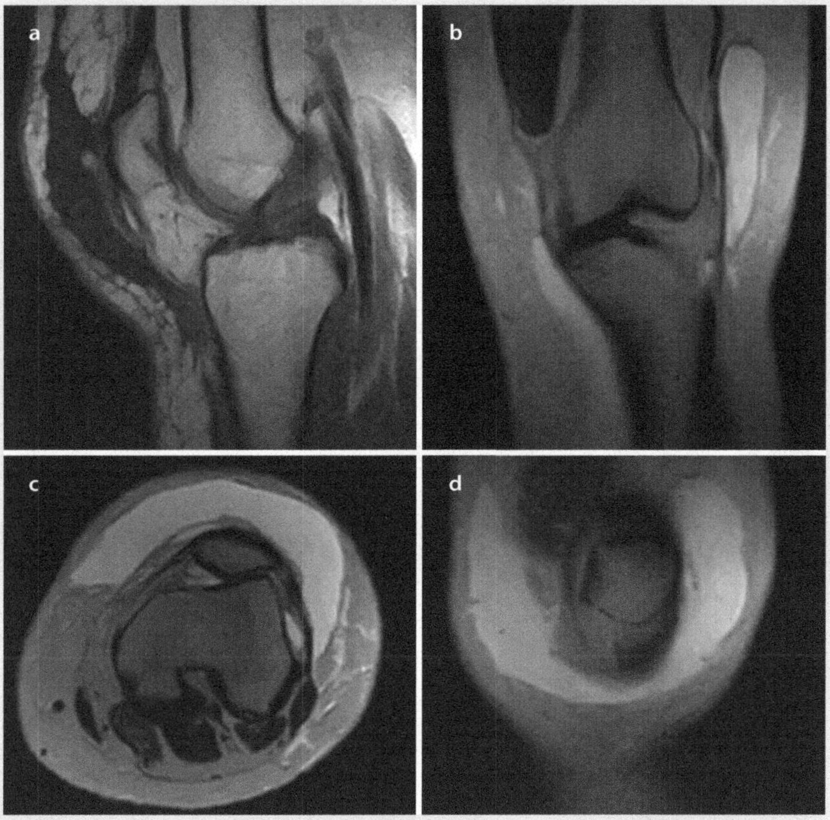

◘ A 38-year-old male with a history of a motorcycle accident 2 months back presented with gradually enlarging swelling associated with pain in the anterolateral aspect of the thigh extending to the knee joint

S. Saran et al., *101 Knee Imaging Case Series*, 101 MSK Imaging 1,
https://doi.org/10.1007/978-3-032-21567-3_52

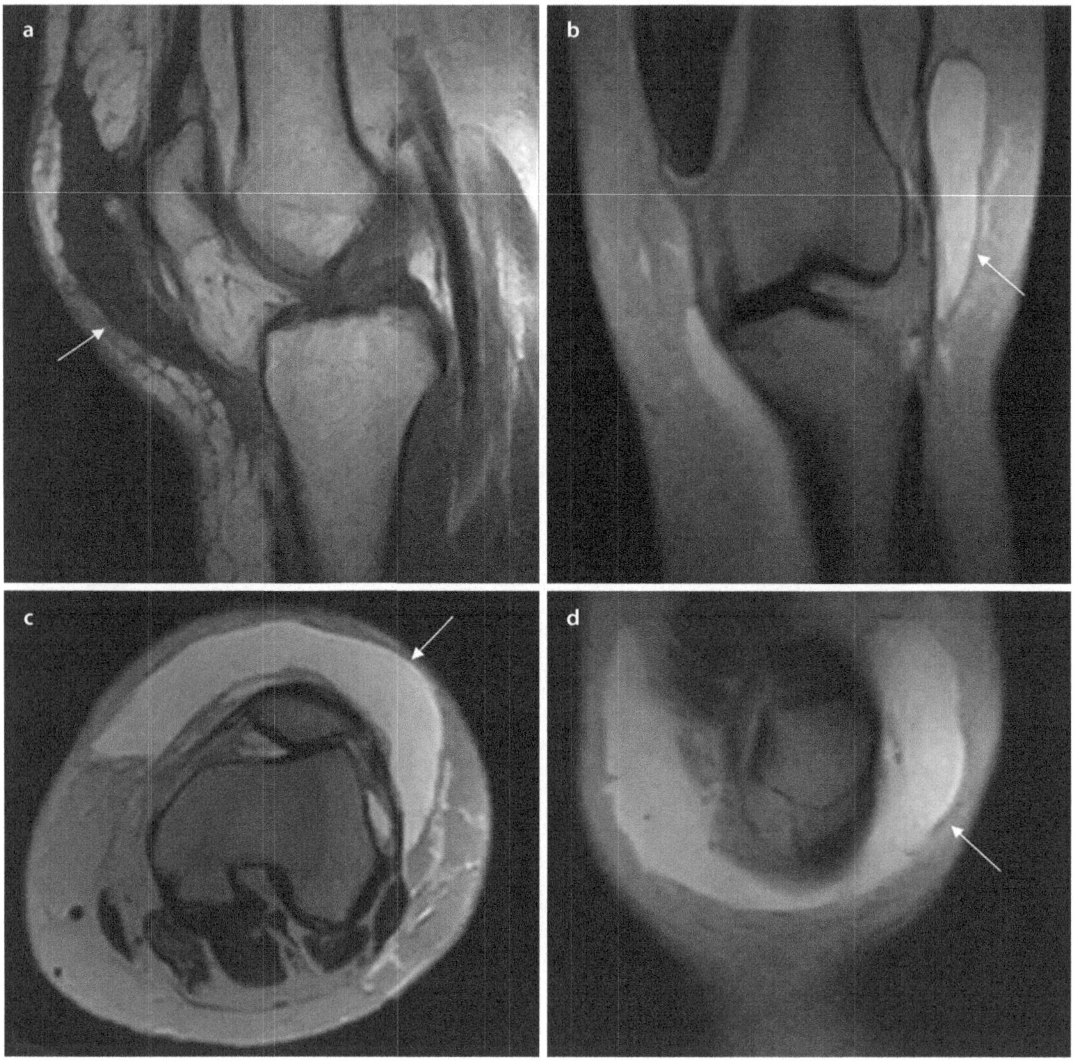

MRI knee **a**–**d** shows the presence of a large area of altered signal intensity (arrows) in the extensor aspect of the knee joint, exhibiting low signal on the T1-weighted sagittal sequence **a** and high signal on the T2-weighted coronal (**b** and **d**) and T2-weighted axial **c** sequences, localised predominantly in the subcutaneous plane. MRI findings in the context of clinical history point towards Morel-Lavallee lesion

Morel-Lavallée Lesion

Definition & Pathophysiology

- A Morel-Lavallée lesion is a closed, degloving soft-tissue injury resulting from a sudden, severe shear force (typically tangential and rotational) that traumatically separates the skin and subcutaneous tissue from the underlying fascia (typically the deep fascia overlying muscle). This disruption shears the perforating blood vessels and lymphatics, leading to a cavity that fills with blood and lymph.

Clinical Presentation

- History: Significant trauma, often with associated fractures (e.g., pelvic fractures, proximal tibia fractures).
- Symptoms & signs:
  - Soft, fluctuant, swelling: a large, boggy area of swelling that may be subtly ballotable. It is often non-tender or only mildly tender in the chronic phase.
  - Overlying skin may show ecchymosis and abrasions.
  - The size of the swelling may change, often increasing over time as the collection expands.
  - The lateral thigh (greater trochanter) is the most classic site. Other sites include the lumbosacral region, buttocks, and knee (suprapatellar region).

Imaging Findings

Imaging is crucial for diagnosis, characterisation, and guiding management.

- Ultrasound
  - A hypoechoic, fluid-filled collection in the plane between the subcutaneous fat and the underlying fascia.
  - May appear simple, anechoic or complex with internal septations, debris, and fat globules.
  - Typically shows no internal vascularity, helping to distinguish it from a vascular malformation or tumour.
- MRI
  - T1-weighted: The collection is typically isointense or slightly hyperintense to muscle. High signal may indicate fat globules or subacute blood products.
  - T2-weighted/STIR: The fluid component is markedly hyperintense. Internal low-signal septations are common. A thin, low-signal fibrous capsule is often visible in chronic lesions.
  - T1-weighted post-contrast: The fibrous capsule and internal septations enhance vividly, while the central fluid component does not.

Classification

- Lesions can be characterised based on their chronicity and MRI appearance.

- Acute/subacute: Simple seroma or hematoma.
- Chronic: Organised with a thick, enhancing fibrous capsule.
- Infected: Thick, enhancing wall with surrounding cellulitis/oedema.

Differential Diagnosis

- Hematoma: typically more acute, painful, and will often resolve spontaneously.
- Abscess: presents with signs of infection (fever, erythema, warmth); shows a thick, irregular, enhancing wall and surrounding oedema.
- Bursitis: confined to an anatomical bursa (e.g., trochanteric bursa).
- Soft tissue sarcoma: a solid, enhancing mass, not a simple fluid collection.
- Lymphatic or venous malformation: may look similar but often has more complex vascularity on Doppler.

Management

Management depends on the size, chronicity, and symptomatology of the lesion.

- Conservative management (for small, asymptomatic lesions)
  - Compression bandaging: to collapse the potential space and promote adherence of the tissue layers.
  - Observation: Some small, acute lesions may resolve spontaneously.
- Minimally invasive intervention.
  - Percutaneous aspiration & compression: simple drainage of the collection. However, recurrence is very high due to the persistent potential space and ongoing fluid production.
  - After aspiration, a sclerosing agent (e.g., doxycycline, talc, or absolute alcohol) is injected into the cavity.
  - The sclerosing agent induces an inflammatory reaction, causing the walls of the cavity to scar together and obliterate the space.
  - This is often combined with continuous compression.
- Surgical intervention (for large, chronic, or recurrent lesions)
  - Open debridement and surgical excision.
  - Quilting sutures are often placed to tack the subcutaneous tissue down to the underlying fascia, eliminating the dead space.
  - Post-operative drains are essential.

Suggested Reading

AlJuwied H, AlNajadah D, Mostafa Z, Ashraf A, Jarragh A, Lari A. Missed and mismanaged: severe consequences of Morel Lavallee lesions-a case series. J Surg Case Rep. 2025;2025(9):rjaf731.

Karp JD, Oduwole SO, Nazarian LN. Chronic Morel-Lavallée lesion treated with percutaneous ultrasonic debridement. J Clin Ultrasound. 2025.

Sarani N, Ahluwalia A, Buchanan A, Kartiko S, Quintana MT. Morel-Lavallée lesion: What you need to know. J Trauma Acute Care Surg. 2025.

Case 53

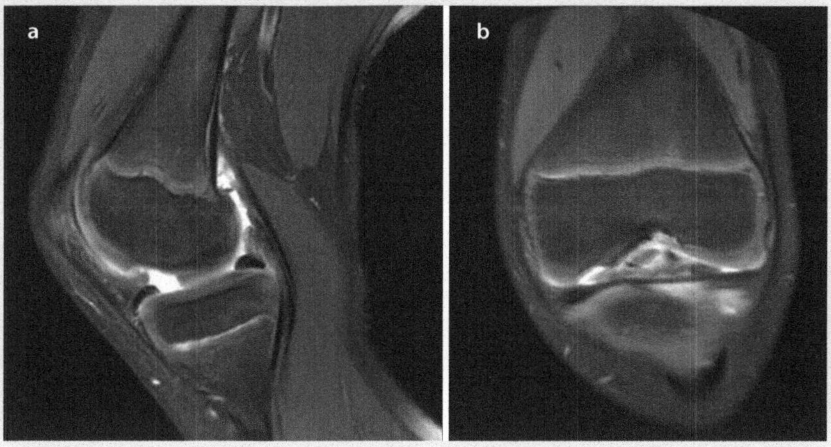

A 12-year-old male presented with knee pain following injury during a football match

S. Saran et al., *101 Knee Imaging Case Series*, 101 MSK Imaging 1,
https://doi.org/10.1007/978-3-032-21567-3_53

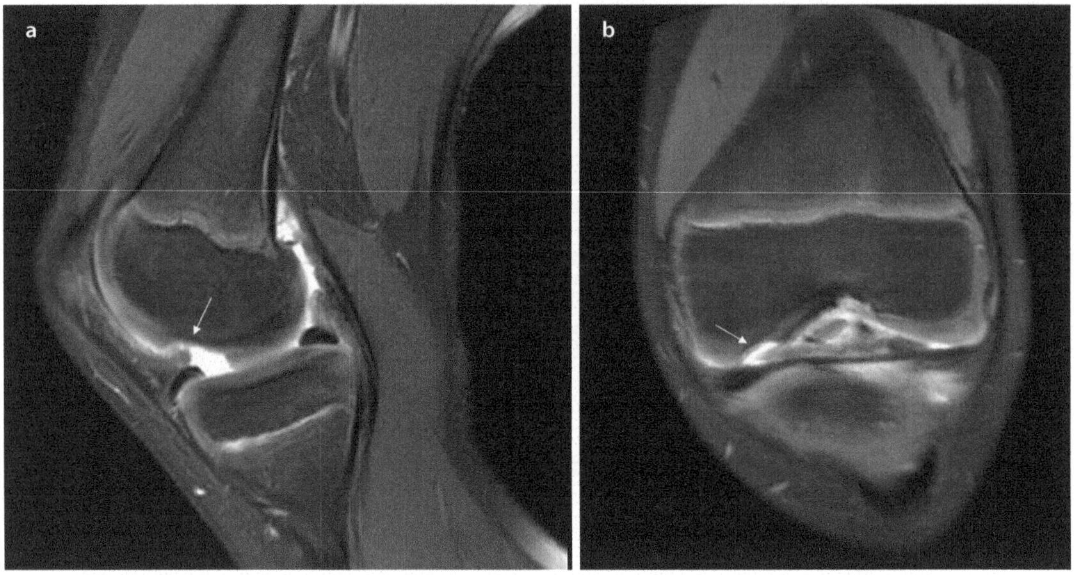

■ MRI **a** (sagittal) and **b** (coronal), PDFS weighted sequences shows the presence of an osteochondral defect in the lateral aspect of the medial femoral condyle (arrows). The donor site is seen; however, no obvious loose body was identified

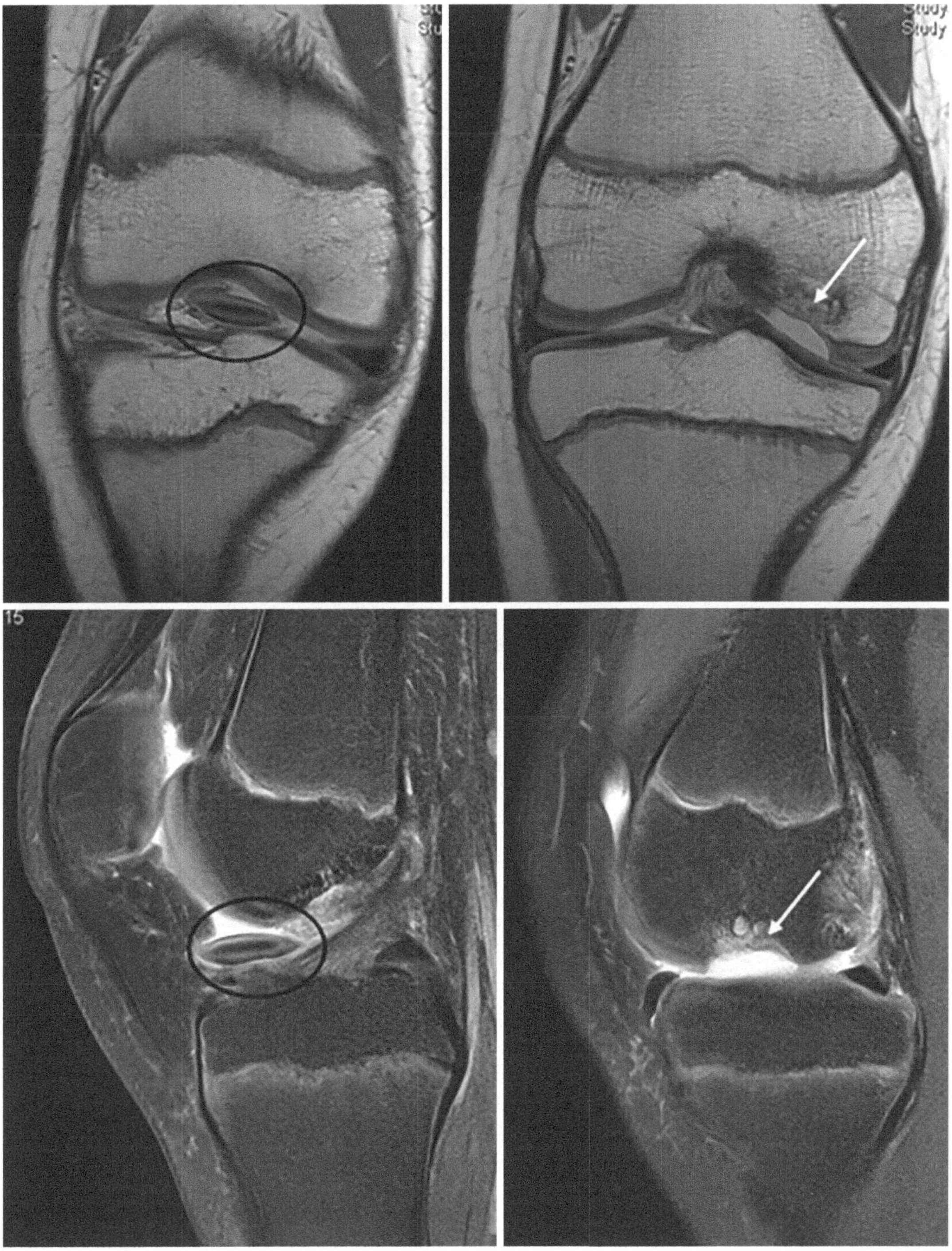

Companion case: Another case of osteochondral defect (arrows) with loose body (circle)

Osteochondral Defect (OCD)

Definition & Pathophysiology

- An osteochondral defect (OCD) refers to a focal injury affecting the articular cartilage and the underlying subchondral bone. In the femoral condyle, it represents a separation of an osteochondral fragment from the joint surface, which can lead to instability, pain, and premature osteoarthritis.
- Location: Most common on the medial femoral condyle (70–80%), typically on the lateral aspect ("classic" site). The lateral femoral condyle is less frequently involved.
- Pathogenesis: The exact cause is multifactorial, likely involving:
  - Repetitive microtrauma: stress on the subchondral bone leading to ischemia and necrosis.
  - Ischemia: compromise of the blood supply to the subchondral bone.

Clinical Presentation

- Demographics: most commonly affects adolescent athletes.
- Symptoms:
  - Vague, poorly localized knee pain, often activity-related.
  - Stiffness, swelling, and catching or locking if the fragment becomes unstable or detached.

Imaging Findings

- Radiography
  - Early stage: may be normal or show a subtle subchondral lucency.
  - Established lesion: shows a well-circumscribed, crescent-shaped area of radiolucency separating the osteochondral fragment from the underlying bone.
  - Advanced stage: a sclerotic rim surrounds the fragment, and a loose body may be visible if detached.
- MRI
  - MRI is essential for evaluating cartilage integrity, bone marrow oedema, and fragment stability—the key factors determining treatment.
  - T1-weighted: The osteochondral fragment is of low signal intensity. Helps define the size and morphology of the fragment.

  - T2-weighted/STIR: Shows high signal intensity (oedema) in the bone marrow. Key signs of an unstable lesion include:
    - Fluid signal intensity completely surrounding the fragment known as the "Rim Sign".
    - Cystic areas >5 mm beneath the fragment.

Differential Diagnosis

- Spontaneous osteonecrosis of the knee (SONK): Typically in older patients (>55 years), acute onset, and involves a larger area of the weight-bearing condyle.

Management

- Treatment is dictated by patient skeletal maturity (open vs. closed growth plates) and lesion stability.
- Conservative management (for stable lesions in skeletally immature patients).
- Surgical intervention: Indicated for failed conservative treatment, unstable lesions, or skeletally mature patients.
  - Arthroscopic drilling
  - Fixation of the fragment
  - Cartilage restoration procedures (for unsalvageable fragments or defects).

Suggested Reading

Accadbled F, Vial J, Sales de Gauzy J. Osteochondritis dissecans of the knee. Orthop Traumatol Surg Res. 2018;104(1S):S97–S105.

Gorbachova T, Melenevsky Y, Cohen M, Cerniglia BW. Osteochondral lesions of the knee: differentiating the most common entities at MRI. Radiographics. 2018;38(5):1478–95.

Case 54

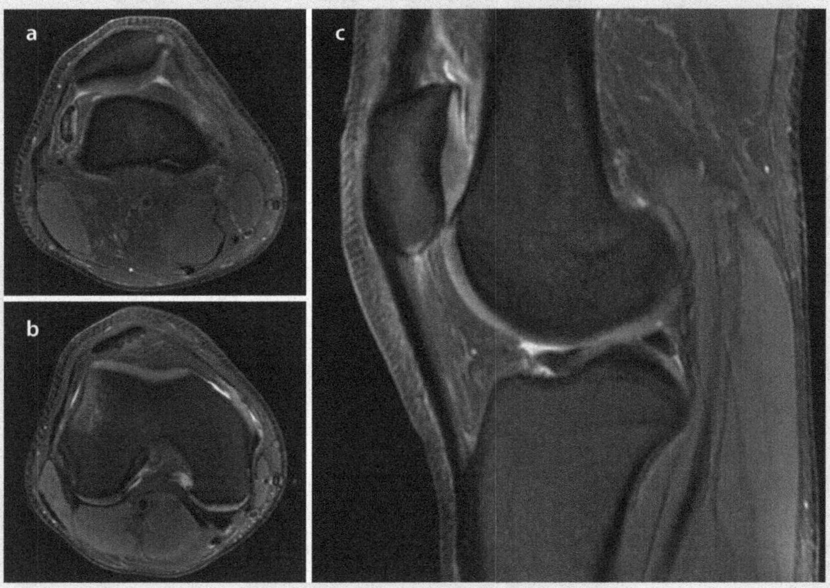

■ A 24-year-old male presents with pain in the extensor aspect of the knee joint following minor trauma

S. Saran et al., *101 Knee Imaging Case Series*, 101 MSK Imaging 1,
https://doi.org/10.1007/978-3-032-21567-3_54

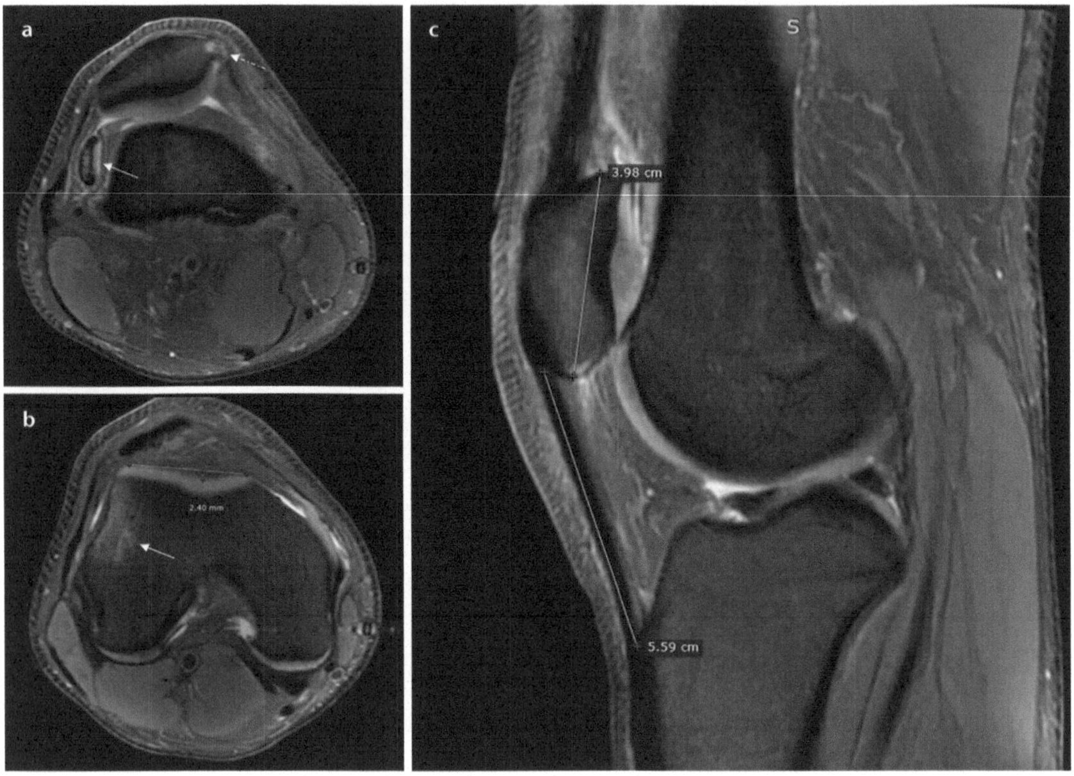

◘ MRI knee, PDFS weighted axial **a**, **b** and sagittal **c** sequences showing an osteochondral fragment (arrow in **a**) in the lateral joint recess with a bony defect at the medial patellar margin at the attachment of the medial patellofemoral ligament (MPFL) (dashed arrow in **a**), suggesting avulsion of MPFL. Marrow contusion (arrow in **b**) is noted in the lateral femoral condyle, suggesting recent impaction injury. The depth of the trochlear groove is 2.4 mm (normal 5 mm), suggesting a flat trochlear groove due to trochlear dysplasia (callipers in **b**). The Insall-Salvati Index, determined by dividing the length of the patellar tendon by the length of the patella, is 1.4 (callipers in **c**), suggesting patella alta. The constellation of findings suggests the possibility of a recent episode of lateral patellar dislocation

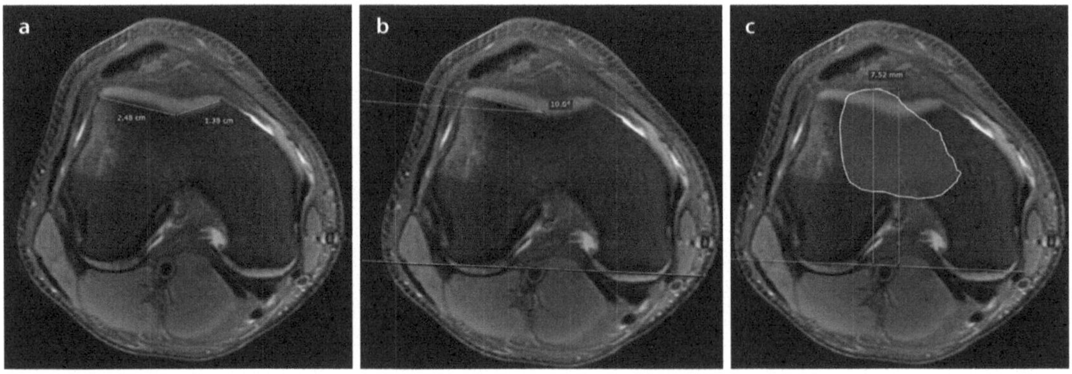

◘ Further measurements taken in the case: **a** Ratio of medial to lateral facet was 55% in this case, which was normal. **b** Lateral trochlear inclination is 10 degrees, suggesting trochlear dysplasia. **c** Distance between the tibial tubercle and the trochlear groove is 7.52 mm, which is normal

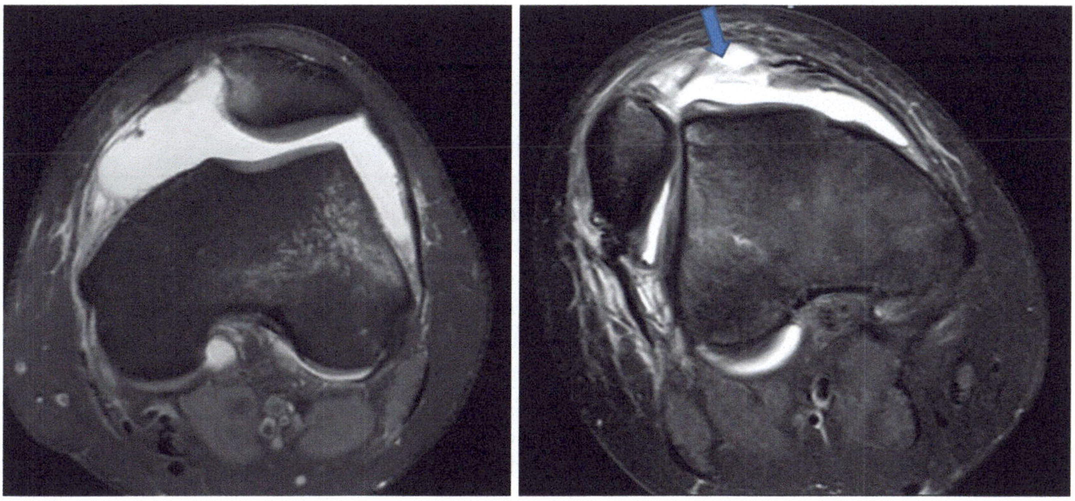

Companion cases: Patellar dislocation with tear of MPFL in two different patients (arrow)

Transient lateral patellar dislocation – Definition & Pathophysiology

- Transient lateral patellar dislocation is a common knee injury where the patella dislocates laterally and then spontaneously reduces immediately after the traumatic event. The patient often does not realise the patella is dislocated.
- A sudden, forceful internal rotation of the femur on a fixed tibia with the knee in slight flexion. This is often a non-contact twisting injury during sports (e.g., cutting, pivoting) or a direct blow to the medial side of the knee.
- The injury causes damage to the medial patellar stabilisers (MPFL and medial retinaculum) and can create bone bruising from the impact of the patella over the lateral femoral condyle.

Clinical Presentation

- A traumatic twisting event followed by immediate pain and a sensation of the knee "popping out of place" or "giving way".
- Medial para-patellar pain. The most specific symptom, caused by tearing of the MPFL—the primary restraint to lateral dislocation.
- Swelling: rapid onset hemarthrosis.
- Tenderness: palpation tenderness over the medial patellar border and adductor tubercle (MPFL attachment site).
- Patellar apprehension test: positive. The clinician attempts to sublux the patella laterally; the patient reacts with guarding and apprehension.

- Positive J-Sign: The patella translates laterally in a "J" path during terminal knee extension, indicating maltracking.

Imaging Findings

- Conventional radiography
  - Often normal as the patella has reduced.
  - May show a small avulsion fracture from the medial patellar border.
  - Assess for underlying anatomic risk factors (e.g., patella alta, trochlear dysplasia).
- MRI
  - Pathognomonic "bone bruise" pattern: This pattern is caused by the impact during reduction ("kissing contusions").
    Oedema in the medial aspect of the patella.
    Oedema in the anterolateral aspect of the lateral femoral condyle.
  - Medial soft tissue injuries: tear of the MPFL: Seen as oedema and discontinuity, typically at its patellar attachment.
  - Sprain/tear of the medial retinaculum.
  - Intra-articular injuries: possible associated osteochondral fractures or meniscal tears.

Anatomical Risk Factors

- Patellofemoral dislocations are rarely caused by trauma alone and almost always occur due to underlying anatomical predispositions. If these predisposing factors are not surgically corrected after a first dislocation, there is a nearly 50% chance of recurrence. This chronic instability leads to significant cartilage damage and severe arthritis. The primary goals of surgery are to repair any immediate damage and to correct these underlying anatomical anomalies.
- Magnetic resonance imaging (MRI) is crucial for identifying and measuring these key risk factors, which include:
  - Trochlear Dysplasia: This is an abnormal flattening or convex shape of the femoral groove that the patella tracks in. It is the most important bony risk factor. Dysplasia is diagnosed by:
    - Sulcus depth (TD): < 3 mm (Normal >5.2 mm).
    - Facet asymmetry (MT/LT): A medial facet length < 40% of the lateral facet length.
    - Lateral trochlear inclination (LTI): < 11 degrees.

- Patella alta: Patella sits too high. It reduces contact area with the femoral groove, especially when the knee is slightly bent, leading to instability. It is measured by the:
  - Insall-Salvati Index: A ratio > 1.3 (PT/PL) indicates patella alta (Normal = 0.8–1.2).
- Tibial tuberosity lateralisation: It is measured by the distance between the tibial tubercle (TT) and the trochlear groove (TG).
  - TT-TG distance: > 20 mm indicates significant lateralisation (Normal <15 mm, Borderline 15–20 mm).

Management

- Acute phase (first 1–3 weeks)
  - Immobilisation: A knee brace locked in extension for 2–3 weeks to allow the medial soft tissues to heal in a reduced position.
  - Weight-bearing: As tolerated with crutches.
  - NSAIDs: For pain and inflammation control.
- Rehabilitation Phase
  - The goal is to correct the underlying muscle imbalances that predispose to dislocation.
  - Vastus medialis obliquus (VMO) strengthening: The key dynamic stabiliser of the patella.
  - Core and hip strengthening: Addressing weak hip abductors and external rotators reduces internal femoral rotation, a major risk factor.
  - Restoring range of motion.
  - Patellar taping/bracing: can help with tracking and provide confidence during rehab.
- Surgical management
  - Indications: large osteochondral fracture with a loose body; recurrent dislocations despite adequate rehabilitation; and persistent instability.
  - Procedures:
    - MPFL reconstruction: The most common procedure, which recreates the main ligamentous checkrein against dislocation.
    - Arthroscopy: to remove loose bodies or repair chondral defects.
    - Realignment procedures (e.g., tibial tubercle osteotomy): reserved for cases with significant underlying bony malalignment.

Prognosis & Risk of Recurrence

- High recurrence rate: Up to 50% after a first-time dislocation, especially in young, active patients with underlying anatomic risk factors.
- Most patients do well with non-operative management focused on comprehensive rehabilitation.

Suggested Reading

Diederichs G, Issever AS, Scheffler S. MR imaging of patellar instability: injury patterns and assessment of risk factors. Radiographics. 2010;30(4):961–81.

Tompkins MA, Rohr SR, Agel J, Arendt EA. Anatomic patellar instability risk factors in primary lateral patellar dislocations do not predict injury patterns: an MRI-based study. Knee Surg Sports Traumatol Arthrosc. 2018;26(3):677–84.

Case 55

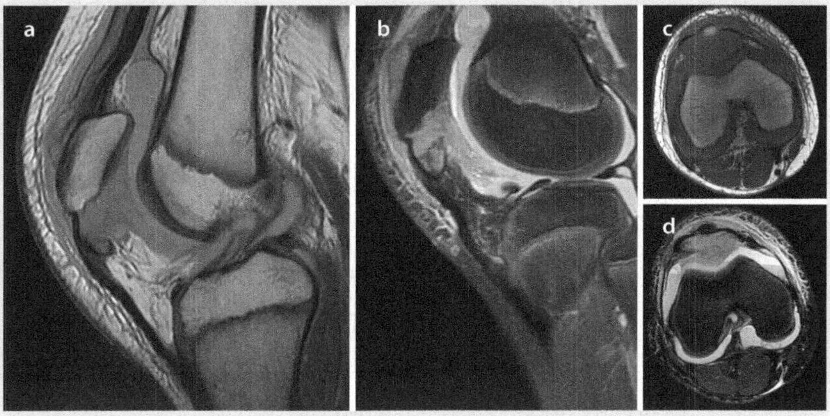

■ A 14-year-old football player presented with a sudden onset of pain in the extensor aspect of the knee with extensor lag

S. Saran et al., *101 Knee Imaging Case Series*, 101 MSK Imaging 1,
https://doi.org/10.1007/978-3-032-21567-3_55

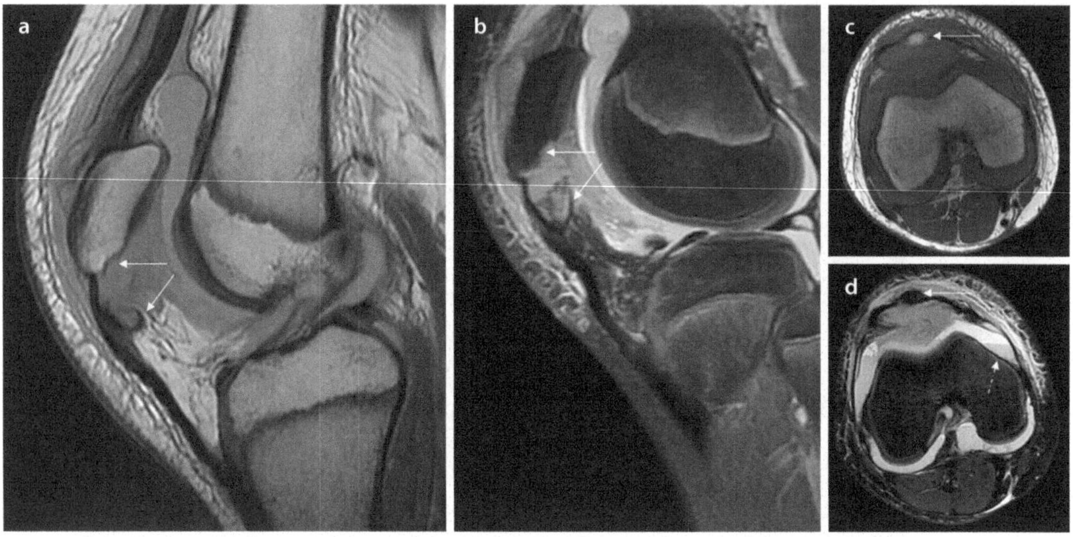

■ MRI knee **a**–**d** (Sagittal PD **a**, PDFS **b**, axial T1 **c** and PDFS **d**) shows the presence of an avulsion fracture from the inferior pole of the patella (arrows) with an extensive amount of oedema in the overlying soft tissue. Patella Alta is noted. Presence of hemarthrosis with layering of fluid in the joint cavity is also seen (dashed arrow in **d**). The diagnosis is patellar sleeve fracture

Patellar Sleeve Fracture

Definition & Pathophysiology

- A patellar sleeve fracture is a unique paediatric injury characterised by an osteochondral avulsion fracture from the inferior pole of the patella. A small fragment of bone is avulsed along with a large "sleeve" of cartilage from the patella.
- Mechanism: A sudden, forceful contraction of the quadriceps against resistance, typically during a jumping or sprinting activity where the child lands awkwardly or attempts a rapid change in direction. This forceful eccentric contraction avulses the immature bone at the patellar tendon attachment.
- Anatomy: In children, the patellar tendon attaches primarily to the patellar cartilage, which is weaker than the bone. The fracture line propagates through the chondro-osseous junction, avulsing a cartilage sleeve with a small, often deceptively small, bony fragment.

Clinical Presentation

- Demographics: Typically occurs in skeletally immature children and adolescents, most commonly between ages 8 and 12.

- Signs and symptoms:
  - Acute anterior knee pain following a jumping or sprinting injury.
  - Immediate inability to bear weight or actively extend the knee.
  - Hemarthrosis.
  - Loss of active knee extension: The patient cannot perform a straight leg raise. This is the cardinal sign and indicates disruption of the extensor mechanism.
  - Tenderness at the inferior pole of the patella.
  - High-riding patella (patella alta) if the fragment is significantly displaced.

Imaging Findings

- Radiography
  - A small, fleck-like bony fragment avulsed from the inferior pole of the patella. This fragment may be subtle and easily missed.
  - Patella alta: A high-riding patella indicates proximal retraction by the quadriceps.
  - Abnormal patellar contour: A "drooping" or irregular inferior pole.
  - The radiograph dramatically underestimates the size of the avulsed fragment, which includes a large portion of the articular cartilage.
- Ultrasound
  - Can dynamically visualise the osteo-cartilaginous fragment and the discontinuity in the extensor mechanism.
- MRI
  - MRI is crucial for visualising the cartilage and planning surgery, as it reveals the true size of the injury. It demonstrates the large, cartilaginous fragment involving the articular surface, which is not visible on the radiograph.
  - T1-weighted: Shows the avulsed bony fragment. The cartilaginous sleeve is an intermediate signal.
  - T2-weighted/PD FS/STIR: The cartilaginous sleeve is hyperintense. A fluid-filled gap is seen between the fragment and the patella. There is extensive bone marrow oedema in the patella.

Differential Diagnosis

- Sinding-Larsen-Johansson syndrome: A chronic traction apophysitis of the inferior patellar pole. It presents with an insidious onset of pain and no disruption of the extensor mechanism.

- Jumper's knee: pain at the patellar tendon origin, but without a fracture fragment or acute extensor mechanism disruption.
- Bipartite patella: a normal variant with a smooth, rounded ossification centre at the superolateral pole, not the inferior pole. It is asymptomatic and not associated with trauma.
- Patellar tendon rupture: more common in adults; the defect is in the tendon substance, and the patella is high riding, but no bony fragment is avulsed.

Management

- Treatment depends entirely on the displacement of the fragment and the integrity of the extensor mechanism.
- Non-surgical management: only for truly non-displaced fractures with an intact extensor mechanism (patient can perform a straight leg raise).
  - Treatment: Immobilisation in a knee extension brace or cylinder cast for 4–6 weeks, followed by progressive rehabilitation.
  - Surgical Intervention: for any displacement of the fragment or disruption of the extensor mechanism (inability to perform a straight leg raise).
  - Procedure: open reduction and internal fixation (ORIF).
  - The fracture is reduced anatomically, restoring the articular surface.
  - Fixation is achieved using two parallel Kirschner wires (K-wires) with a tension band wire in a figure-of-eight configuration. This converts the distracting forces of the quadriceps into compressive forces at the fracture site.
  - Sutures through the cartilage sleeve may also be used.
  - Goal: To achieve a stable, anatomical reduction that allows for early protected motion and prevents long-term complications like patellofemoral arthritis and extensor lag.

Complications

- The displaced bone-forming tissue can continue to grow and ossify, enlarging and possibly duplicating the patella.

Suggested Reading

Hua YF, Zhang YR, Guo L. Retrospective study of patellar fractures and damage of accessory soft tissue based on MRI. PLoS One. 2024;19(3):e0295671.

Shimasaki K, Uesugi M, Kobayashi T, Tanaka H, Ichimura H. Inferior pole sleeve fracture of the patella in an adolescent: a case report. Cureus. 2023;15(1):e33494.

Case 56

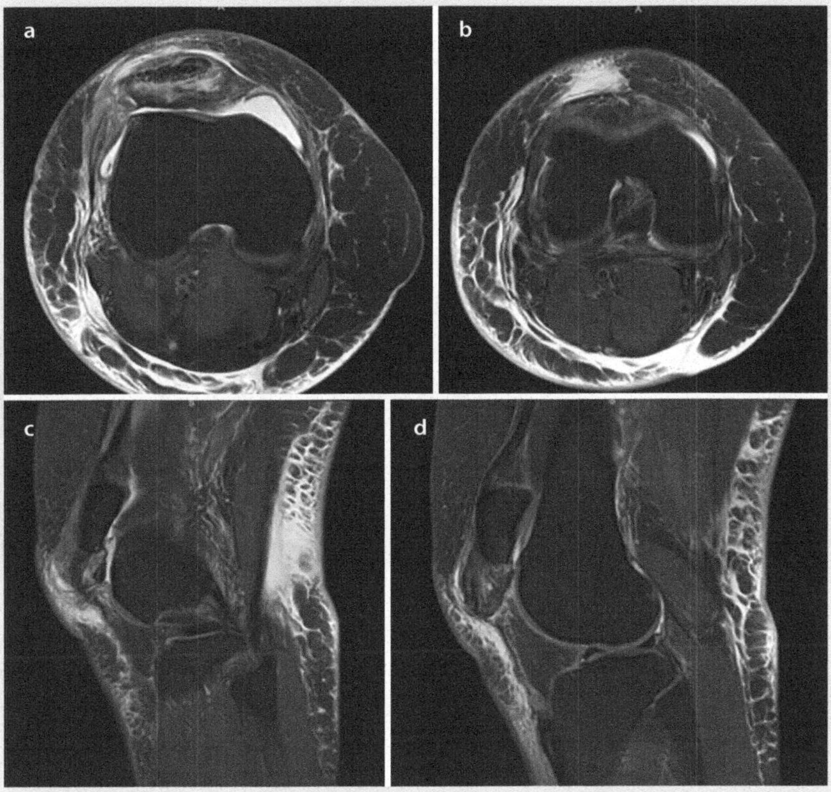

■ A 24-year-old male presented with severe pain, swelling and loss of extension of the right knee following trauma to the extensor aspect of the knee

S. Saran et al., *101 Knee Imaging Case Series*, 101 MSK Imaging 1,
https://doi.org/10.1007/978-3-032-21567-3_56

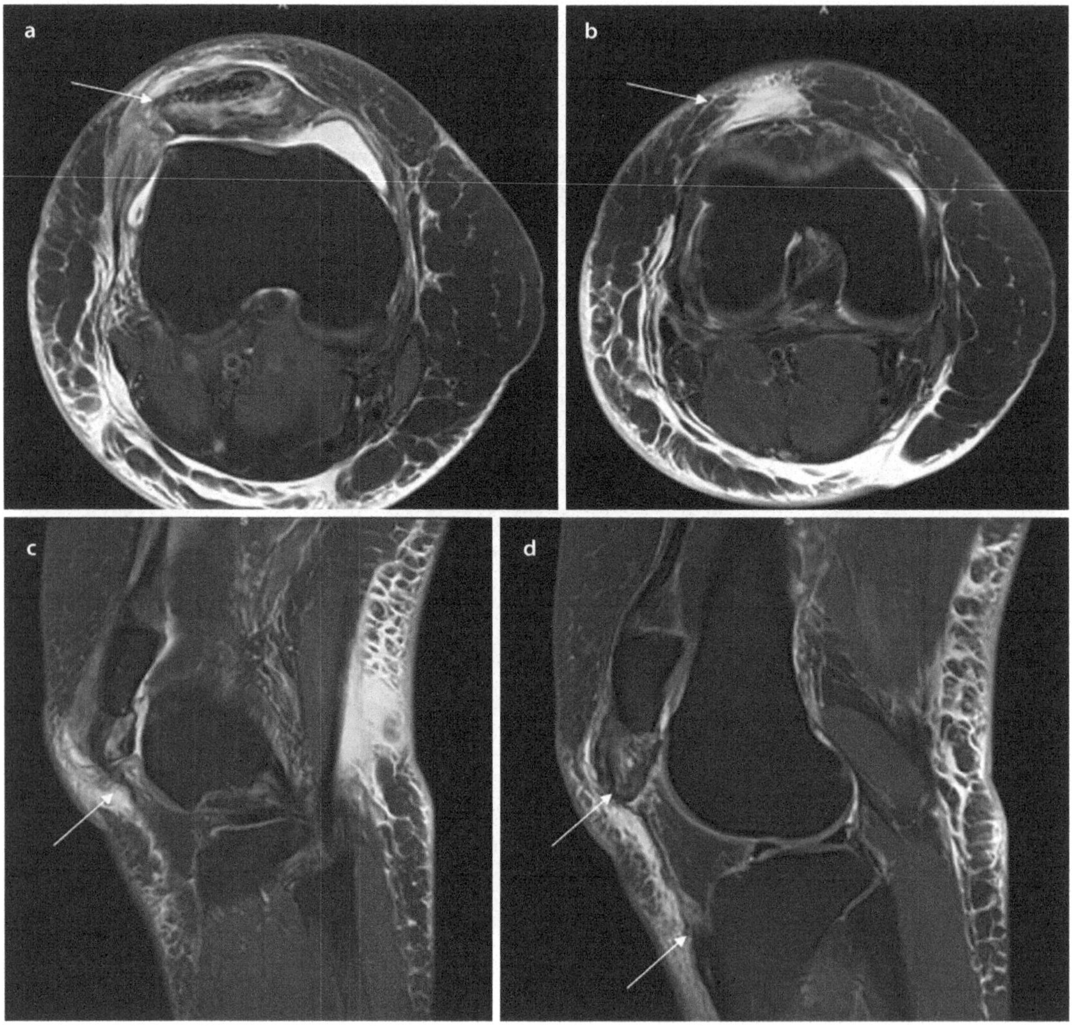

◘ MRI knee **a**–**d** (PDFS axial **a**, **b**, and sagittal **c**, **d**) sequences show a full-thickness rupture of the patellar tendon in the mid-part with retraction of torn edges (arrow). An overlying prepatellar collection is also seen, along with patella alta

Patellar Tendon Rupture

Definition & Pathophysiology

- A patellar tendon rupture is a disruptive injury involving the complete or near-complete tear of the tendon connecting the patella to the tibial tuberosity. This injury disrupts the knee's extensor mechanism, rendering active knee extension impossible or severely weakened.
- Typically occurs due to a sudden, forceful contraction of the quadriceps against a fixed load, often with the knee in a partially flexed position. Common scenarios include:

- A misstep or fall
- Jumping and landing awkwardly
- Direct laceration to the tendon
- Location: Most ruptures occur at the proximal (patellar) attachment of the tendon.

Risk Factors

- Pre-existing tendinopathy ("jumper's knee").
- Systemic diseases (e.g., diabetes mellitus, rheumatoid arthritis, chronic renal failure).
- Corticosteroid use (systemic or local injections).
- Previous surgery (e.g., ACL reconstruction with patellar tendon autograft).

Clinical Presentation

- Acute history: A traumatic event often accompanied by an audible "pop" or tearing sensation.
- Immediate, severe anterior knee pain.
- Inability to bear weight.
- Significant swelling and bruising.
- Physical exam findings:
  - Palpable defect: a noticeable gap in the infrapatellar region.
  - High-riding patella (patella alta).
  - Loss of active knee extension.
  - Positive extensor lag.

Imaging Findings

- Radiography
  - Patella alta: The patella is positioned abnormally high. This is assessed using indices like the Insall-Salvati ratio (where a ratio > 1.2 suggests patella alta).
  - Bony avulsion: In some cases, a small bone fragment may be avulsed from the inferior pole of the patella or the tibial tuberosity.
- Ultrasound
  - Can dynamically visualise a complete tendon discontinuity with a fluid-filled gap.
  - Useful for assessing retraction of the patella.
- MRI
  - Complete tear: full-thickness fluid signal disrupting all tendon fibres.
  - Retraction: the degree of proximal retraction of the patella.

  - Tendon quality: assesses the condition of the remaining tendon stump for repair.
  - Associated injuries: evaluates for damage to the menisci, cartilage, or other structures.

Classification

- Acute vs. chronic (>4–6 weeks old). Chronic tears are more challenging to repair due to tendon retraction and scarring.
- Complete vs. partial: Complete tears require surgery; high-grade partial tears (>50% thickness) are often also repaired surgically.

Management

Complete ruptures are virtually always treated surgically to restore extensor mechanism function.

- Surgical repair
  - Ideally performed within 2 weeks of injury before significant scarring and contracture occur.
  - Strong, non-absorbable sutures are passed through the tendon and secured to the patella via transosseous tunnels or suture anchors.
  - Reinforcement (augmentation): in cases of poor tissue quality or delayed repair, the construct may be reinforced with a cerclage wire or heavy suture passed around the patella and through the tibial tuberosity (a "tension band" technique).
- Post-operative rehabilitation
  - Rehabilitation is prolonged and carefully staged to protect the repair.
- Return to sport: typically takes 6–9 months or longer.

Complications

- Re-rupture
- Knee stiffness
- Extensor lag
- Post-traumatic arthritis
- Infection

Prognosis

With timely surgical repair and strict adherence to rehabilitation, most patients achieve good-to-excellent outcomes, regaining functional range of motion and strength. However, a full return to high-level sports is not guaranteed, and some residual weakness or stiffness is common.

Suggested Reading

Fazal MA, Moonot P, Haddad F. Radiographic features of acute patellar tendon rupture. Orthop Surg. 2015;7(4):338–42.

Hosalkar HS, Cheung-Moore E, Atanda A Jr, Ogilvie C, Lackman RD. An undescribed cause of patellar tendon rupture. Am J Orthop (Belle Mead NJ). 2005;34(7):333–6.

Tandberg AN, Grindem H, Wiig C, Figved W. Knee sliced open by skate blade: complete patellar tendon rupture in an elite long track speed skater. BMJ Case Rep. 2019;12(4):e228611.

Case 57

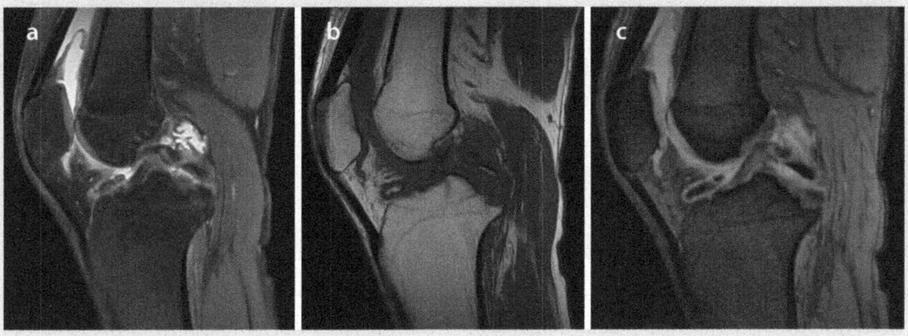

◘ A 24-year-old male suffered a dashboard injury in the right knee and presented with severe pain and swelling

S. Saran et al., *101 Knee Imaging Case Series*, 101 MSK Imaging 1,
https://doi.org/10.1007/978-3-032-21567-3_57

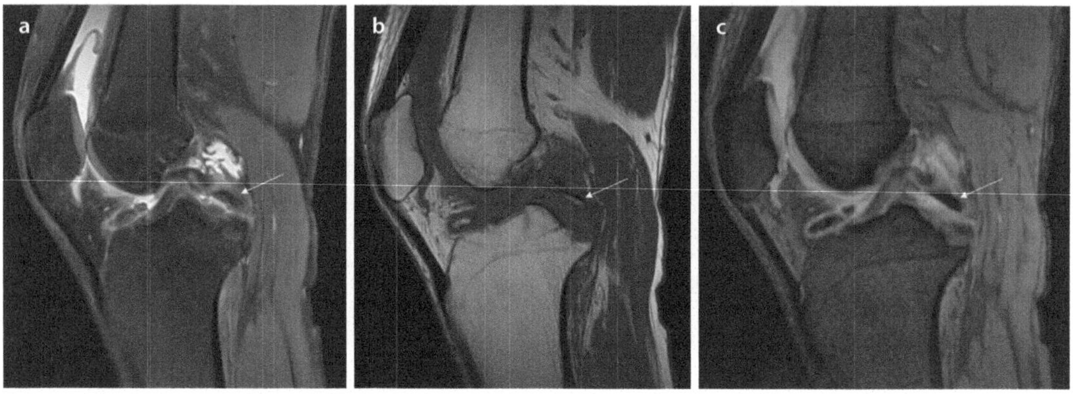

MRI knee sagittal plane PDFS **a**, T1 **b** and GRE **c** sequences show separation of the bony fragment (arrows) from the tibial insertion of the posterior cruciate ligament (PCL). It is a PCL avulsion fracture. A few other small osseous fragments are displaced anteriorly behind Hoffa's fat pad

Posterior Cruciate Ligament (PCL) Avulsion Fracture

Definition & Pathophysiology

- A PCL (posterior cruciate ligament) avulsion fracture is a bony injury where the PCL, with a fragment of its tibial attachment site, is pulled away from the bone. This is distinct from a mid-substance ligament tear.
- It represents the most common isolated ▶ PCL lesion.
- Mechanism: Typically caused by a high-energy traumatic event that places excessive stress on the PCL. The classic mechanisms include "dashboard injury" and hyperextension injury.

Clinical Presentation

- Posterior knee pain.
- Swelling and effusion.
- Instability: a feeling of the knee "giving way", especially during descending stairs or deceleration.
- Posterior drawer test: positive, demonstrating excessive posterior translation of the tibia.
- Posterior sag sign (Godfrey's test): with the hip and knee flexed, the tibia sags posteriorly relative to the femur due to gravity.

Imaging Findings

- Radiography
  - Shows a bony fragment avulsed from the posterior tibial plateau, often best seen on a well-penetrated lateral view.
- Computed tomography
  - Essential for pre-operative planning.
  - Precisely defines the size, location, and degree of displacement of the avulsed fragment.
  - Assesses for comminution (fragmentation) of the fracture bed.
- MRI
  - While the fracture is visible, MRI's primary role is to evaluate the entire ligament and other structures.
  - Crucial for identifying concurrent damage to the ACL, menisci, posterolateral corner (PLC), and cartilage.

Classification

- Type I: Minimally displaced fragment.
- Type II: Partially displaced fragment with a hinge.
- Type III: Completely displaced fragment, often with rotation.

Management

The decision between surgical and non-surgical management depends primarily on the displacement and rotation of the fragment.

- Non-surgical management (conservative)
  - Indication: for minimally displaced or non-displaced fractures (type i).
  - Immobilisation in a knee brace locked in extension for 4–6 weeks to reduce tension on the PCL.
  - Protected weight-bearing with crutches.
  - Physical therapy: focused on restoring the range of motion and quadriceps strengthening after the immobilisation period.
- Surgical intervention (open reduction and internal fixation—ORIF)
  - The fragment is reduced (placed back into its anatomical position) and fixed using cannulated screws or a suture anchor technique.
  - Goal: To restore the normal anatomy and tension of the PCL, thereby restoring knee stability.

Prognosis & Complications

- Excellent prognosis with anatomical surgical reduction and fixation.
- Outcomes are generally better than for mid-substance PCL tears because the ligament itself is healthy; the bone-to-bone healing is more predictable.

Suggested Reading

Chipman DE, Cirrincione PM, Mintz DN, DiFelice GS, Warren RF, Green DW. Posterior cruciate ligament femoral avulsion fractures in pediatric patients: a report of 2 interesting surgical cases. JBJS Case Connect. 2023;13(3).

Katsman A, Strauss EJ, Campbell KA, Alaia MJ. Posterior cruciate ligament avulsion fractures. Curr Rev Musculoskelet Med. 2018;11(3):503–9.

Case 58

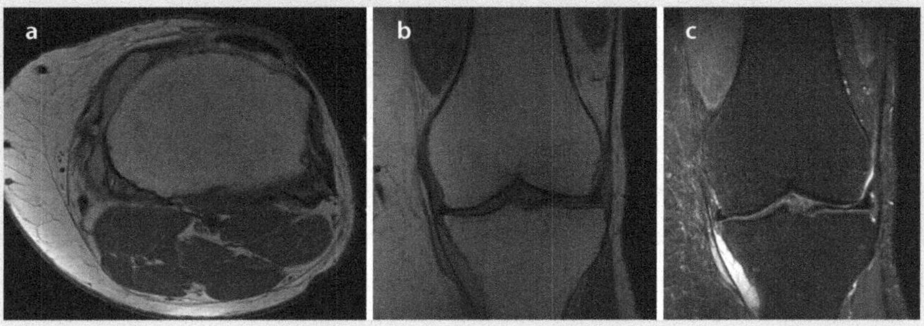

▪ A 56-year-old female presented with pain, tenderness and soft swelling in the medial aspect of the knee joint

S. Saran et al., *101 Knee Imaging Case Series*, 101 MSK Imaging 1,
https://doi.org/10.1007/978-3-032-21567-3_58

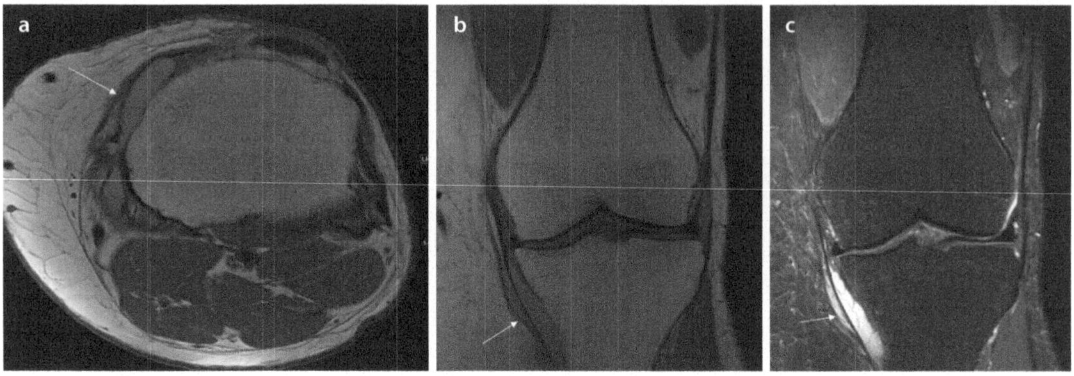

MRI knee **a**–**c** (PD axial **a**, PD coronal **b** and PDFS coronal **c**) shows the presence of a well-defined lesion (arrows) with fluid signals noted along the tendons of sartorius, gracilis and semitendinosus near their combined insertion on the anteromedial tibia. The characteristic location and imaging features are of Pes anserine bursitis

Pes Anserine Bursitis

Definition & Pathophysiology

- Pes anserine bursitis is the inflammation of the pes anserine bursa, a fluid-filled sac located on the medial side of the knee, approximately 5–6 cm below the joint line. It lies between the tibia and the conjoined tendons of three muscles: the sartorius, gracilis, and semitendinosus (the "pes anserinus" or "goose's foot").
- Function: The bursa reduces friction between these tendons and the underlying bone.
- Mechanism of inflammation: caused by repetitive stress or friction from the overlying tendons, leading to microtrauma, inflammation, and fluid accumulation within the bursa.

Clinical Presentation

- Demographics: more common in middle-aged women, overweight individuals, and athletes (especially runners, swimmers).
- Common associations include osteoarthritis of the knee, obesity, rheumatoid arthritis and valgus knee deformity.
- Symptoms:
  - Pain: Insidious onset of pain and tenderness on the medial side of the proximal tibia, well below the joint line. Pain worsens with activities.
  - Swelling: A soft, palpable swelling may be present at the site.
  - Stiffness: Especially after periods of inactivity.

Imaging Findings

- Ultrasound
  - Shows a fluid-filled, compressible, anechoic or hypoechoic collection superficial to the tibia and deep to the pes anserine tendons.
  - Doppler: May show hyperaemia in the surrounding soft tissues, indicating active inflammation.
  - Allows for dynamic assessment and is excellent for guiding diagnostic and therapeutic injections.
- MRI
  - The fluid-filled bursa appears as a well-defined, fluid signal intensity collection superficial to the tibia and deep to the pes anserine tendons.

Differential Diagnosis

- Medial collateral ligament (MCL) bursitis: typically located between the superficial and deep components of MCL.

Management

- Treatment is primarily conservative and focuses on reducing inflammation and addressing underlying biomechanical factors.
- Conservative management:
  - Activity modification, pain killers and physical therapy.
- Image-guided intervention:
  - Ultrasound-guided corticosteroid injection: A highly effective treatment. Under ultrasound guidance, a mixture of a corticosteroid and a local anaesthetic is injected directly into the bursa. This provides both diagnostic confirmation (immediate pain relief) and therapeutic relief by reducing inflammation.

Suggested Reading

Rennie WJ, Saifuddin A. Pes anserine bursitis: incidence in symptomatic knees and clinical presentation. Skeletal Radiol. 2005;34(7):395–8.

Sekkat A, Chaouche I, Alami Bassim G, Akammar A, El Bouardi N, Haloua M, Alaoui Lamrani MY, Boubbou M, Maaroufi M, Alami B. Pes anserine bursitis as a complication of tibial osteochondroma. Radiol Case Rep. 2024;19(9):3752–6.

Case 59

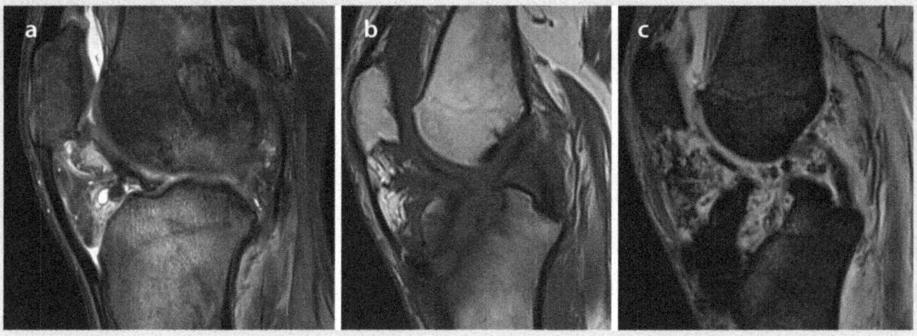

■ A 32-year-old male patient presented with pain and swelling in the knee, 2 months post-ACL reconstruction

S. Saran et al., *101 Knee Imaging Case Series*, 101 MSK Imaging 1,
https://doi.org/10.1007/978-3-032-21567-3_59

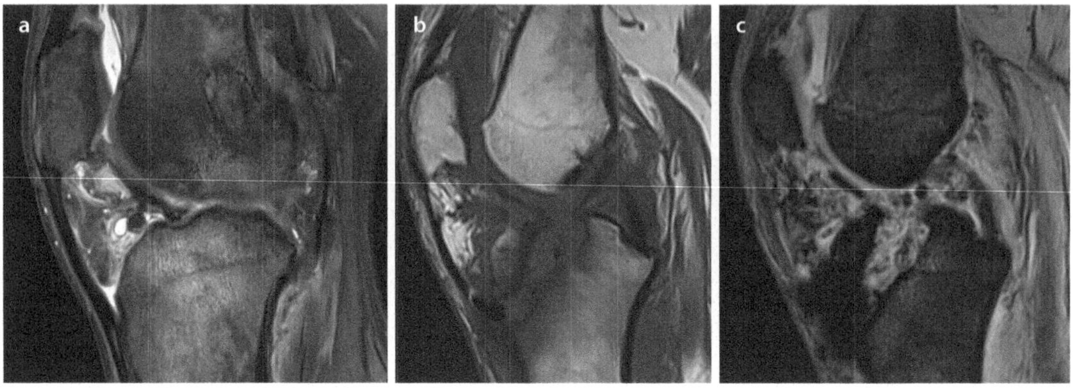

▣ MRI knee, PDFS weighted sagittal **a**, T1 weighted sagittal **b** and GRE sagittal **c** sequences showing status post-ACL reconstruction with the presence of effusion in the suprapatellar recess, Hoffa fat pad oedema and oedema in the femur and tibia with widening of tunnels and joint space narrowing, suggesting the development of infective arthritis

Post-ACL Reconstruction Infective Arthritis

Definition & Pathophysiology

- This is a serious and devastating complication characterised by a bacterial infection within the knee joint following ACL reconstruction surgery. It is considered a surgical emergency.
- Incidence: Rare, occurring in approximately 0.2–1.7% of cases.
- Source of Infection: Bacteria can be introduced during surgery (despite sterile technique) or, rarely, haematogenously (via blood) from a distant site in the days/weeks following surgery.

Clinical Presentation

Symptoms typically present within 2–4 weeks post-operatively, but can occur later.

- Cardinal signs:
  - Significant, worsening pain out of proportion to expected post-op pain.
  - Large, tense knee effusion (swelling).
  - Persistent fever (>38.5 °C / 101.3 °F) and chills.
  - Redness (erythema), warmth, and exquisite tenderness around the knee.
  - Significant stiffness and inability to tolerate the range of motion.

  - Key differentiator from normal post-op course: Normal post-op pain and swelling should gradually improve. In an infection, there is a dramatic escalation of symptoms.

Diagnostic Workup

- Blood tests: elevated white blood Cell (WBC) count (though not always reliable). Erythrocyte sedimentation rate (ESR) and C-reactive protein (CRP) are expected to be elevated post-op but should trend downward. A rising or persistently high ESR/CRP after 5–7 days is highly suspicious for infection.
- Knee aspiration and analysis of synovial fluid.

Imaging Findings

- Radiography: Usually normal initially, but can show rapid joint space loss if diagnosis is delayed.
- MRI: Can show extensive synovitis, effusion, and soft tissue oedema, but is not necessary for diagnosis and can delay definitive treatment.

Management

The goal is to eradicate the infection, salvage the graft if possible, and preserve joint function.

- Surgical debridement: Arthroscopic Irrigation and Debridement is the standard.
- Graft retention vs. removal:
  - Graft retention is attempted if the graft appears healthy and intact. This is the preferred outcome.
  - Graft removal is necessary if the graft is necrotic, loose, or extensively involved. This is a worst-case scenario, often requiring a two-stage revision reconstruction later.
- Antibiotic therapy.

Prognosis & Outcomes

- Graft salvage rate: successful graft retention is achieved in approximately 60–80% of cases with prompt treatment.
- Functional outcomes: even with successful infection eradication, patients often have:
  - Residual stiffness (arthrofibrosis) and loss of motion.
  - Higher risk of osteoarthritis due to cartilage damage from the infection.
  - Weaker functional scores compared to uncomplicated ACL reconstructions.

Suggested Reading

Barbara K, Alan I, Goran V, Saša J. Knee infection following anterior cruciate ligament reconstruction: a cohort study of one thousand, eight hundred and ninety one patients from the single-centre database. Int Orthop. 2020;44(5):869–75.

Geethan I, Easwaran R, Sahanand S, Sivaraman A, Gupta A, Devgan A, et al. Management guidelines for infection after ACL reconstruction: expert opinion statement based on the modified Delphi Survey of Indian Arthroscopy Surgeons. Indian J Orthop. 2021;55(2):342–51.

Scully WF, Fisher SG, Parada SA, Arrington EA. Septic arthritis following anterior cruciate ligament reconstruction: a comprehensive review of the literature. J Surg Orthop Adv. 2013;22:127–33.

Case 60

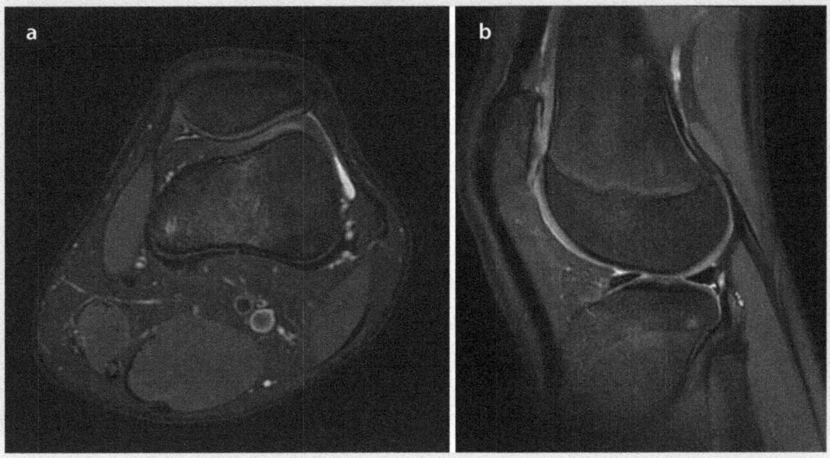

■ A 27-year-old male presented with anterior knee pain exacerbated by hyperextension

S. Saran et al., *101 Knee Imaging Case Series*, 101 MSK Imaging 1,
https://doi.org/10.1007/978-3-032-21567-3_60

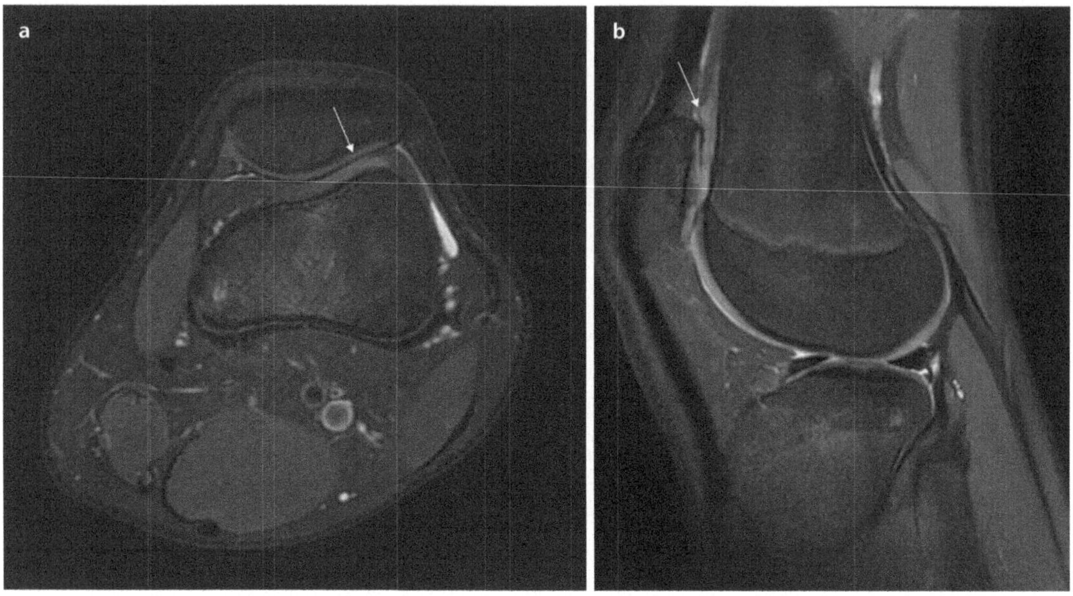

■ MRI knee PDFS axial **a**, sagittal **b** shows oedema and enlargement of the pre-femoral fat pad (arrows) with high signal intensity, suggestive of pre-femoral fat pad impingement syndrome

Pre-femoral Fat Pad Impingement Syndrome (Supratrochlear Fat Pad Impingement)

Definition & Pathophysiology

- Pre-femoral fat pad impingement syndrome is a distinct form of anterior knee pain caused by mechanical entrapment and inflammation of the pre-femoral (supratrochlear) fat pad, located between the anterior femoral cortex and the suprapatellar bursa.

Clinical Presentation

- Symptom: Anterior knee pain.
- Pain is consistently worsened by knee hyperextension, which directly compresses the fat pad between the femur and the patella/quadriceps mechanism.

MRI Findings

- MRI is essential for confirming the diagnosis, identifying the oedema pattern, and revealing the underlying cause.

- T2-weighted/STIR (fat-saturated): Focal high signal intensity (oedema) within the pre-femoral fat pad. The fat pad may also appear enlarged.
- T1-weighted: The normal bright fat signal is replaced by intermediate-to-low signal intensity in the affected area.

Management

- Conservative management: Activity modification and physical therapy
- Image-guided intervention: ultrasound-guided corticosteroid injection can provide significant diagnostic confirmation and therapeutic relief by reducing inflammation within the fat pad.
- Surgical intervention (for refractory cases): arthroscopic debridement.

Suggested Reading

Dheur S, Lorthioir F. Prefemoral fat pad impingement syndrome: correlation between ultrasonography and magnetic resonance imaging. J Belg Soc Radiol. 2024;108(1):61.

Lyu L, Li Y, Zhong J, Yao W. Association among peripatellar fat pad edema and related patellofemoral maltracking parameters: a case-control magnetic resonance imaging study. BMC Musculoskelet Disord. 2023;24(1):678.

Case 61

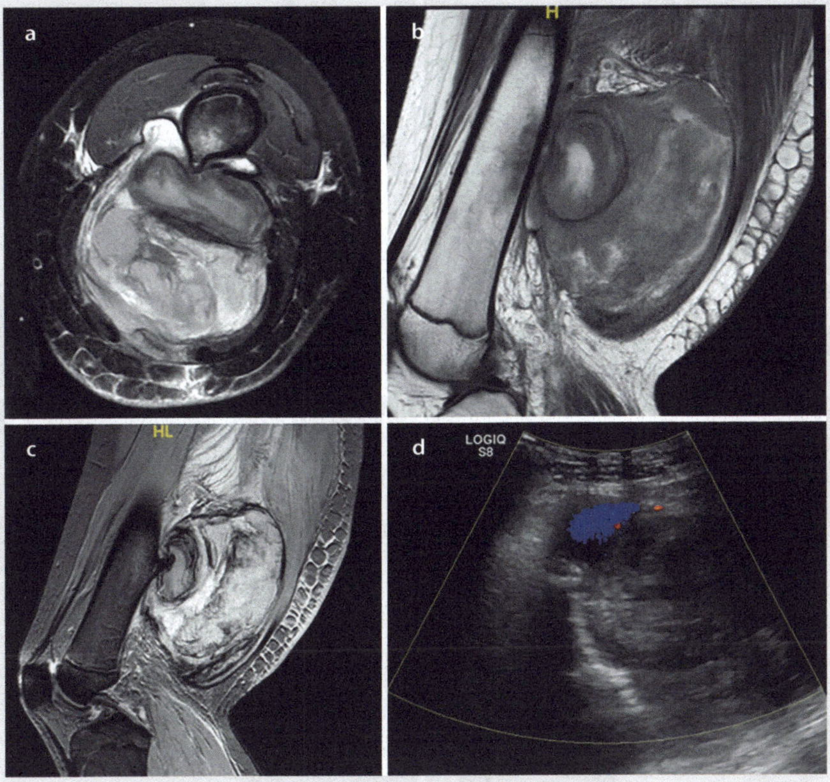

▪ A 13-year-old boy presented with progressive pulsatile swelling in the posterior aspect of the knee

S. Saran et al., *101 Knee Imaging Case Series*, 101 MSK Imaging 1,
https://doi.org/10.1007/978-3-032-21567-3_61

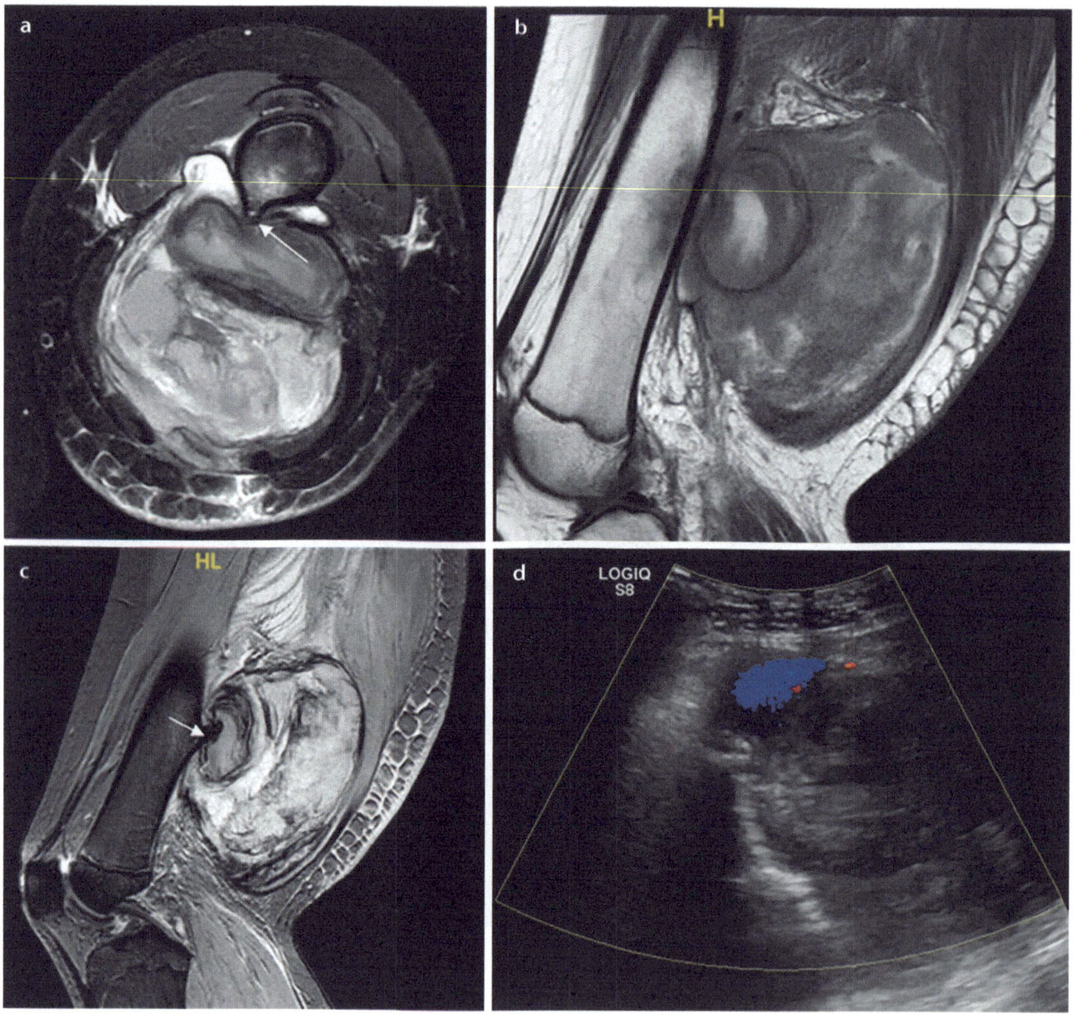

■ MRI Knee **a**–**c** (PDFS axial **a**, T1 sagittal **b**, T2 medic gradient echo sagittla **c**) reveals a pedunculated bony outgrowth from the posterior femoral cortex with marrow continuity, indicative of an exostosis (arrows). The overlying soft tissue exhibits a large heterogeneous area showing variable signal intensity and layering appearing predominantly hyperintense on T1-weighted sequence **b** and shows a peripheral rim of blooming on GRE **c**. Ultrasound **d** shows colour Doppler activity in the centre of the lesion and communication with the popliteal artery. The case was diagnosed as a popliteal artery pseudoaneurysm as a result of pressure effect and trauma by posterior femoral exostosis

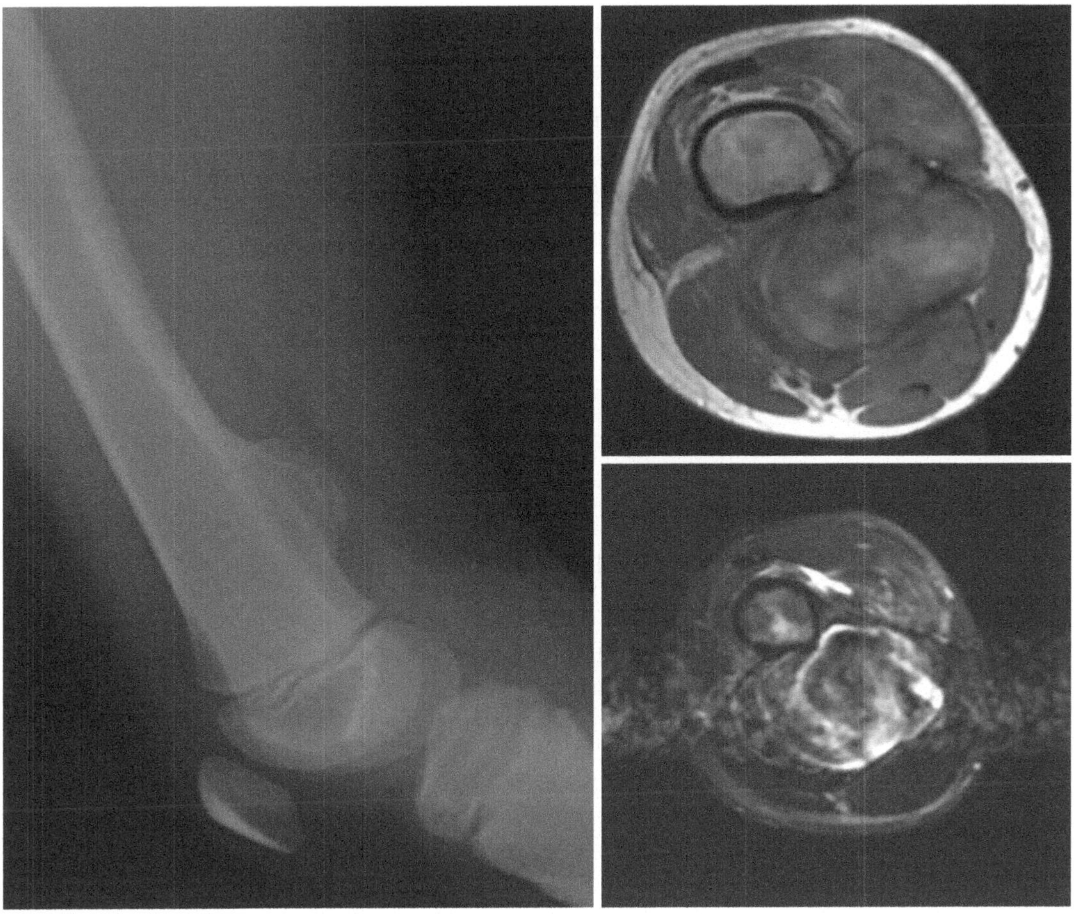

Companion case: Another case of osteochondroma in the posterior femoral cortex with popliteal artery pseudoaneurysm

Popliteal Artery Pseudoaneurysm Secondary to Distal Femoral Exostosis

Definition & Pathophysiology

- This condition involves the formation of a pseudoaneurysm of the popliteal artery, caused by chronic, repetitive mechanical irritation from a bony outgrowth (exostosis or osteochondroma) on the distal femur.
- Pseudoaneurysm vs. true aneurysm:
  - True aneurysm: Involves a localised dilation of all three layers of the arterial wall (intima, media, adventitia).
  - Pseudoaneurysm: A “false” sac formed when a hole in the arterial wall allows blood to leak out, contained only by the surrounding adventitia, connective tissue, and hematoma. This is the typical mechanism in this scenario.

Clinical Presentation

- Patient profile: typically a child, adolescent, or young adult (the demographic for osteochondromas).
- Symptoms:
  - Pulsatile mass: a palpable, often painful, pulsating swelling in the popliteal fossa.
  - Pain: deep, localised pain behind the knee.
  - Lower limb ischemia: coolness, pallor, or claudication in the calf/foot due to compromised blood flow.
  - Neurological symptoms: numbness, tingling, or weakness in the leg/foot from compression of the adjacent tibial nerve.
  - Venous congestion: swelling and oedema from compression of the popliteal vein.

Imaging Findings

- Ultrasound with Colour Doppler
  - B-Mode: Shows a complex, cystic or solid-appearing mass adjacent to the artery.
  - Colour Doppler: Reveals the classic "yin-yang" sign—a swirling pattern of blood flow into the pseudoaneurysm sac during systole and out during diastole.
  - Spectral Doppler: Can identify the "to-and-fro" waveform in the neck of the pseudoaneurysm.
- CT angiography (CTA)
  - CTA provides a comprehensive "roadmap" by visualising both the bone and vascular pathology in one study.
  - Exquisitely demonstrates the pedunculated exostosis projecting from the distal femur and its direct mechanical contact with the artery.
  - Clearly delineates the saccular outpouching from the popliteal artery, its size, and its relationship to the parent vessel.
- MRI/MRA
  - Excellent for visualising the exostosis and its cartilage cap.
  - MRA can confirm the vascular lesion without ionising radiation, which is beneficial in younger patients.
- Conventional angiography
  - Remains the gold standard for diagnosis and allows for immediate endovascular intervention if needed.

Management

- Endovascular repair (stent graft):
  - A covered stent is placed across the neck of the pseudoaneurysm to exclude it from the circulation.

- Advantage: less invasive.
- Disadvantage: less ideal in young patients due to long-term durability concerns and the need for lifelong surveillance. It also remains vulnerable to repeat injury if the bony spike is not removed.

- Vascular repair (addressing the pseudoaneurysm): the goal is to exclude the pseudoaneurysm and restore normal blood flow. Resection and bypass is the standard treatment. The damaged segment of the popliteal artery (including the pseudoaneurysm) is resected and bypassed using an autologous vein graft (e.g., great saphenous vein).
- Surgical excision of the exostosis: the bony spur is meticulously removed at its base to prevent recurrence. This is crucial to prevent future damage to the vascular repair or recurrence of the pseudoaneurysm.

Suggested Reading

Huang H, Zhang X, Wang Y, Tang H, Huang X, Zhang H, Li D. Popliteal artery pseudoaneurysm and secondary ipsilateral deep vein thrombosis caused by an exostosis in a mature adult. J Vasc Surg Cases Innov Tech. 2023;10(1):101375.

Syed W, Bhat MA, Ashraf HZ, Ganie F, Ahmad F. Popliteal artery pseudoaneurysm due to femur exostosis. Asian Cardiovasc Thorac Ann. 2019;27(1):39–41.

Vanhegan IS, Shehzad KN, Bhatti TS, Waters TS. Acute popliteal pseudoaneurysm rupture secondary to distal femoral osteochondroma in a patient with hereditary multiple exostoses. Ann R Coll Surg Engl. 2012;94(3):e134–6.

Case 62

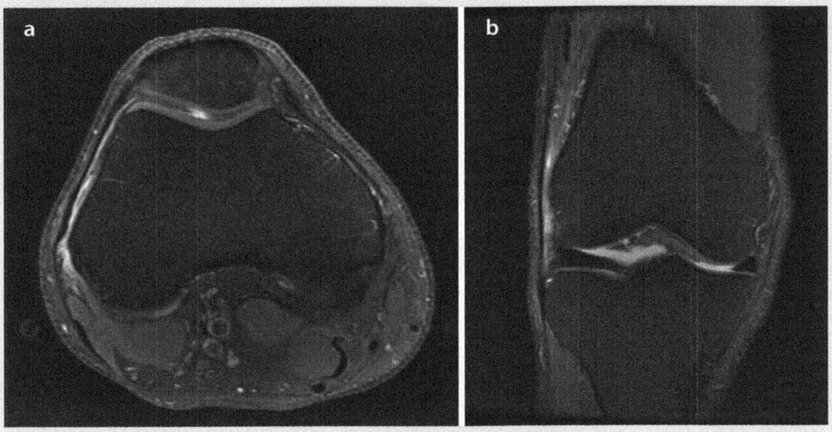

■ A 23-year-old marathon runner presented with pain in the lateral aspect of the knee joint

S. Saran et al., *101 Knee Imaging Case Series*, 101 MSK Imaging 1,
https://doi.org/10.1007/978-3-032-21567-3_62

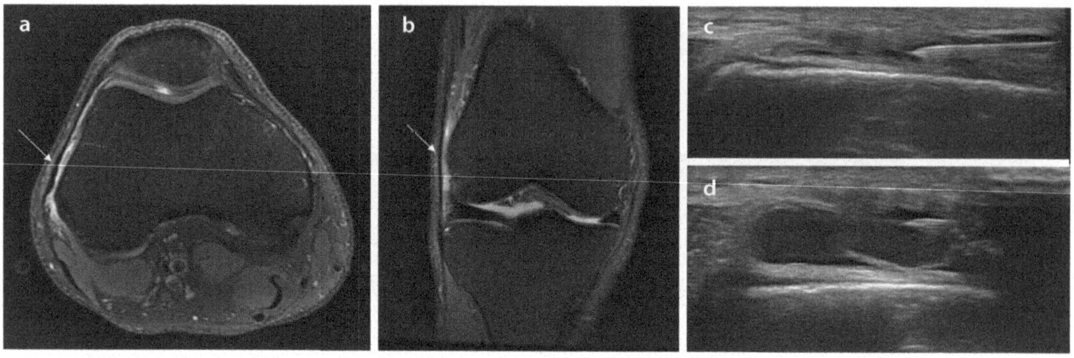

■ MRI knee PDFS axial **a**, PDFS coronal **b** shows the presence of hyperintense signal intensity interposed between the iliotibial band and the lateral femoral condyle (arrow), appearances are of Iliotibial band friction syndrome. Ultrasound-guided steroid injection was performed in this patient, which provided long-lasting pain relief (**c** and **d**)

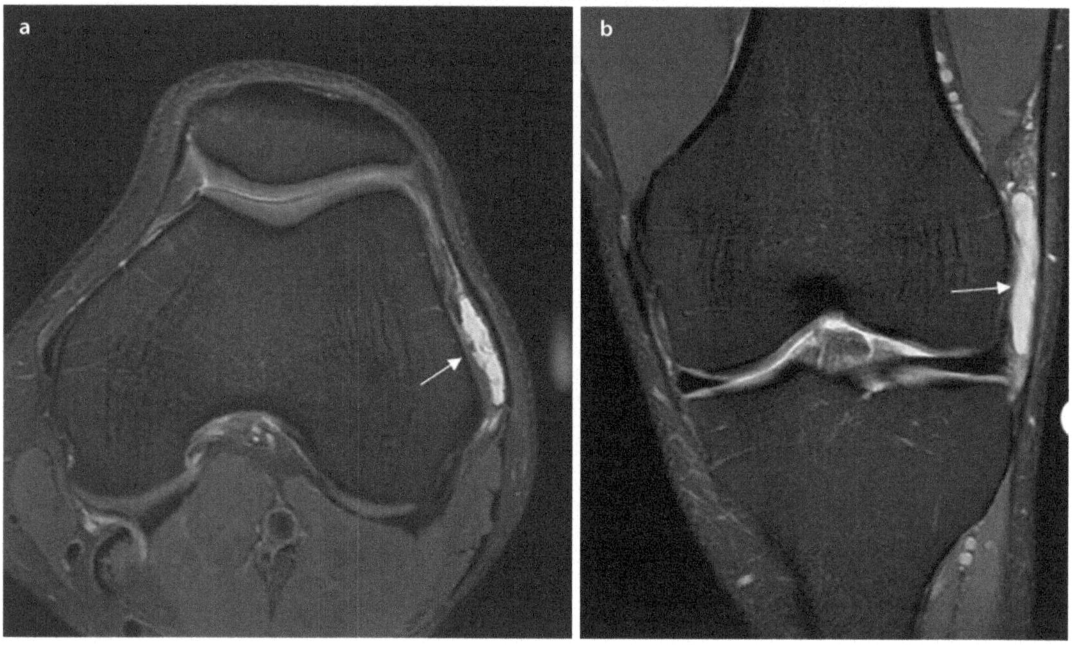

■ Companion case: MRI knee PDFS axial **a** and coronal sequence **b** showing a well-defined cystic lesion (arrows) in the interface between the lateral femoral condyle and iliotibial band (ITB), appearances are of ganglion cyst due to ITB friction syndrome

Iliotibial Band (ITB) Friction Syndrome

Definition & Pathophysiology

- Iliotibial Band (ITB) friction syndrome is a common overuse injury and a primary cause of lateral knee pain, particularly in runners and cyclists. It is an extra-articular, non-inflammatory condition characterised by friction-

induced irritation of the distal iliotibial band and the underlying tissues.
- The ITB is a thick band of fascia that runs from the hip (tensor fascia lata and gluteus maximus) to the lateral tibia (Gerdy's tubercle).
- Site of impingement: The primary site of pathology is where the ITB slides over the lateral femoral epicondyle, approximately 30 degrees of knee flexion.

Clinical Presentation

- Demographics: Common in runners, cyclists, military personnel, and athletes involved in sports requiring repetitive knee flexion.
- Symptoms: sharp, burning lateral knee pain localised precisely to the lateral femoral epicondyle. Pain may radiate up the thigh or down the shin.
- Sometimes a mild, localised swelling is palpable over the lateral epicondyle.

Physical Exam Findings

- Point tenderness: exquisite tenderness to palpation directly over the lateral femoral epicondyle, about 2–3 cm proximal to the joint line.
- Noble compression test: the clinician applies pressure over the lateral femoral epicondyle while passively extending the patient's knee from a flexed position. Pain at approximately 30 degrees of flexion is a positive test.

Imaging Findings

Imaging is typically used to rule out other causes of lateral knee pain rather than to diagnose ITBS, as findings can be subtle.

- Ultrasound
  - Can show a thickened, heterogeneous, and hypoechoic ITB over the lateral femoral epicondyle with the presence of fluid and increased vascularity deep to the ITB.
- MRI
  - T2-weighted/STIR (fat-saturated): Ill-defined high signal intensity in the fat tissue between the ITB and the lateral femoral epicondyle with thickening of the distal ITB and fluid deep to the ITB, representing a secondary bursitis.

Differential Diagnosis

- Lateral meniscal tear: pain is typically at the joint line and may be associated with mechanical symptoms (locking, catching).
- Lateral collateral ligament sprain: pain is more proximal, and instability may be present.

Management

- Conservative management
  - Activity modification: the cornerstone of treatment. This includes relative rest (reducing mileage, avoiding downhill running, and cross-training) and identifying & correcting training errors.
  - Physical therapy: Stretching focused on the ITB, tensor fascia lata, gluteus maximus, and hip flexors. Strengthening is the most critical component. Targeting hip abductors and external rotators (gluteus medius and minimus) to improve pelvic stability and reduce strain on the ITB.
  - NSAIDs: For short-term pain and inflammation control.
- Corticosteroid Injection: An ultrasound-guided steroid injection into the inflamed tissue deep to the ITB can provide diagnostic confirmation and significant therapeutic relief for refractory cases.
- Surgical intervention (refractory cases)

Suggested Reading

Everhart JS, Kirven JC, Higgins J, Hair A, Chaudhari AAMW, Flanigan DC. The relationship between lateral epicondyle morphology and iliotibial band friction syndrome: a matched case-control study. Knee. 2019;26(6):1198–203.

Kim JK, Kim T, Lee HS, Kim DK. Feasibility and reliability of various morphologic features on magnetic resonance imaging for iliotibial band friction syndrome. Korean J Pain. 2023;36(2):208–15.

Case 63

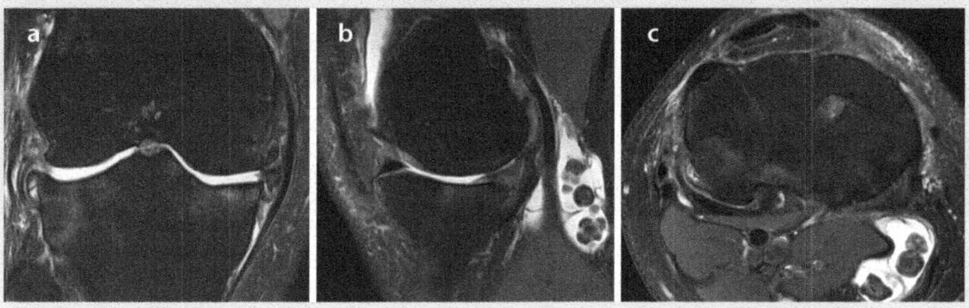

■ A 65-year-old female with chronic pain in bilateral knee joints presented with locking and catching of the right knee

S. Saran et al., *101 Knee Imaging Case Series*, 101 MSK Imaging 1,
https://doi.org/10.1007/978-3-032-21567-3_63

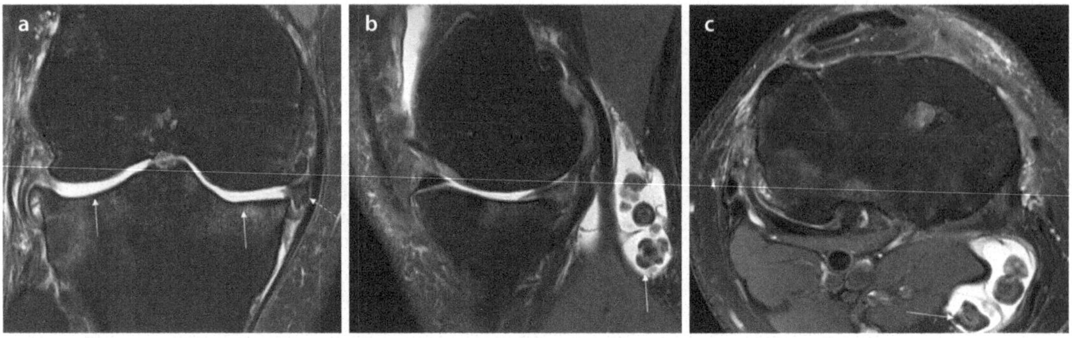

◘ MRI knee PDFS coronal **a**, sagittal **b** and axial **c** shows severe degenerative changes in the knee joint marked by complete loss of articular cartilage in the medial and lateral tibio-femoral joint (arrows in **a**) with extrusion of the medial meniscus (dashed arrow). **b**, **c** demonstrate the presence of multiple loose bodies (arrows) of varying sizes in the baker's cyst. The constellation of findings supports the diagnosis of secondary osteochondromatosis in the setting of severe osteoarthritis

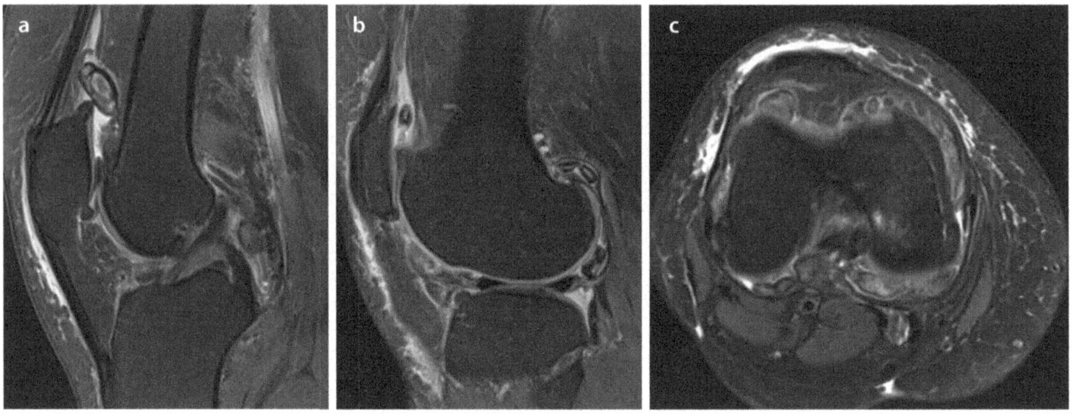

◘ Companion case: MRI knee shows severe degenerative changes in the knee joint with the presence of multiple loose bodies of varying sizes in the joint

Secondary Synovial Osteochondromatosis in the Setting of Severe Osteoarthritis

Definition & Pathophysiology

- Secondary synovial osteochondromatosis is a metaplastic and calcific process of the synovial membrane, characterised by the formation of multiple cartilaginous loose bodies within the joint. Unlike the primary (idiopathic) form, it occurs secondarily in response to chronic joint degeneration or irritation, most commonly in the setting of severe osteoarthritis.
- Mechanism: chronic joint inflammation and mechanical wear in severe osteoarthritis stimulate the synovial lining to undergo metaplasia, transforming into cartilage-forming

cells (chondrocytes). These cartilage nodules form, detach, and can later calcify or ossify, becoming visible on imaging as loose bodies.

Clinical Presentation

- Patients have established symptoms of severe, chronic osteoarthritis like pain, stiffness, crepitus, and reduced range of motion.
- Superimposed symptoms from loose bodies: locking, catching, or giving way as loose bodies become interposed between the articular surfaces.

Imaging Findings

- Imaging reveals features of both severe osteoarthritis and the characteristic loose bodies of osteochondromatosis.
- Radiography: findings of severe osteoarthritis.
  - Marked joint space narrowing.
  - Subchondral sclerosis (increased bone density).
  - Large osteophytes.
  - Subchondral cysts (geodes).
  - Findings of osteochondromatosis: Multiple, round/oval intra-articular opacities of varying sizes. The loose bodies are often numerous but fewer than in the primary disease and show less uniform size and shape.
- MRI.
  - MRI is superior for visualising non-calcified cartilage nodules and the extent of synovial disease.
  - T1-weighted: loose bodies appear as multiple low to intermediate signal intensity nodules within the joint. The synovium may appear thickened.
  - T2-weighted/PD FS/STIR: The cartilage nodules are hyperintense. If ossified, they will have a central fat signal surrounded by a low-signal cortical rim.
  - Gradient-Echo (GRE) Excellent for detecting calcifications.

Differential Diagnosis

- Primary synovial osteochondromatosis: occurs in a younger demographic (30–50 yrs) in an otherwise normal joint. Loose bodies are typically more uniform in size and much more numerous.
- Pigmented villonodular synovitis (PVNS): Causes synovial thickening and nodules, but these are dark on T2-weighted images due to hemosiderin deposition.
- Inflammatory arthritis with rice bodies.

Management

Treatment is directed at the underlying osteoarthritis and the mechanical symptoms caused by the loose bodies.

- Conservative management (for mild symptoms or poor surgical candidates)
  - Osteoarthritis management: analgesics, activity modification, physical therapy for strengthening, and weight loss.
  - Intra-articular injections: corticosteroid injections can help reduce synovitis and pain, but do not address the loose bodies.
- Surgical management (definitive treatment)
  - Procedure: arthroscopic debridement & synovectomy.
  - Loose body removal: All identifiable loose bodies are removed from the joint.
  - Synovectomy: The metaplastic synovium is debrided to reduce the source of new loose body formation.
  - Treatment of underlying osteoarthritis: Concurrent procedures may include chondroplasty (smoothing damaged cartilage), meniscal debridement, and removal of offending osteophytes.
  - Definitive procedure: total joint arthroplasty.

Suggested Reading

La QD, Baloch A, Ayub M, Ahmed S, La HB, Rahman R, Pryor F, Mansoor M. Extensive synovial osteochondromatosis secondary to avascular necrosis of the femoral head: a case of multifocal extra-articular involvement. Cureus. 2025;17(9):e91715.

Turan A, Çeltikçi P, Tufan A, Öztürk MA. Basic radiological assessment of synovial diseases: a pictorial essay. Eur J Rheumatol. 2017;4(2):166.

Case 64

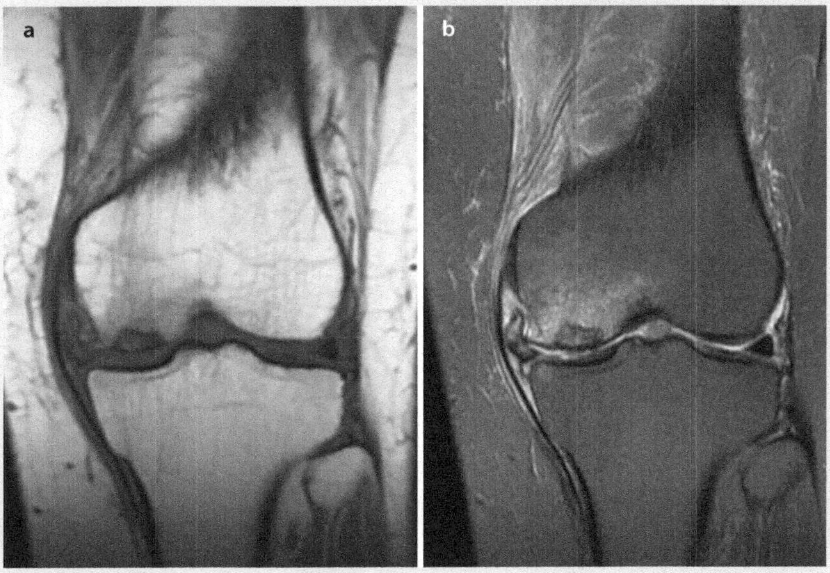

A 55-year-old female presented with an acute onset of pain in the knee joint

S. Saran et al., *101 Knee Imaging Case Series*, 101 MSK Imaging 1,
https://doi.org/10.1007/978-3-032-21567-3_64

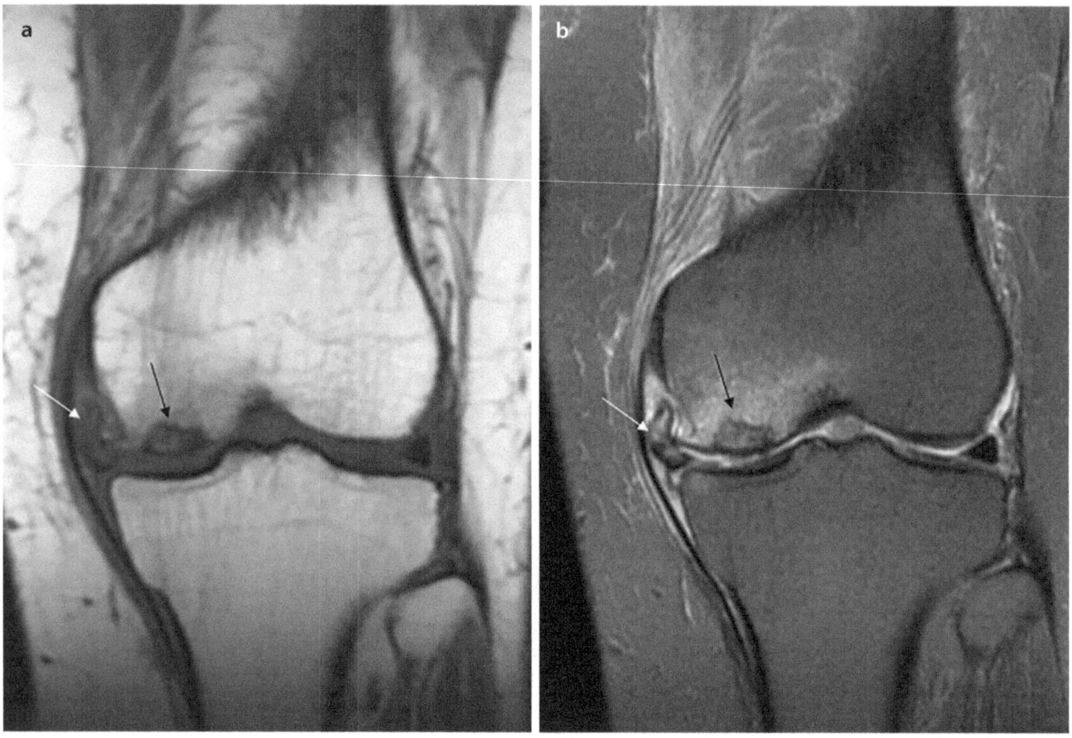

▪ MRI knee, T1 weighted **a** and PDFS **b** coronal sequences showing a geographic, serpiginous area of low signal intensity in the subchondral bone of the medial femoral condyle (black arrow) with oedema surrounding it, suggesting a subchondral insufficiency fracture. Overlying cartilage shows collapse and degeneration along with extrusion of the medial meniscus (white arrow), pointing towards the meniscal root tear and degenerative knee arthritis. Metaphyseal burst sign, indicated by soft tissue oedema surrounding the meta-epiphyseal region of the affected condyle, is also seen

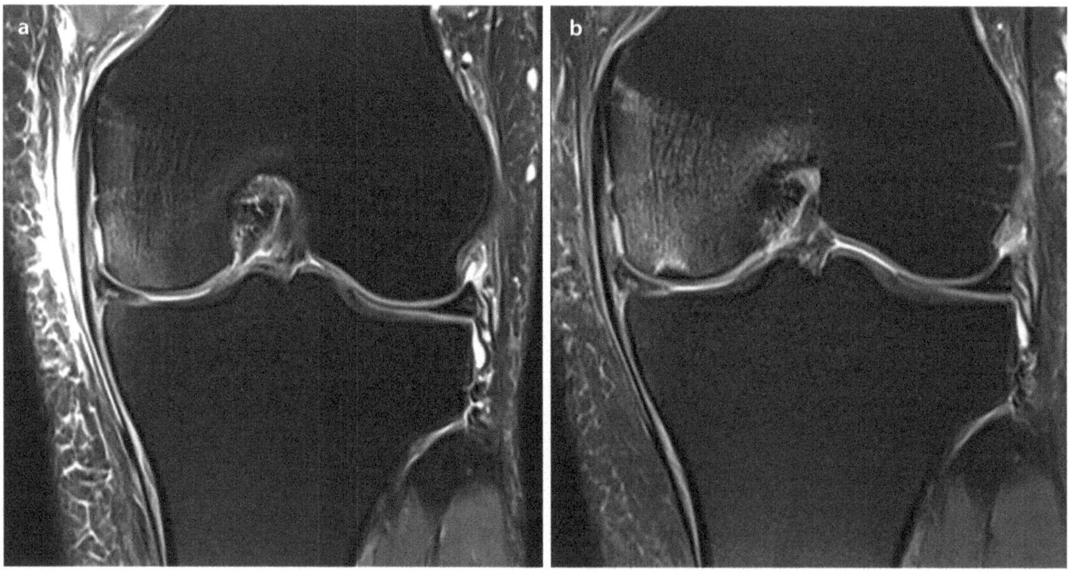

▪ Companion case: Developing subchondral insufficiency fracture in the medial femoral condyle, evident as marrow oedema **a** in an MRI, followed by well-developed serpiginous hypointense fracture line evident on MRI **b** done one month after the first scan

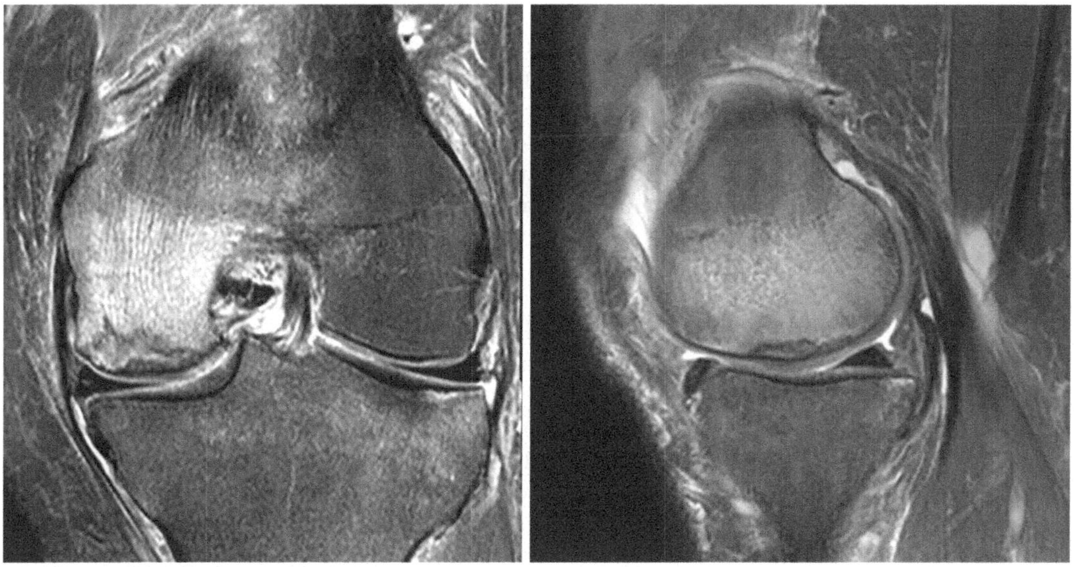

Companion case: another case of subchondral insufficiency fracture in the medial femoral condyle with intense marrow oedema and metaphyseal burst sign

Subchondral Insufficiency Fracture

Definition & Pathophysiology

- A subchondral insufficiency fracture is a type of stress fracture that occurs in the weight-bearing portion of the bone, just beneath the cartilage (subchondral bone). It is caused by normal or physiological stress applied to bone with diminished elastic resistance.
- Mechanism: Unlike an acute traumatic fracture, it results from cumulative microtrauma in weakened bone. The subchondral bone plate fails due to repetitive loading, which it can no longer absorb.
- Risk factors: Severe osteoporosis is the most common underlying cause. Other factors include vitamin D deficiency, rheumatoid arthritis, and corticosteroid use.
- Consequence: The fracture disrupts the structural support for the overlying articular cartilage, leading to rapid joint collapse and secondary osteoarthritis if not properly managed.

Clinical Presentation

- Typically occurs in elderly patients (70+ years), more commonly in postmenopausal women with osteoporosis. It can also be seen in younger patients with metabolic bone disease.

- Symptoms:
  - Acute or subacute onset of medial knee pain.
  - Pain is mechanical: worse with weight-bearing and relieved by rest.
  - Often, no significant trauma is recalled, or a history of a minor twist or stumble.
  - Limited range of motion and joint effusion may be present.

Imaging Findings

- Radiography
  - Early stages: often normal.
  - Later findings: a faint, crescent-shaped lucent line beneath the articular surface ("crescent sign")—indicating fracture and impending collapse. Flattening or collapse of the femoral condyle. Rapidly progressive joint space narrowing due to cartilage collapse.
- MRI: MRI is exquisitely sensitive for detecting bone marrow oedema and the fracture line long before it is visible on radiograph.
  - T1-weighted: Geographic, serpiginous area of low signal intensity in the subchondral bone of the medial femoral condyle.
  - T2/PD-weighted FS/STIR: Extensive high signal intensity oedema surrounding the fracture. Fracture line is seen as a low-signal intensity line within the edematous bone, parallel and adjacent to the articular surface.
  - Metaphyseal burst sign: Vidoni et al described a novel indirect sign. This sign represents oedema of the tissues overlying the metaphyseal region of the affected condyle, where the nutrient vessels enter the bone to provide blood supply to the adjacent bone.
  - May appear normal initially but can show degeneration or collapse as the disease progresses.

Differential Diagnosis

- Spontaneous osteonecrosis of the knee: Now widely believed to be the same entity or a sequelae of a subchondral insufficiency fracture. The "necrosis" is likely secondary to the fracture disrupting the blood supply.
- Osteochondral lesion: typically seen in younger, active patients.

Management

The goal is to unload the affected condyle to allow the fracture to heal and prevent collapse.

- Conservative management.
  - Strict unloading: Non-weight-bearing or toe-touch weight-bearing for 6–8 weeks with crutches. This is the most critical component.
  - Bracing: The use of an unloader brace that shifts weight away from the medial compartment.
  - Analgesics for pain control.
  - Osteoporosis treatment: Calcium, Vitamin D, and Bisphosphonates to address the underlying bone quality issue.
  - Physical therapy: Focus on non-weight-bearing range of motion and strengthening exercises for the hip and quadriceps.
- Surgical intervention: Surgery is considered if conservative treatment fails or if there is significant collapse.
  - Joint-preserving procedures: Arthroscopic drilling (subchondroplasty) to stimulate healing and inject a bone substitute material to support the subchondral bone.
  - Joint-replacing procedures: Unicompartmental knee arthroplasty, if only the medial compartment is affected. This is often the ideal solution.
  - Total knee arthroplasty, for older patients with more widespread arthritis.

Prognosis

- Guarded. The outcome depends on the size of the lesion and the degree of collapse at the time of diagnosis.
- With strict adherence to non-weight-bearing, smaller fractures can heal without sequelae.
- Larger fractures often progress to collapse and secondary osteoarthritis, necessitating knee replacement surgery.

Suggested Reading

Malghem J, Lecouvet F, Vande Berg B, Kirchgesner T, Omoumi P. Subchondral insufficiency fractures, subchondral insufficiency fractures with osteonecrosis, and other apparently spontaneous subchondral bone lesions of the knee-pathogenesis and diagnosis at imaging. Insights Imaging. 2023;14(1):164.

Ochi J, Nozaki T, Nimura A, Yamaguchi T, Kitamura N. Subchondral insufficiency fracture of the knee: rcview of current concepts and radiological differential diagnoses. Jpn J Radiol. 2022;40(5):443–57.

Vidoni A, Shah R, Mak D, Beale D, Beale S, James S, Botchu R. Metaphyseal burst sign: a secondary sign on MRI of subchondral insufficiency fracture of the knee. J Med Imaging Radiat Oncol. 2018;62(6):764–8.

Case 65

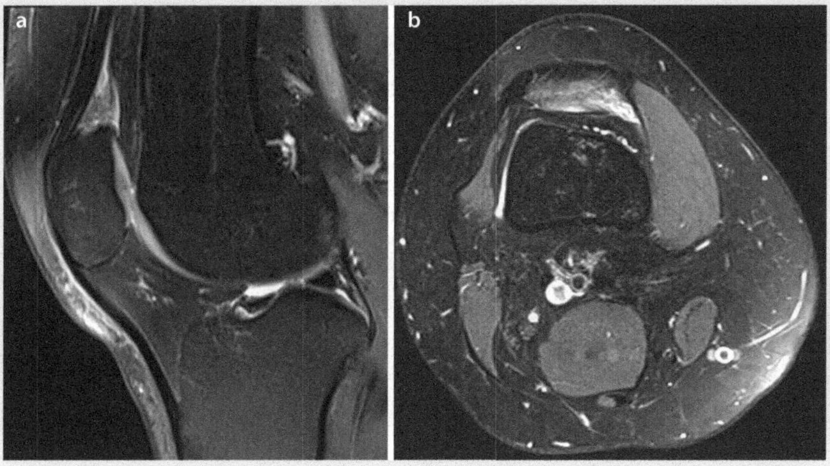

A 25-year-old male presented with anterior knee pain and tenderness at the superior pole of the patella

S. Saran et al., *101 Knee Imaging Case Series*, 101 MSK Imaging 1,
https://doi.org/10.1007/978-3-032-21567-3_65

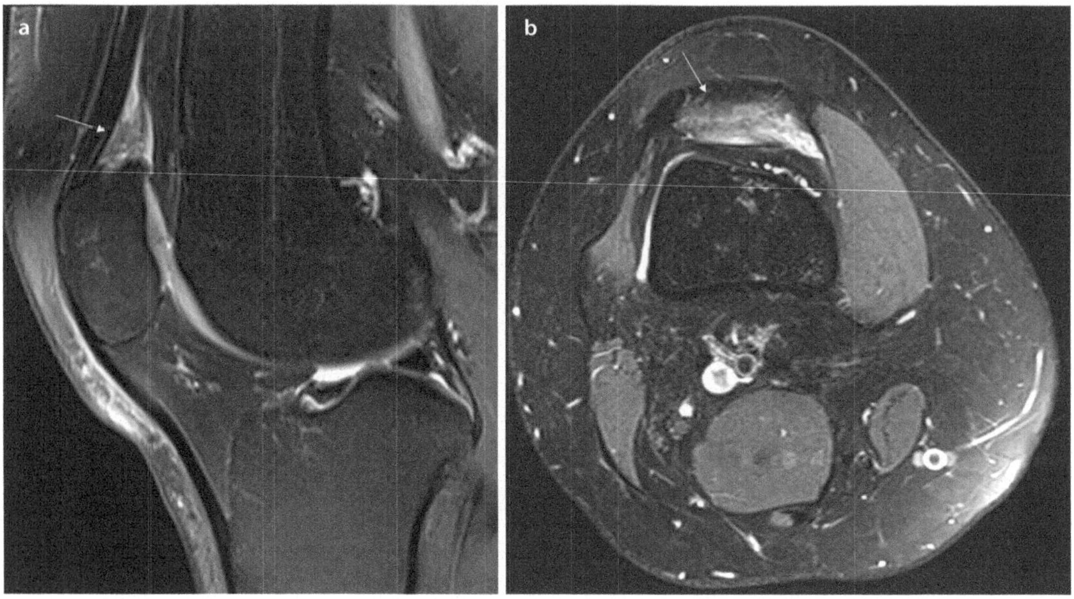

■ MRI knee PDFS sagittal **a** and axial **b** shows oedema in the suprapatellar fat pad (arrows) with a mass effect on the adjacent suprapatellar recess. Findings are suggestive of suprapatellar fat pad impingement syndrome

Suprapatellar Fat Pad Impingement Syndrome

Definition & Pathophysiology

- Anterior suprapatellar fat pad impingement syndrome is a proposed and controversial cause of anterior knee pain. It is characterized by edema and enlargement of the fat pad located posterior to the quadriceps tendon and superior to the patella.
- Controversy: The MRI findings of fat pad edema are frequently incidental or considered an anatomical variant. A diagnosis cannot be made on imaging findings alone and requires a strict correlation with specific clinical signs and symptoms.
- Aetiology: The cause is unclear. The leading theory is repetitive microtrauma leading to fibrosis and haemorrhage within the fat pad.

Clinical Presentation

- Symptoms: anterior knee pain.
- Point tenderness: maximal at the superior pole of the patella (distinguishing it from Hoffa's syndrome, which is inferior).
- Pain exacerbation: pain is worsened by deep knee flexion, which is thought to pinch the fat pad between the patella and femur.

MRI Findings

- The following findings are suggestive but non-specific:
- T1-weighted: Low signal intensity within the anterior suprapatellar fat pad (replacing the normal bright fat signal).
- T2-weighted/STIR: High signal intensity within the fat pad.
- T1 C+ (Gd): Enhancement of the inflamed fat pad.
- Enlargement: Anteroposterior (AP) diameter ≥10 mm.
- Mass effect: the fat pad has a convex border, exerting mass effect on the suprapatellar recess and the quadriceps tendon.

Differential Diagnosis & Diagnostic Caution

- The primary challenge is distinguishing a symptomatic fat pad from an incidental finding.
- Incidental fat pad edema: the most likely scenario. The radiologist must avoid over-calling this finding without the specific clinical context of superior patellar pain worsened by deep flexion.

Management

- Conservative management
  - Activity modification: avoidance of deep flexion activities.
  - Anti-inflammatory medications.
  - Physical therapy: to address strength and flexibility imbalances.
- Image-guided intervention (diagnostic and therapeutic)
  - Ultrasound-guided injection: an injection of a local anaesthetic and corticosteroid into the fat pad is a critical step.
- Surgical intervention
  - Arthroscopic resection: considered only in cases with persistent, debilitating symptoms that fail conservative and injection therapy. Involves debridement or partial resection of the fibrotic fat pad.

Suggested Reading

Bas A, Tutar O, Yanik I, Samanci C. Quadriceps fat-pad impingement syndrome: MRI findings. BMJ Case Rep. 2012;2012:bcr2012007643.

Yuksel Y, Ergun T, Torun E, Unal M, Sonnow L, Kose O. The relationship between quadriceps fat pad syndrome and patellofemoral morphology: a case-control study. J Orthop Traumatol. 2021;22(1):17.

Case 66

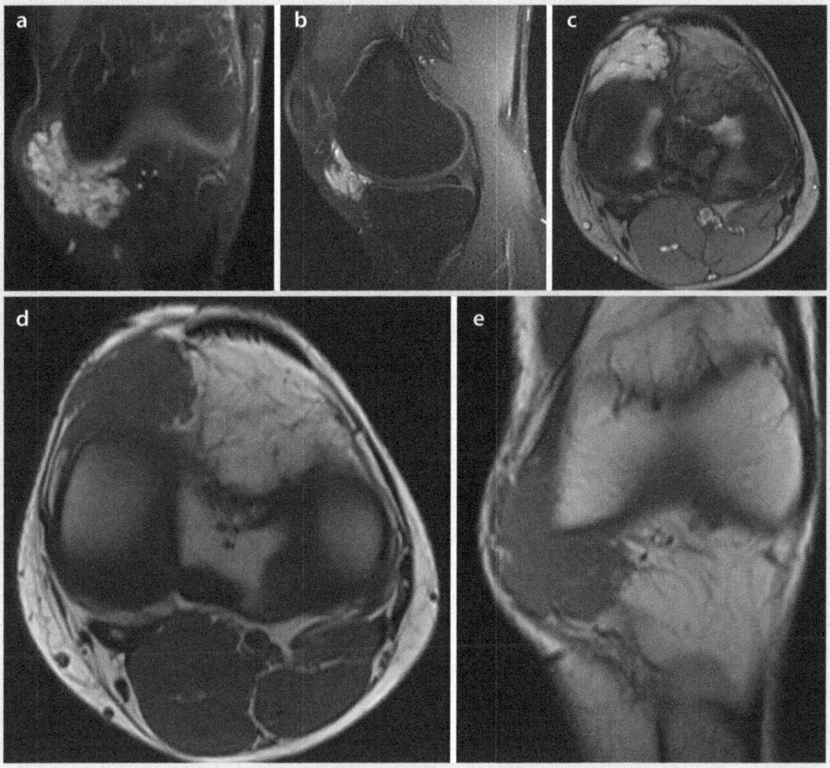

A 20-year-old male patient presented with pain and swelling in the knee joint

S. Saran et al., *101 Knee Imaging Case Series*, 101 MSK Imaging 1,
https://doi.org/10.1007/978-3-032-21567-3_66

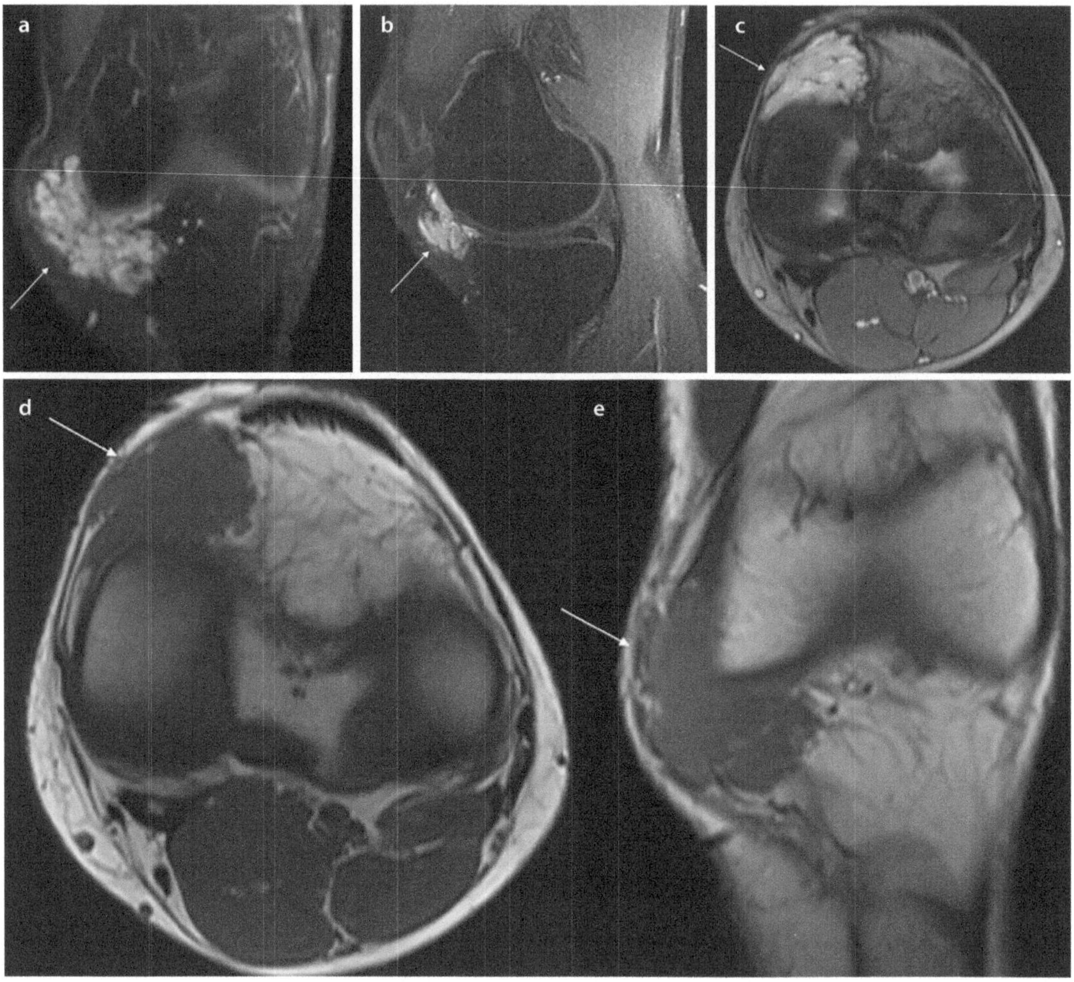

■ MRI knee, PDFS weighted coronal **a**, sagittal **b**, and axial **c** sequences, and T1 weighted axial **d** and coronal **e** sequences showing a well-defined lobulated lesion (arrows) appearing hyperintense on PDFS and intermediate signal intensity on T1-weighted images with thin, serpentine septa showing signal intensity of fat. Imaging findings are consistent with synovial hemangioma of the knee joint

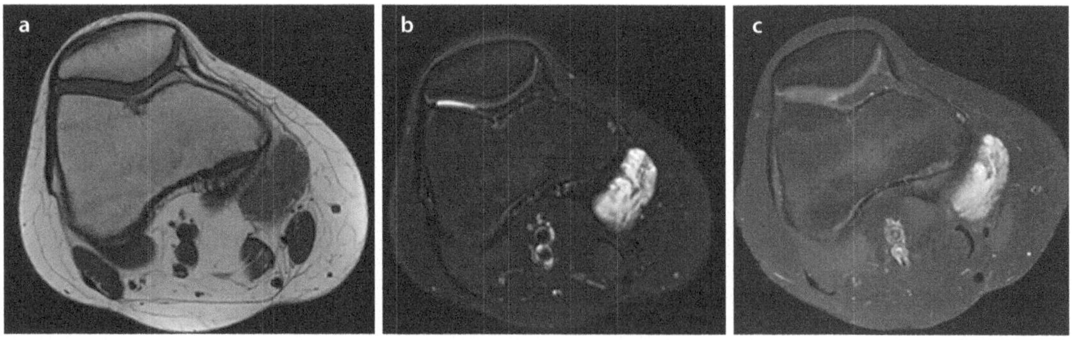

■ Companion case: A case of haemangioma in the juxta-articular region closely related to the joint capsule of the knee

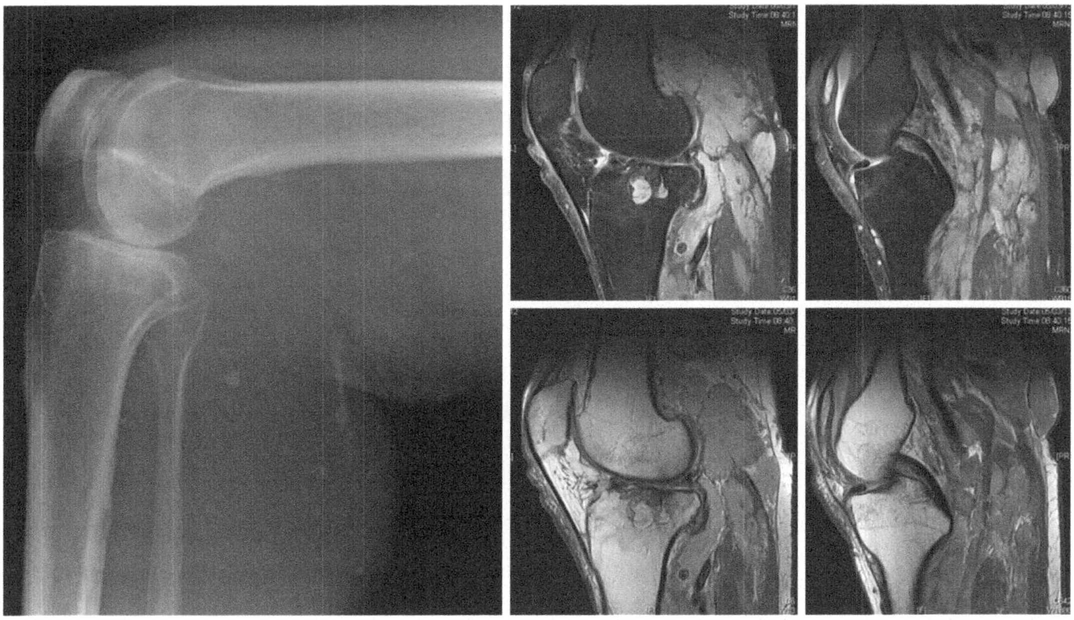

Companion case: Soft tissue hemangioma in the popliteal region with phleboliths and intraarticular extension

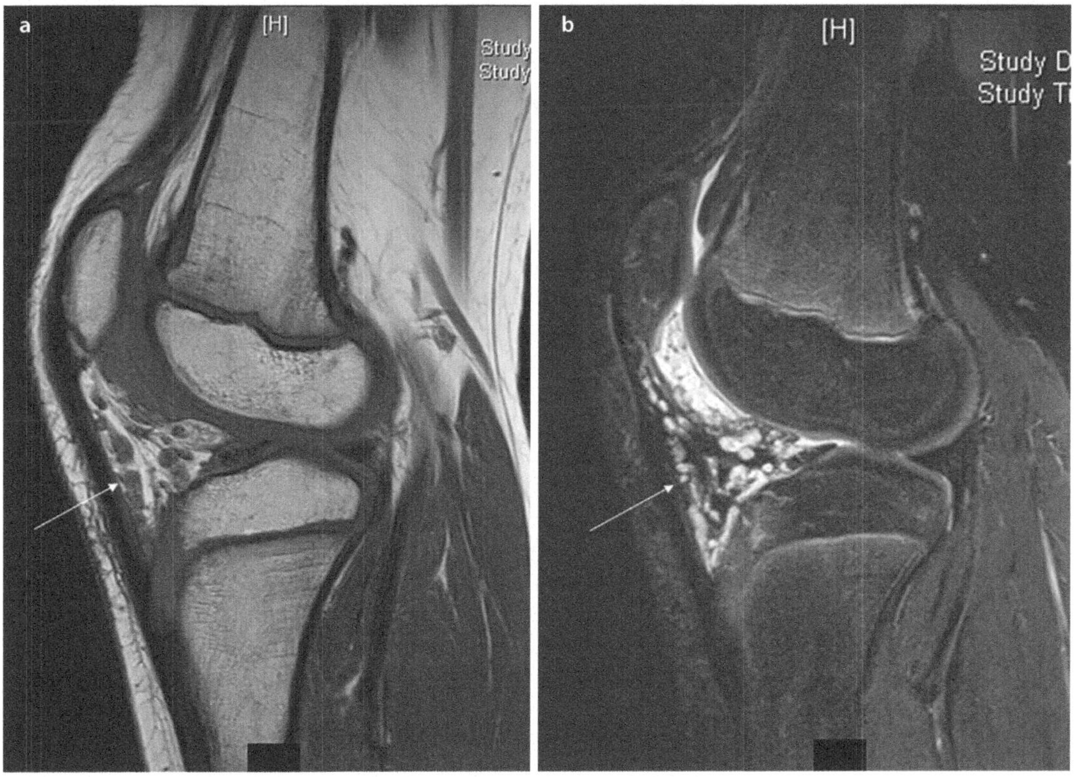

Companion case: Synovial hemangioma (arrows) in the Hoffa's fat pad

Synovial Hemangioma of the Knee Joint

Definition & Epidemiology

- A rare, benign, hamartomatous proliferation of blood vessels arising from the subsynovial mesenchymal tissue.
- Constitutes <1% of all haemangiomas.
- The knee joint is the most common site (>95% of cases).

Clinical Presentation

- Primarily affects children and young adults, often leading to a significant diagnostic delay.
- Pain and swelling: the most common symptoms.
- Recurrent hemarthrosis: spontaneous or minor-trauma-induced bloody joint effusions. This is a major red flag.
- Decreased range of motion: often with tenderness and quadriceps atrophy.

Classification

Synovial haemangiomas are classified based on their anatomical extent.

- Articular: Confined within the joint capsule.
- Juxta-articular: Involving the periarticular soft tissues.
- Both: A combination of both intra- and extra-articular components.

MRI Findings

- T1-weighted: Intermediate signal intensity. Helps distinguish it from fat-containing lesions (e.g., lipoma arborescens).
- T2-weighted/STIR: Markedly hyperintense ("light-bulb bright") with serpentine, flow-void septa.
- Post-Contrast (T1+C): Intense, homogeneous enhancement. Confirms the highly vascular nature of the lesion.
- Additional signs:
  - Phleboliths (signal voids on all sequences)
  - joint effusion
  - synovial hypertrophy
  - hemosiderin deposits suggesting recurrent intra-articular haemorrhage

Differential Diagnosis

- Pigmented villonodular synovitis (PVNS): Typically shows "blooming" artifact on gradient-echo sequences due to hemosiderin deposition.
- Synovial sarcoma: A malignant tumour that may contain calcifications and is often more aggressive/infiltrative.
- Lipoma arborescens: Has a fat signal on all sequences.
- Synovial osteochondromatosis: Shows numerous intra-articular loose bodies, which may be calcified.
- Hemophilic arthropathy: Clinical history of a bleeding disorder is key.

Management

Treatment is indicated for symptomatic relief and prevention of degenerative joint disease from recurrent hemarthrosis.

- Sclerotherapy: a minimally invasive alternative to surgery
- Complete surgical excision:
  - Arthroscopic or open synovectomy with complete removal of the hemangioma.
  - High recurrence rate is common with incomplete resection due to the lesion's infiltrative nature.
  - Pre-operative angiography & embolisation: May be used for large, complex lesions to reduce intraoperative bleeding.

Suggested Reading

Guler I, Nayman A, Koplay M, Paksoy Y. Synovial hemangioma of the knee joint: magnetic resonance imaging findings. Pol J Radiol. 2015;80:450–2.

Hernández-Hermoso JA, Moranas-Barrero J, García-Oltra E, Collado-Saenz F, López-Marne S. Location, clinical presentation, diagnostic algorithm and open vs. arthroscopic surgery of knee synovial haemangioma: a report of four cases and a literature review. Front Surg. 2021;8:792380.

Kankane A, Rustagi A, Jain U, Krishna L, Talwar J. Juxta-articular synovial hemangioma of the ankle: a rare benign tumor. Cureus. 2025;17(4):e81596.

Lopez-Oliva CL, Wang EH, Cañal JP. Synovial haemangioma of the knee: an under recognised condition. Int Orthop. 2015;39(10):2037–40.

Case 67

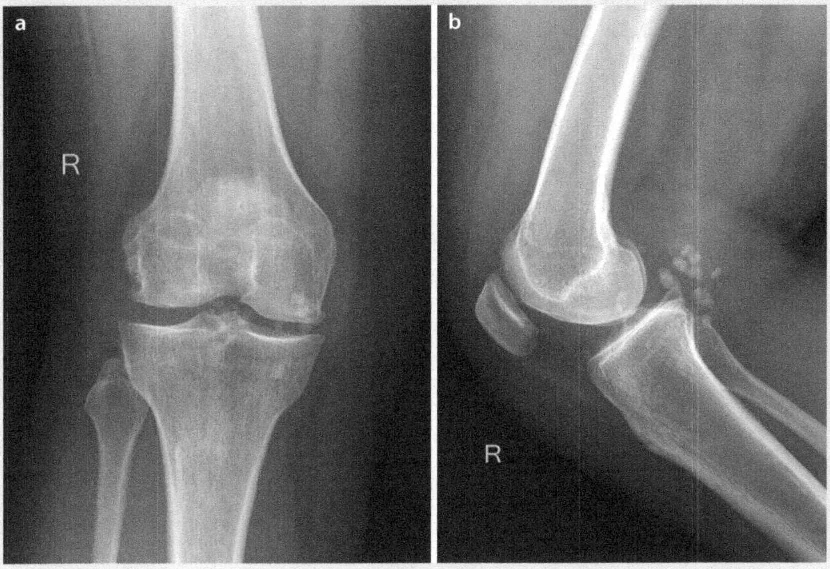

■ A 30-year-old female with a history of knee pain and locking

S. Saran et al., *101 Knee Imaging Case Series*, 101 MSK Imaging 1,
https://doi.org/10.1007/978-3-032-21567-3_67

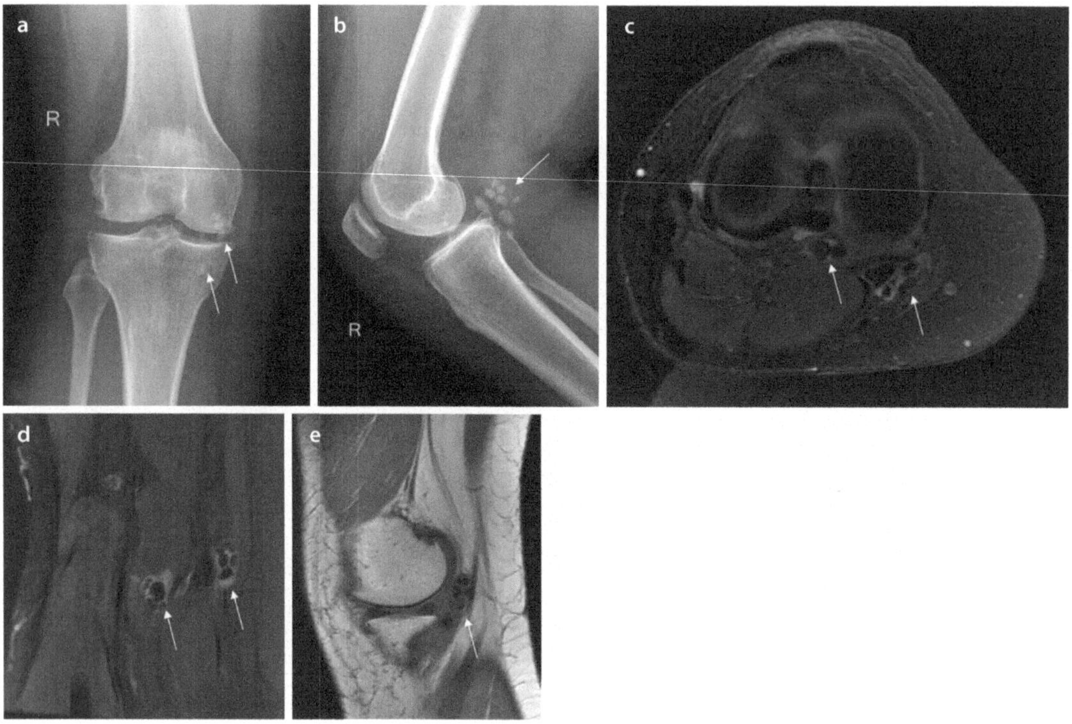

■ Anteroposterior **a**, lateral **b** radiographs showing multiple ossified loose bodies (arrows) occupying the posteromedial aspect of the joint space and adjacent soft tissue. MRI knee, PDFS weighted axial **c**, coronal **d**, and sagittal T1 weighted **e** sequences showing multiple ossified loose bodies (arrows) occupying the posteromedial aspect of the joint space and adjacent bursa. The loose bodies do not show the presence of internal marrow signals in this case. Imaging findings suggest the possibility of primary synovial osteochondromatosis

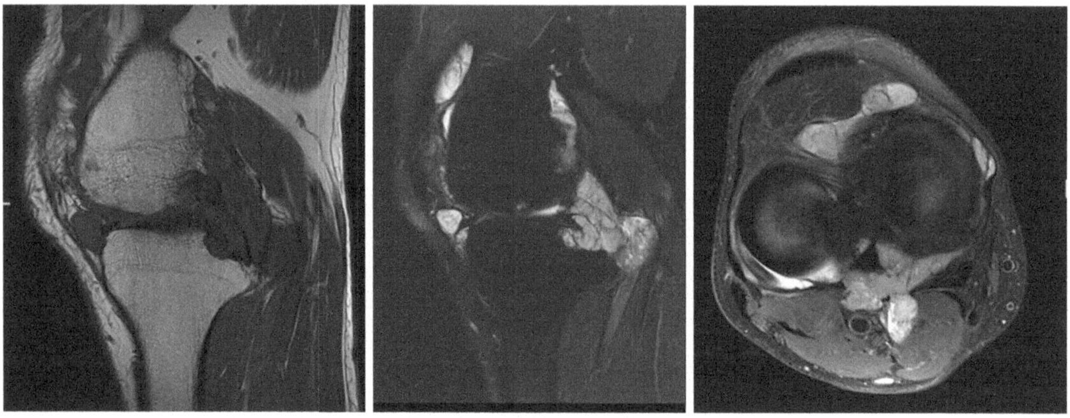

■ Companion case: Another case of primary synovial chondromatosis in the knee joint

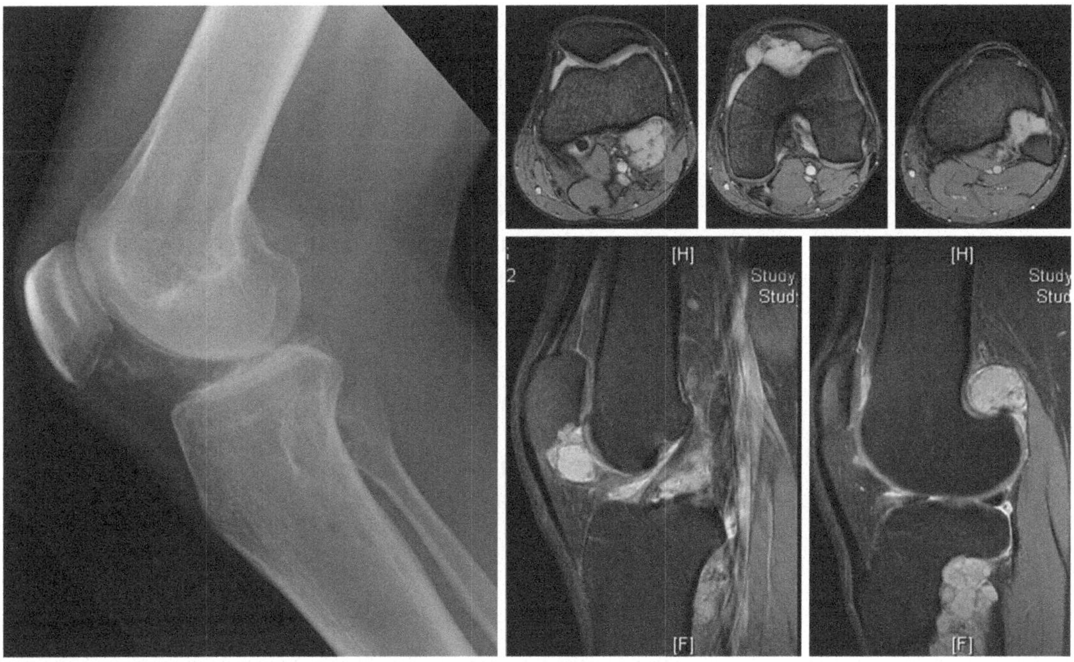

■ Companion case: Another case of primary synovial chondromatosis in the knee joint with chondroid calcifications on radiograph and hyperintense signals on PDFS weighted sequences. The pathology is also extending to involve the superior tibio-fibular joint

Primary Synovial Osteochondromatosis

Definition & Pathophysiology

- A benign, monoarticular neoplastic-like condition characterised by metaplastic proliferation of synovial tissue, leading to the formation of multiple cartilaginous nodules within the joint, bursa, or tendon sheath.
- Cartilage nodules detach, calcify/ossify, and form loose bodies ("joint mice").
- Aetiology: Unknown, but thought to arise from synovial mesenchymal cell metaplasia (not true neoplasia).
- Malignant transformation is rare (<5%, typically to synovial chondrosarcoma).

Clinical Presentation

- Age: Most common in 30- to 50-year-olds (M > F).
- Joints affected: Knee (most common, ~50%). Hip, shoulder, elbow and ankle are other joints which can be involved.
- Symptoms: Pain, swelling, stiffness (chronic, progressive); mechanical symptoms (locking, clicking, reduced range of motion); and palpable nodules (in superficial joints).

Imaging Findings

- Conventional radiographs:
  - Early stage: May appear normal (nodules not yet calcified).
  - Classic findings: Multiple round/oval calcified/ossified loose bodies (uniform size, "cluster of pearls").
  - No underlying joint degeneration (helps distinguish from secondary synovial osteochondromatosis).
- MRI
  - Non-mineralised nodules: T1: intermediate signal; T2/PD: hyperintense (cartilage signal).
  - Mineralised nodules: T1/T2: hypointense (due to calcification).
  - Post-contrast: peripheral synovial enhancement.
  - Synovial thickening & effusion.

Management

- Observation: Asymptomatic cases (if no mechanical symptoms).
- Surgical treatment (definitive): Arthroscopic or open synovectomy + loose body removal (treatment of choice).
- Recurrence rate: ~10–20% (incomplete synovectomy).
- Malignant suspicion: If rapid growth, bone destruction, or pain at rest → biopsy to rule out synovial chondrosarcoma.

Differential Diagnosis

- Secondary synovial osteochondromatosis: Due to osteoarthritis/trauma; fewer loose bodies, irregular sizes.
- Pigmented villonodular synovitis: Hemosiderin deposition (T2 hypointensity), no calcifications.

Prognosis

- Good after complete synovectomy (most patients regain full function).
- Recurrence is possible if residual disease remains.

Suggested Reading

Alamiri N, Alfayez SM, Marwan Y, Groszman L, Al Farii H, Burman M. Arthroscopic management of knee synovial chondromatosis: a systematic review of outcomes and recurrence. Int Orthop. 2025;49(5):1037–45.

Janssen A, Odekerken G. L'image du mois. L'ostéochondromatose synoviale [Synovial chondromatosis]. Rev Med Liege. 2023;78(10):533–4. French. PMID: 37830315.

Shafie M, Babaei Aghdam Z, Shirzad Moghaddam Z, Ayati Firoozabadi M, Emami Razavi SZ, Hosseini M, Azadvari M. Bilateral primary synovial chondromatosis in the knee joint. Clin Case Rep. 2022;10(12):e6618.

Most Difficult Cases

Contents

Case 68

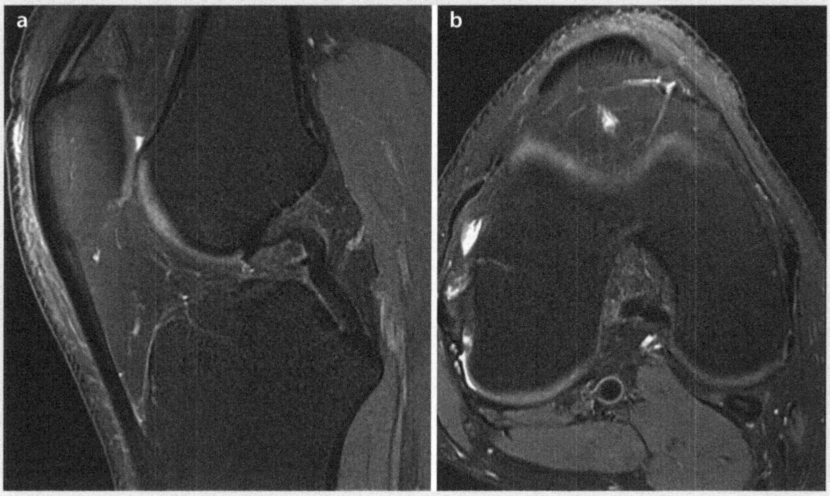

■ A 24-year-old male with no previous history of twisting knee injury

S. Saran et al., *101 Knee Imaging Case Series*, 101 MSK Imaging 1,
https://doi.org/10.1007/978-3-032-21567-3_68

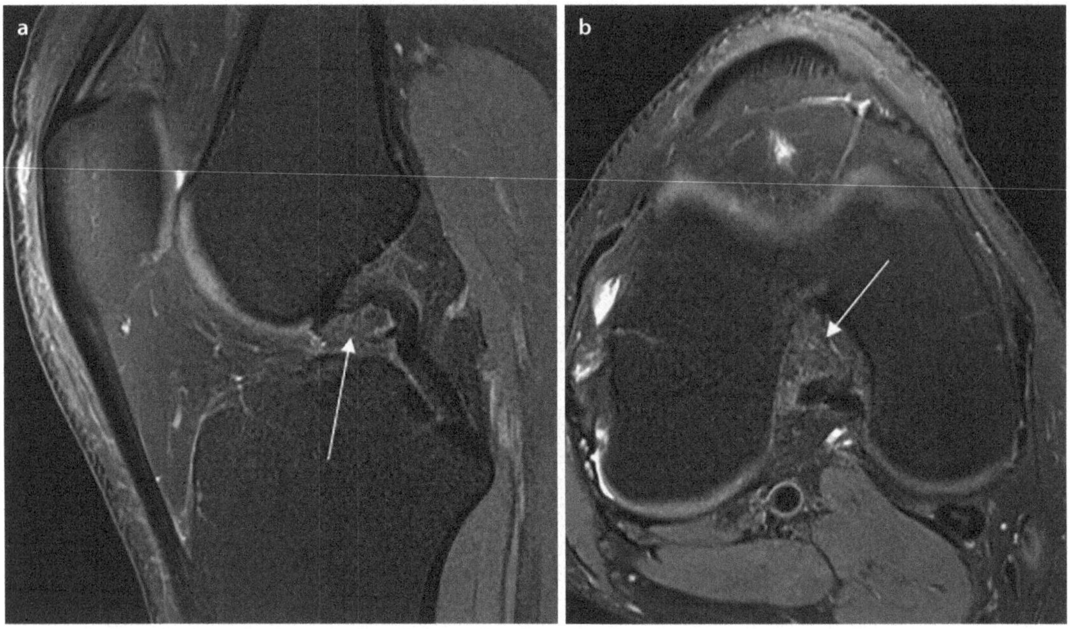

■ MR knee PDFS sagittal **a** and axial images **b**. There is non-visualisation of the anterior cruciate ligament in its expected location (arrows) with an intact posterior cruciate ligament

Congenital Absence of the Anterior Cruciate Ligament

Definition & Pathophysiology

- Congenital absence of the anterior cruciate ligament (ACL) is an uncommon condition, often associated with other developmental anomalies such as:
  - Congenital absence of the menisci
  - Congenital dislocation of the knee
  - Congenital short femur
- The ACL serves as the primary restraint against anterior tibial translation during knee hyperextension. Its absence can lead to altered knee biomechanics, though the long-term consequences remain unclear.
- Johansson and Aparisi's study observed that older patients with congenital ACL absence often remained asymptomatic, with no signs of instability or degenerative joint changes. However, a small subset of patients who experienced traumatic knee injuries developed instability and subsequent osteoarthritis, evident as joint space narrowing on radiographs.

- Noble's case report of an 81-year-old man with congenital ACL absence and a ring meniscus demonstrated no arthritic changes, suggesting that some individuals may adapt well over time.

Implications and Management

- Asymptomatic cases may not require intervention, as they can remain stable for decades.
- Symptomatic patients (e.g., those with instability or prior trauma) may benefit from ligament reconstruction or bracing to prevent secondary osteoarthritis.

Further research is needed to understand the biomechanical adaptations and optimal management strategies for this rare condition.

Given its association with other congenital anomalies, thorough clinical and imaging evaluation is essential for accurate diagnosis and personalized treatment planning.

Suggested Reading

Johansson E, Aparisi T. Missing cruciate ligaments in congenital short femur. J Bone Joint Surg Am. 1983;65:1109–15.

Murali J, Monchik K, Fadale P. Congenital absence of the anterior cruciate ligament. Am J Orthop (Belle Mead NJ). 2015;44(8):E283–5. PMID: 26251945.

Noble J. Congenital absence of the anterior cruciate ligament associated with a ring meniscus. J Bone Joint Surg Am. 1975;57:1165–6.

Case 69

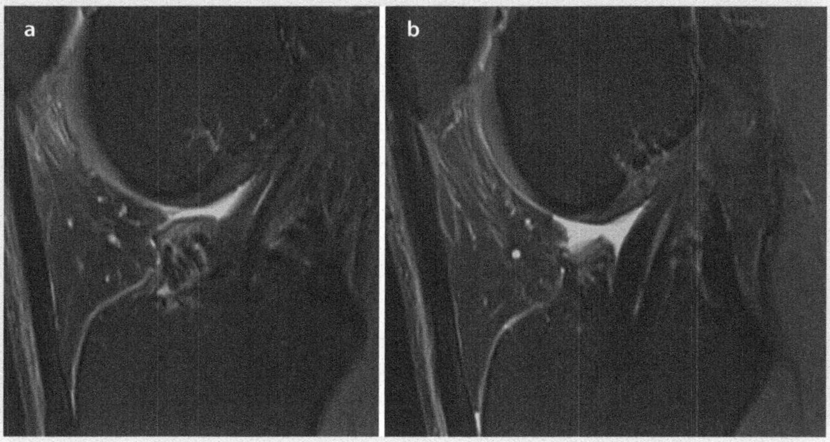

◘ A 27-year-old male presented for an MRI post-ACL reconstruction

S. Saran et al., *101 Knee Imaging Case Series*, 101 MSK Imaging 1,
https://doi.org/10.1007/978-3-032-21567-3_69

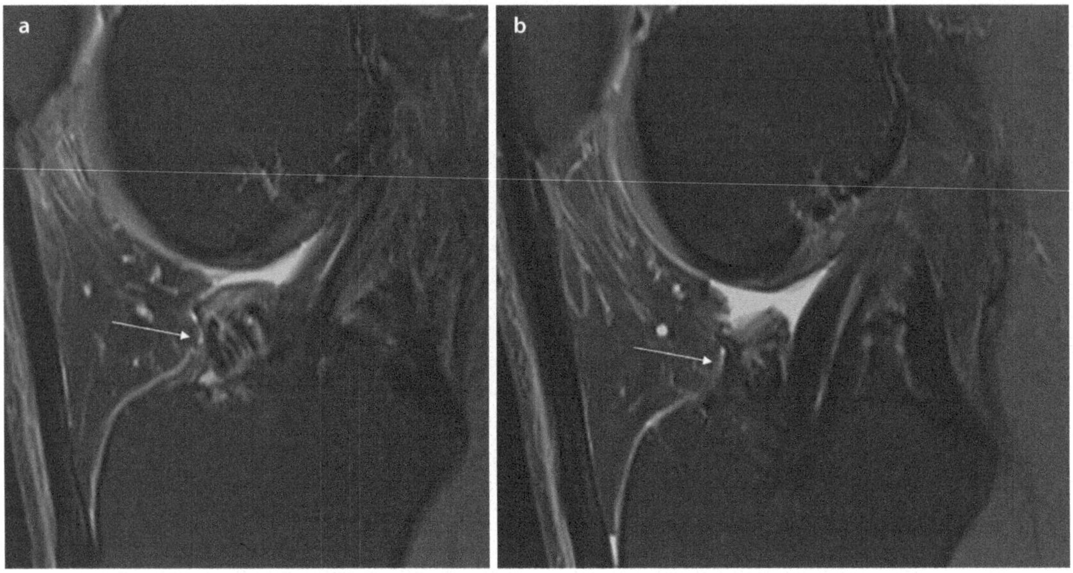

■ MRI knee, PDFS weighted sagittal **a**, **b** sequences showing Anterior cruciate ligament stump preservation (arrows) with reconstruction by graft

Anterior Cruciate Ligament Stump Preservation

Definition & Rationale

- Definition: ACL stump preservation is a surgical technique where the remnants of the torn native ACL are preserved and incorporated into the new graft during an ACL reconstruction.
- Philosophical shift: this moves away from the traditional method of complete debridement (removing the torn stump back to the anatomic footprints) towards a more biologically focused approach.

Theoretical Rationale for Preservation

- Enhanced proprioception:
  - The native ACL stump contains mechanoreceptors (e.g., Ruffini endings, Golgi tendon organs) that provide the brain with sensory feedback about knee position and movement (kinesthesia).
  - Preserving the stump may help restore this "sixth sense" of joint position, potentially improving dynamic stability and reducing re-injury rates.

- Improved vascularity and graft healing (ligamentisation):
  - The remnant tissue has a blood supply. Preserving it may act as a biological scaffold to support revascularisation and cellular repopulation of the new graft. Enhance the "ligamentisation" process, where the graft transforms into a structure resembling a native ligament.
- Biomechanical advantages: The preserved stump may act as a smooth, biological sleeve around the graft, reducing the risk of cyclops lesion formation (a common cause of post-op extension loss caused by scar tissue impingement). It may help seal the joint, potentially reducing fluid extravasation during surgery.
- Guidance for anatomic tunnel placement: The tibial stump can serve as a reliable visual guide for placing the tibial tunnel in the exact anatomic footprint of the native ACL.

Ideal Scenario: A proximal ("mid-substance" or femoral-side) tear where a robust, well-vascularized tibial stump remains.

Controversies and Limitations

- "Envelope of motion" vs. impingement: There is a concern that excessive remnant tissue could cause graft impingement against the intercondylar notch or PCL, leading to loss of motion or graft failure. Careful notchplasty may still be required.
- Lack of conclusive high-level evidence: While biomechanical and histological theories are strong, large-scale randomised controlled trials have not consistently shown a definitive clinical superiority of preservation techniques over standard reconstruction in terms of functional scores or stability.
- Not always possible: The technique is not suitable for all tear patterns, for example, tibial avulsion fractures, chronic, atrophied stumps and completely shredded, non-identifiable remnants.

Suggested Reading

Cho E, Chen J, Xu C, Zhao J. Remnant preservation may improve proprioception after anterior cruciate ligament reconstruction. J Orthop Traumatol. 2022;23(1):22.

Dhillon MS, Bali K, Vasistha RK. Immunohistological evaluation of proprioceptive potential of the residual stump of injured anterior cruciate ligaments (ACL). Int Orthop. 2010;34(5):737–41.

Sha L, Xie G, Zhao S, Zhao J. A morphologic and quantitative comparison of mechanoreceptors in the tibial remnants of the ruptured human anterior cruciate ligament. Medicine (Baltimore). 2017;96(5):e6081.

Case 70

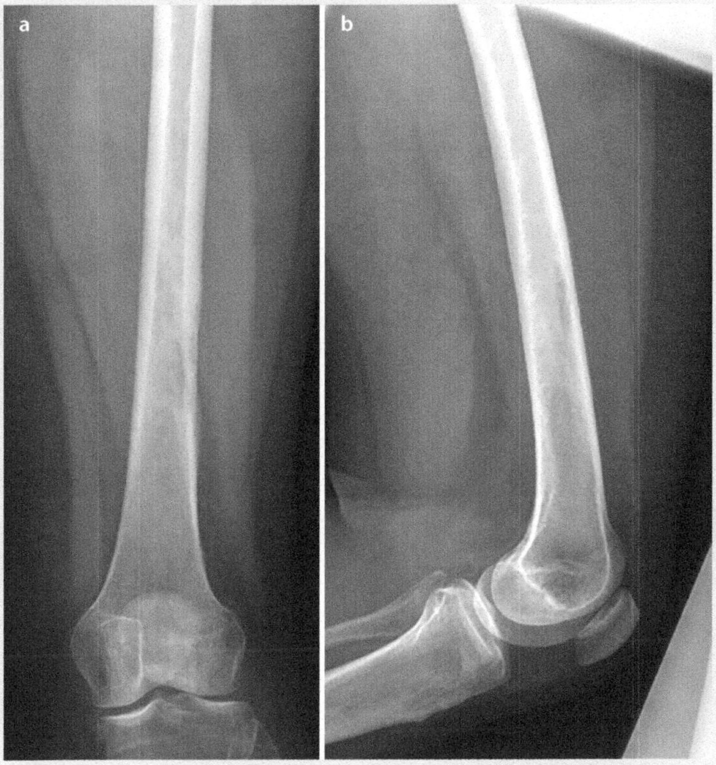

A 56-year-old male presented with pain in the mid-thigh region

S. Saran et al., *101 Knee Imaging Case Series*, 101 MSK Imaging 1,
https://doi.org/10.1007/978-3-032-21567-3_70

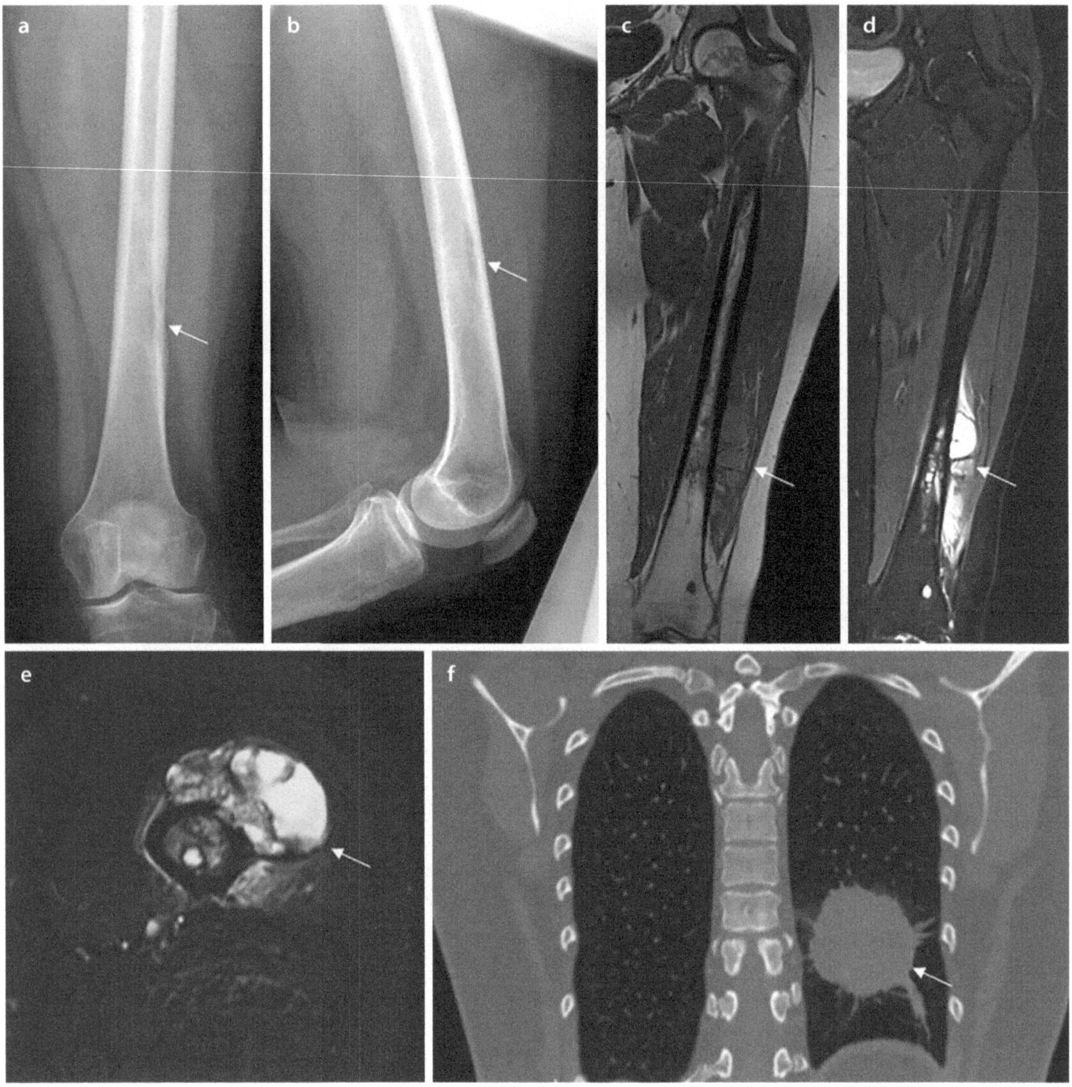

■ Radiographs anteroposterior **a** and lateral **b** show the presence of an ill-defined osteolytic lesion with a permeative pattern of bone destruction and a wide zone of transition involving mid-femoral diaphysis (arrows) with areas of cortical breach. Radiographic feature in this age group raises the suspicion of an aggressive bone tumour with the possibility of metastasis most likely. MRI thigh coronal T1 **c**, STIR **d** and STIR axial **e** was performed next, which showed the extent of the lesion (arrows) with hypointense signals on T1-weighted sequence **c** and hyperintense signals on STIR **d**, **e** images. A CECT thorax **f** performed in search for the primary, identified a large mass lesion (arrow) in the left lung with speculated margins

Cookie-Bite Metastasis

Definition & Pathophysiology

- "Cookie-bite" metastasis is associated with lung cancer metastases. The appearance describes a sharply demarcated, round or oval, purely lytic lesion that resembles a bite taken out of the bone. In the context of lung cancer, this pattern often indicates a bulky, rapidly growing metastasis.

Clinical Presentation

- Typically seen in a patient with a known history of lung carcinoma (often squamous cell or adenocarcinoma). It may also be the first presenting sign of an occult lung primary, especially in a smoker.
- Symptoms:
  - Deep, localised bone pain, often worse at night and may precede radiographic changes.
  - High risk of pathologic fracture due to the significant cortical destruction, especially in weight-bearing bones like the femur.
  - Constitutional symptoms like weight loss, fatigue, and cough may be present.

Imaging Findings

- Radiograph
  - A single, large, "punched-out" lytic lesion with an ill-defined, non-sclerotic margin and a wide zone of transition.
  - Shows focal, complete destruction—the "bite." The lesion often appears expansile, ballooning the bone.
  - Associated soft tissue component may be present.
- CT
  - Confirms the purely lytic nature and precisely defines the extent of cortical breach.
  - Essential for assessing the risk of impending fracture.
  - A CT of the chest will typically identify the primary lung tumour.
  - MRI
  - MRI defines the full intramedullary and soft tissue extent, which is often larger than apparent on a radiograph.

Differential Diagnosis

- Plasmacytoma/multiple myeloma: Can be identical. Differentiated by serum/urine electrophoresis and bone marrow biopsy.
- Primary bone sarcoma: Such as a lytic osteosarcoma or fibrosarcoma, though these are typically associated with a larger soft tissue component.

Management

- Management is palliative, focusing on local control, symptom relief, and systemic treatment.
- Surgical intervention may be needed for an impending pathologic fracture.

Suggested Reading

Greenspan A, Norman A. Osteolytic cortical destruction: an unusual pattern of skeletal metastases. Skeletal Radiol. 1988;17(6):402–6.

Ho HH, Hsu YC, Hsu HH, Huang GS. Cookie bite cortical osteolytic lesions: a hint of skeletal metastasis from bronchogenic carcinoma. QJM. 2015;108(12):975–6.

Case 71

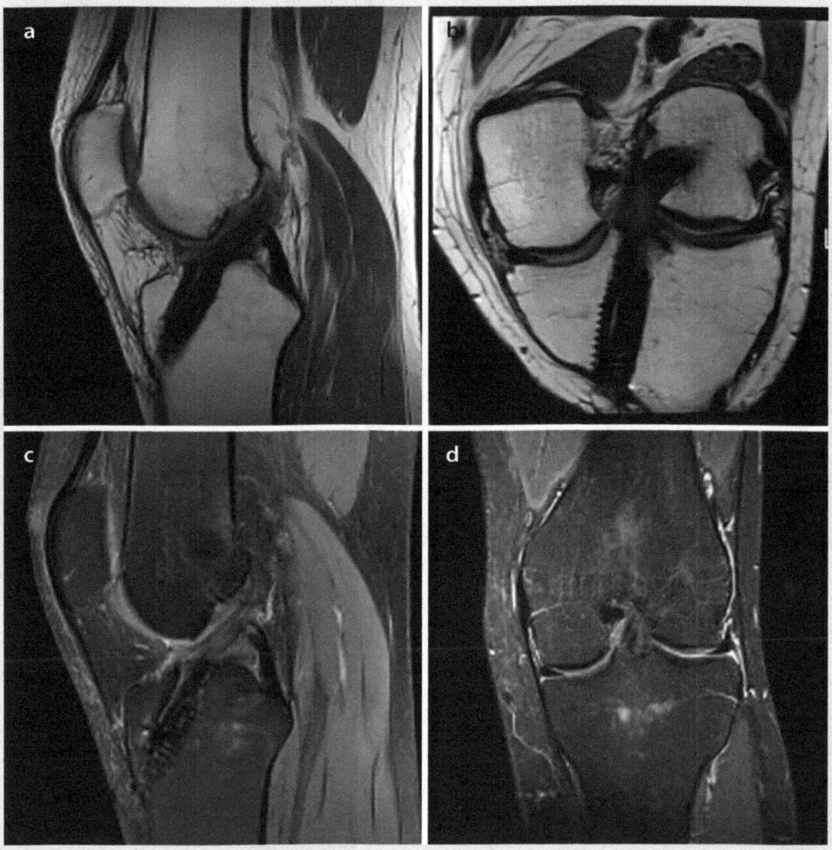

◘ A 35-year-old male with pain and limited range of motion after 2 years of ACL graft placement

S. Saran et al., *101 Knee Imaging Case Series*, 101 MSK Imaging 1,
https://doi.org/10.1007/978-3-032-21567-3_71

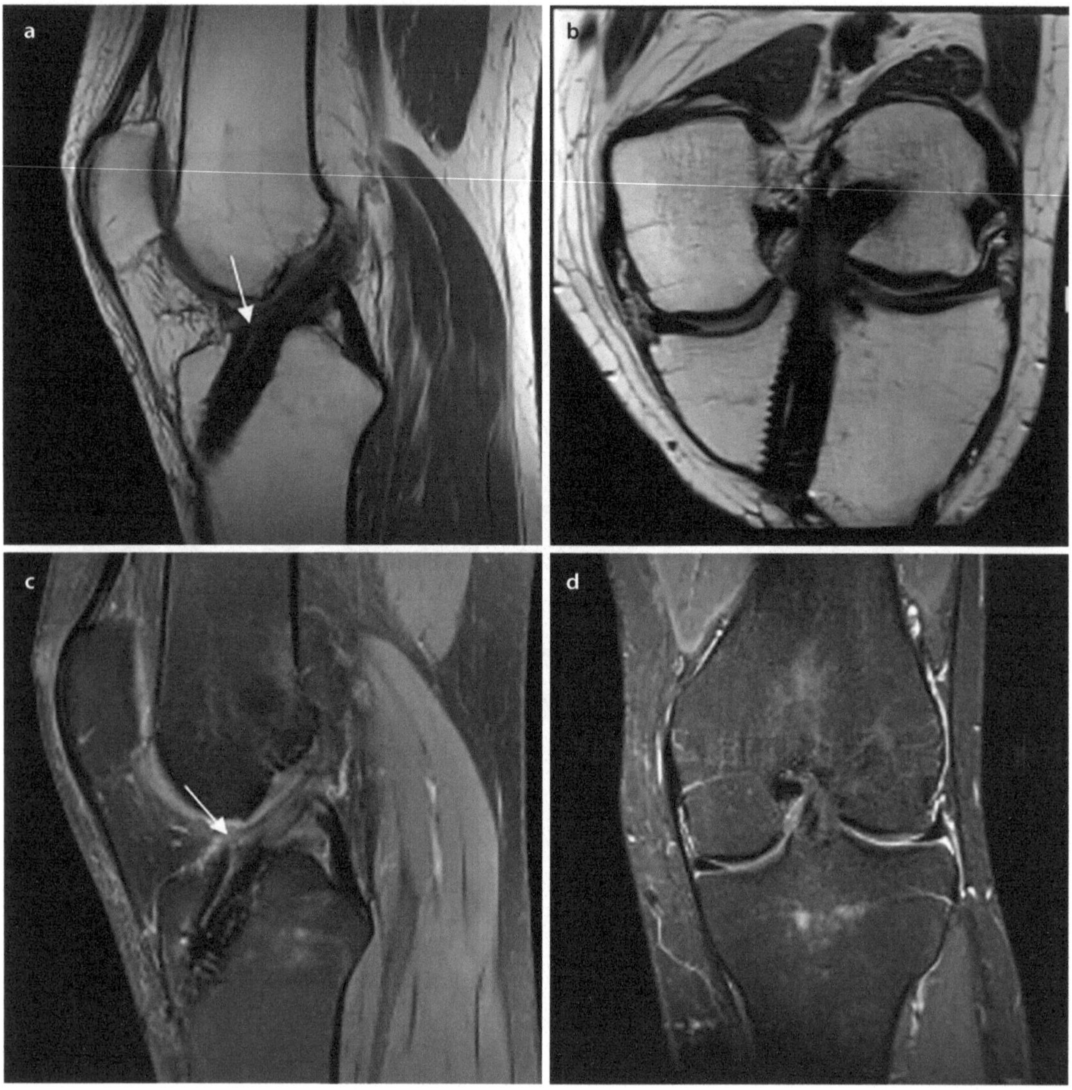

■ MRI knee T1 weighted sagittal **a**, coronal **b**, PDFS sagittal **c** and coronal **d** sequence showing fraying of the anterior distal graft with oedema and focal tear (arrows) with the anterior graft in contact with the femoral roof

ACL Graft Roof Impingement

Roof impingement occurs when an anteriorly placed ACL graft contacts the intercondylar notch (femoral roof) during knee extension, leading to:

1. Graft abrasion/attenuation → Increased risk of failure.
2. Cyclops lesion formation → Extension deficit.
3. Pain and limited ROM (especially terminal extension).

Primary Causes

1. Non-anatomic graft placement:
   - Tibial tunnel too anterior (violates the "quadrant rule").
   - Graft verticalization (excessive coronal angle).
2. Inadequate notchplasty: narrow intercondylar notch impinges on the graft.
3. Graft hypertrophy: post-surgical swelling/scarring exacerbates contact.

MRI

1. Direct signs:
   - Graft signal hyperintensity at the notch (focal oedema/tear).
   - Bone oedema in the femoral roof (chronic friction).
2. Indirect signs:
   - Cyclops lesion (nodular fibrosis anterior to the graft).
   - Graft thickening/loss of tension in extension.

Prognosis & Complications

- Early intervention leads to excellent outcomes.
- Delayed treatment leads to Graft failure (up to 15% revision rate).

Suggested Reading

Mann O, Al-Dadah O. Anterior cruciate ligament reconstruction: Effect of graft tunnel position on early to mid-term clinical outcomes. World J Orthop. 2024;15(8):744–53.

Udagawa K, Niki Y, Enomoto H, Toyama Y, Suda Y. Factors influencing graft impingement on the wall of the intercondylar notch after anatomic double-bundle anterior cruciate ligament reconstruction. Am J Sports Med. 2014;42(9):2219–25.

Case 72

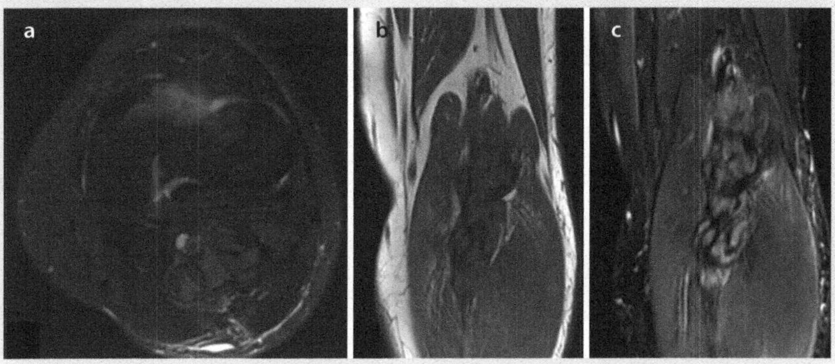

A 37-year-old male presented with hard, painless swelling in the popliteal region

S. Saran et al., *101 Knee Imaging Case Series*, 101 MSK Imaging 1,
https://doi.org/10.1007/978-3-032-21567-3_72

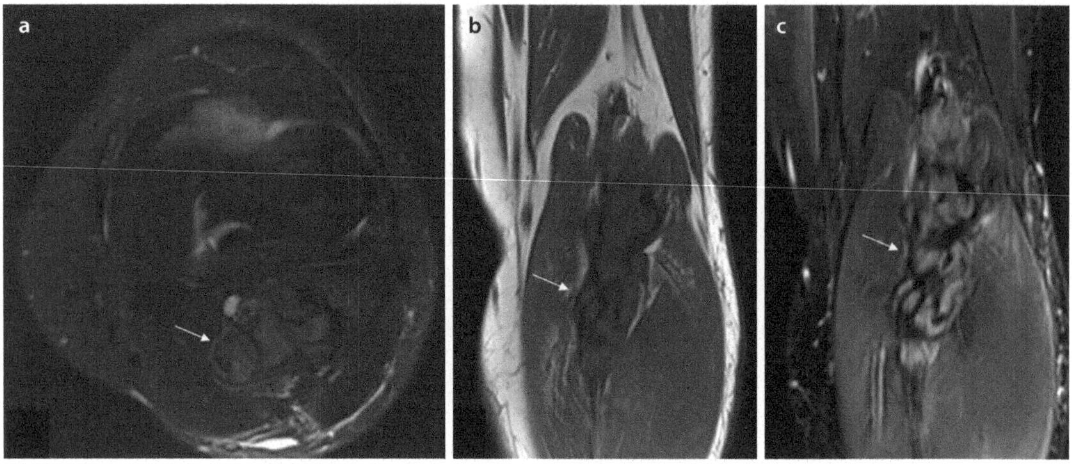

■ MRI knee **a**–**c** shows the presence of an ill-defined infiltrative lesion (arrows) showing mixed signal intensity appearing predominantly hypointense on both PDFS **a**, **c** and T1 **b** weighted sequences. Infiltrative nature with hypointense signal bands and fascial tails in keeping with fibromatosis

Fibromatosis

Definition & Pathophysiology

- Fibromatosis, also known as a desmoid-type fibromatosis or an aggressive fibromatosis, is a rare, benign, but locally aggressive soft tissue tumour. It arises from the musculo-aponeurotic structures—specifically the fascial sheaths and connective tissue within muscles.
- Pathology: It is composed of proliferating, well-differentiated fibroblasts and myofibroblasts within a collagenous stroma. It is clonally derived but lacks the ability to metastasise, placing it in a borderline category between benign and malignant.
- It is characterised by an infiltrative growth pattern and a high rate of local recurrence after surgery, but it does not metastasise.

Clinical Presentation

- Demographics: Most common in adults aged 20–40 years, with a slight female predominance. It can also occur in children.
- The popliteal fossa is an uncommon but well-documented site.

- Symptoms:
  - A firm, fixed, deep-seated mass that is often painless initially.
  - Pain or discomfort can develop as the lesion enlarges and compresses adjacent nerves (e.g., tibial nerve) or vessels.
  - Limited joint movement.

Imaging Findings

- Imaging is crucial for defining the extent of this infiltrative lesion and guiding management.
- MRI
  - MRI is the most important modality, showing characteristic features of a fibrous tumour.
  - T1-weighted: The lesion is typically isointense or slightly hypointense to skeletal muscle. It appears as an ill-defined, infiltrative mass.
  - T2-weighted / STIR: The signal is heterogeneous. Cellular areas are moderately hyperintense, while the abundant collagenous components are hypointense. This "band-like" or "stringy" low T2 signal is a classic feature.
  - T1-weighted post-contrast: Shows variable, often moderate to marked enhancement. The enhancement pattern can be heterogeneous.
  - The lesion does not have a capsule and often shows "fascial tail signs"—finger-like projections extending along muscle septa and fascia.
- Ultrasound
  - Shows a heterogeneous, hypoechoic mass with irregular borders.
  - Doppler may show internal vascularity.

Differential Diagnosis

- Nodular fasciitis: A benign, reactive lesion that grows rapidly and often has a more defined margin. It may be categorised as myxoid, cellular, or fibrous. This histologic diversity likely accounts for the variable MR imaging appearance of the lesions.
- Schwannoma: A benign nerve sheath tumour that is well-circumscribed, often shows a "target sign" on T2, and is associated with a nerve.
- Synovial sarcoma: A malignant tumour that can occur in young adults. It is often more heterogeneous, may contain calcifications, and can be more well-defined.

- Pigmented villonodular synovitis (PVNS): Arises from the joint lining and is characteristically dark on T1 and T2 due to hemosiderin.
- Myxofibrosarcoma: A malignant sarcoma with an infiltrative growth pattern, but it typically has a prominent myxoid (very bright T2) component.

Management

- Management of desmoid-type fibromatosis has evolved significantly away from immediate, aggressive surgery due to high recurrence rates. A multidisciplinary team approach is essential.
- Radiation therapy: Effective for local control in symptomatic, progressive lesions that are not amenable to surgery or systemic therapy. Cryotherapy is now the preferred treatment for fibromatosis.
- Surgical intervention: for symptomatic lesions, progressive growth despite medical therapy, or lesions causing significant functional impairment.
  - Procedure: wide local excision. The goal is to remove the tumour with a margin of normal tissue to reduce the risk of recurrence.

Suggested Reading

Handa S, Prajapati T, Phulware RH, Saran S. Periosteal desmoid tumor: a benign-appearing lesion manifesting as smooth metaphyseal scalloping of the femur on plain radiography. Indian J Musculoskelet Radiol. 2025;7:210–3.

Murphey MD, Ruble CM, Tyszko SM, Zbojniewicz AM, Potter BK, Miettinen M. From the archives of the AFIP: musculoskeletal fibromatoses: radiologic-pathologic correlation. Radiographics. 2009;29(7):2143–73.

Walker EA, Petscavage JM, Brian PL, Logie CI, Montini KM, Murphey MD. Imaging features of superficial and deep fibromatoses in the adult population. Sarcoma. 2012;2012:215810.

Case 73

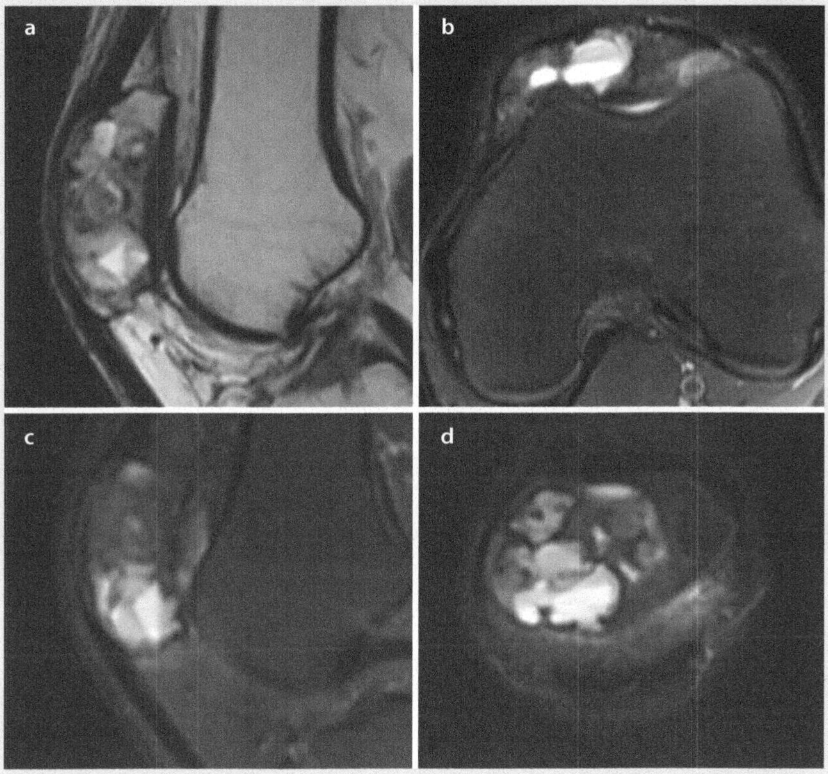

A 32-year-old male presented with pain and swelling in the patella

S. Saran et al., *101 Knee Imaging Case Series*, 101 MSK Imaging 1,
https://doi.org/10.1007/978-3-032-21567-3_73

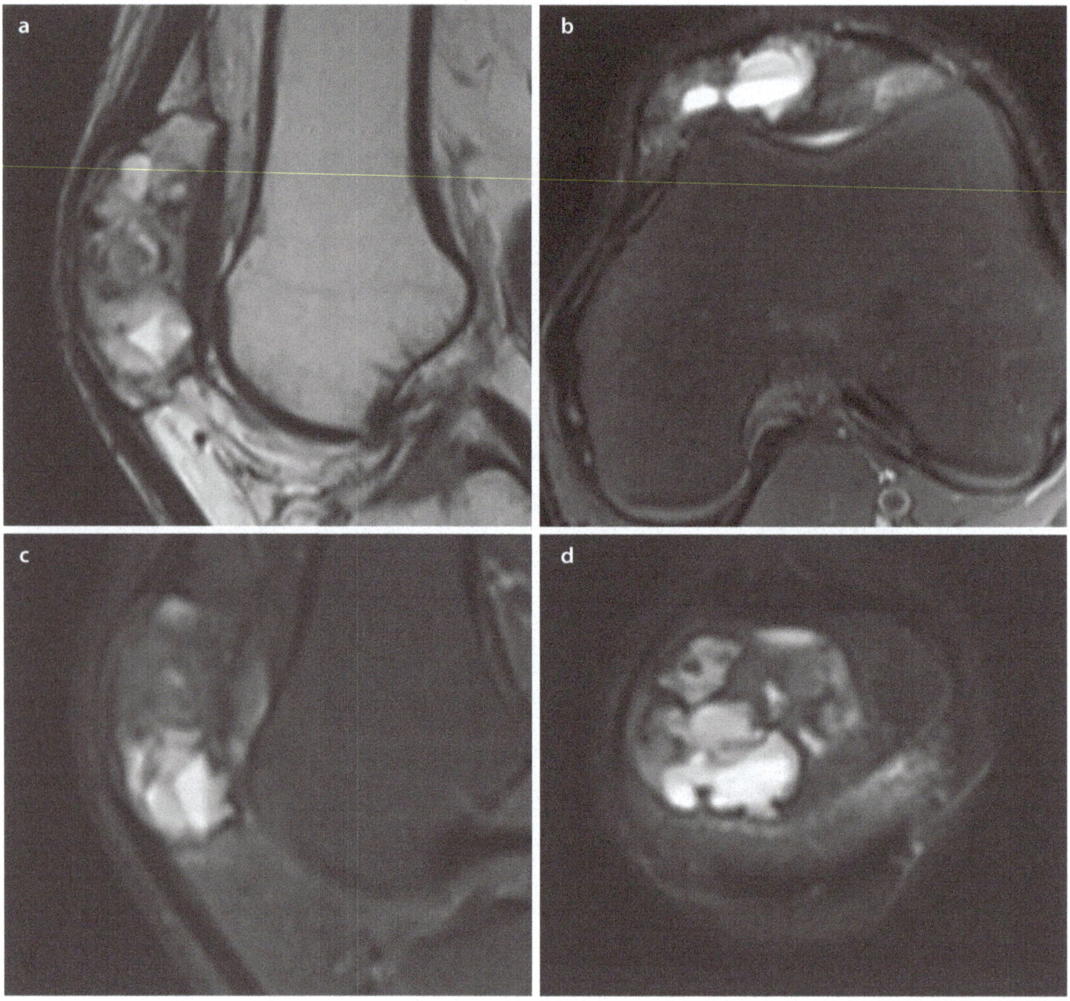

■ MRI PD sagittal **a**, axial PDFS **b**, sagittal PDFS **c** and coronal PDFS **d**. A well-defined PDFS hyperintense expansile lytic lesion with fluid levels seen in the patella. MRI findings are of a giant cell tumour with secondary aneurysmal bone cyst

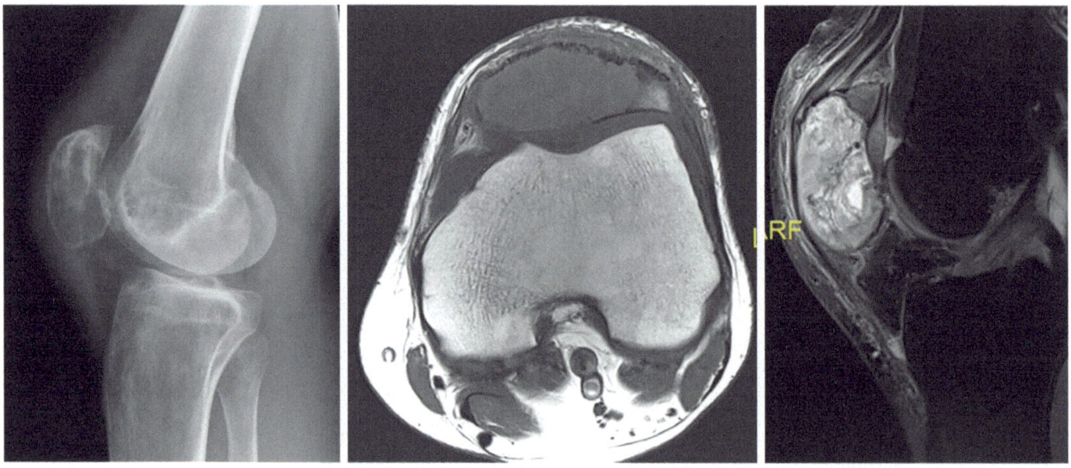

■ Companion case: Another case of GCT in the patella

Giant Cell Tumour of Bone with Secondary Aneurysmal Bone Cyst

Definition & Pathophysiology

- This is a rare and complex lesion where a primary, benign but locally aggressive Giant cell tumour (GCT) of the patella develops a secondary Aneurysmal Bone Cyst (ABC) component within it. The GCT is the driving neoplasm, while the ABC represents a reactive, hemodynamic phenomenon within the tumour.

Clinical Presentation

- Demographics: skeletally mature adults aged 20–45 years.
- Location: The patella is a very rare site for GCT (<1% of cases), making this an unusual presentation.
- Symptoms:
  - Anterior knee pain: worsens with activity, especially climbing stairs or kneeling.
  - Swelling and tenderness: over the patella.
  - Palpable mass: a firm, expanded patella may be palpable.
  - Effusion: due to intra-articular irritation.
  - Pathologic fracture: possible due to bony destruction.

Imaging Findings

- Imaging reveals a mixed solid and cystic, expansile lesion of the patella.
- Radiography
  - A lytic, expansile lesion with a "soap-bubble" or trabeculated appearance.
  - Cortex: marked cortical thinning and expansion. The periphery may show a thin, intact shell of bone or a breached cortex.
  - Matrix: no internal mineralisation.
- MRI
  - T2-weighted/STIR: Heterogeneously low to intermediate signal (a key feature of GCT due to hemosiderin and collagen). Multiple, hyperintense cystic cavities with fluid-fluid levels—the hallmark of the ABC component.
  - The combination of a solid, enhancing tissue mass (GCT) with internal cystic cavities showing fluid-fluid levels (ABC) is highly suggestive of this diagnosis.

Differential Diagnosis

- Primary ABC: Would not have a dominant solid, enhancing component. It is almost purely cystic.
- Chondroblastoma: Occurs in a younger age group (10–25 years) with open physes. Typically shows chondroid matrix calcification ("ring-and-arc") on CT, which GCT lacks.
- Patellar intraosseous ganglion: A purely cystic lesion without a solid, enhancing component.
- Brown tumour of hyperparathyroidism: Radiographically and histologically identical to GCT. Diagnosis is made by checking serum calcium and PTH levels.
- Lymphoma or metastasis: Rare in the patella; typically more permeative and destructive.

Management

- Management is challenging due to the patella's function and the aggressive nature of GCT. The goal is complete removal while preserving extensor mechanism function.

Suggested Reading

Jadhav S, Rathod YS, Rathod SR. Giant cell tumor of the patella: a case report. Cureus. 2024;16(9):e68590.

Shibata T, Nishio J, Matsunaga T, Aoki M, Iwasaki H, Naito M. Giant cell tumor of the patella: aAn uncommon cause of anterior knee pain. Mol Clin Oncol. 2015;3(1):207–11.

Singh J, James SL, Kroon HM, Woertler K, Anderson SE, Jundt G, Davies AM. Tumour and tumour-like lesions of the patella--a multicentre experience. Eur Radiol. 2009;19(3):701–12. https://doi.org/10.1007/s00330-008-1180-x.

Case 74

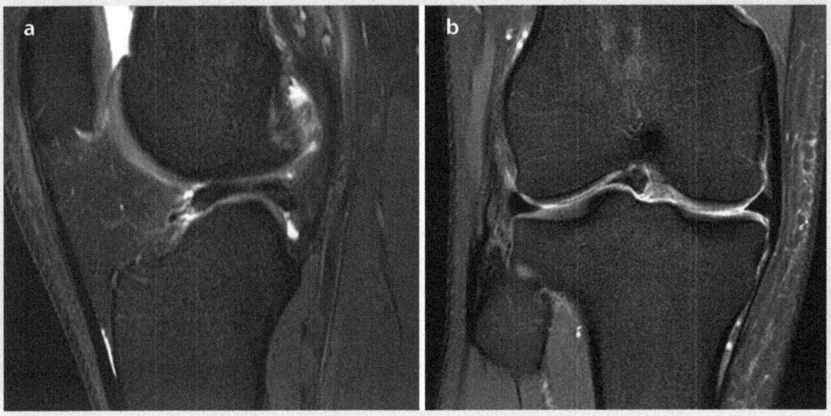

■ A 23-year-old male with a locking sensation in the knee

S. Saran et al., *101 Knee Imaging Case Series*, 101 MSK Imaging 1,
https://doi.org/10.1007/978-3-032-21567-3_74

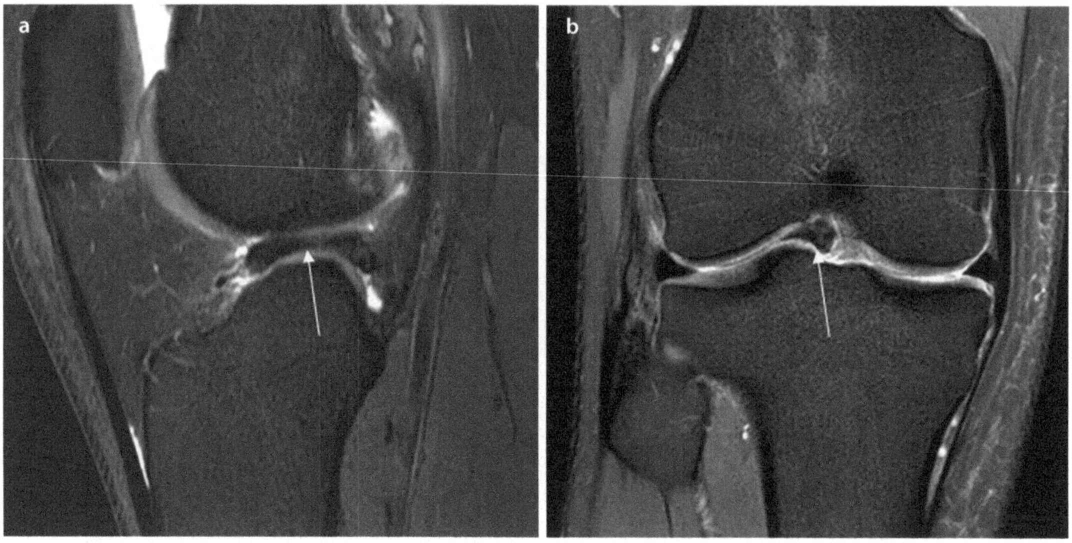

■ MRI knee, PDFS weighted sagittal **a**, and coronal **b** sequence showing a rare congenital anomaly where the lateral meniscus forms a complete ring-like structure (arrow) instead of the normal C-shape, appearances are of a ring-shaped lateral meniscus. Note the "mirror image sign" on the coronal sequence

Ring-Shaped Lateral Meniscus – Definition & Pathophysiology

- A rare congenital anomaly where the lateral meniscus forms a complete or partial ring-like structure instead of the normal C-shape. Its occurrence is relatively rare, with an incidence of up to 2.4%.
- The Watanabe classification categorises lateral meniscus variants into three types: complete discoid, incomplete discoid, and Wrisberg ligament type. Monllau et al. proposed adding the ring-shaped meniscus as a fourth variant within this classification due to its distinct morphology.
- Hypothesised cause: Developmental failure of meniscal embryological regression.

Clinical Features

- Often asymptomatic and an incidental finding on MRI or arthroscopy, but may predispose to meniscal instability or tearing due to abnormal biomechanics.
- If symptomatic: knee pain (especially with activity); clicking, locking, or snapping (due to abnormal motion); and effusion (if secondary tear develops).

MRI Findings

- "Mirror image sign" on coronal images (vs. normal crescentic shape).
- Continuity between anterior and posterior horns (key diagnostic feature).
- Possible hypertrophy (thickened meniscus resembling discoid variant).
- Secondary tear (if present, hyperintense signal on T2/PD).

Differential

Bucket handle meniscal tear: Differentiating a ring-shaped meniscus from a displaced bucket-handle tear can be challenging, but key imaging features help in diagnosis.

- On coronal MRI sequences, the "mirror image sign"—where the intermeniscal bridge mirrors the meniscus body—supports a ring-shaped meniscus.
- Both structures should maintain a smooth, triangular shape, unlike the frayed and irregular appearance of a bucket-handle tear.
- Additionally, the intermeniscal bridge in a ring-shaped meniscus is typically positioned between the femoral and tibial cartilage near the intercondylar eminence, rather than within the intercondylar notch, as seen in displaced bucket-handle tears. This normal variant preserves the meniscus's role in protecting articular cartilage.

Management

- Asymptomatic Cases → No treatment needed.
- Symptomatic or Torn Ring Meniscus → Arthroscopic surgery.

Suggested Reading

Iqbal A, McLoughlin E, Botchu R, James SL. The ring-shaped meniscus: a case series demonstrating the variation of imaging appearances on MRI. Skeletal Radiol. 2020;49(2):281–9.

Mohd Miswan MF, Alsagoff SNA, Yahaya MY, Sikkandar MF, Mohd Khalid MS. A ring-shaped lateral meniscus in an anterior cruciate ligament reconstruction surgery. Cureus. 2025;17(4):e81729.

Monllau JC, León A, Cugat R, Ballester J. Ring-shaped lateral meniscus. Arthroscopy. 1998;14(5):502–4.
Ryu K, Iriuchishima T, Oshida M, Saito A, Kato Y, Tokuhashi Y, Aizawa S. Evaluation of the morphological variations of the meniscus: a cadaver study. Knee Surg Sports Traumatol Arthrosc. 2015;23(1):15–9.
Watanabe M, Takeda S, Ikeuchi H. Tokyo: Igaku-Shoin. Tokyo, Japan: Igaku-Shoin; 1979. Atlas of arthroscopy; p. 156.

Case 75

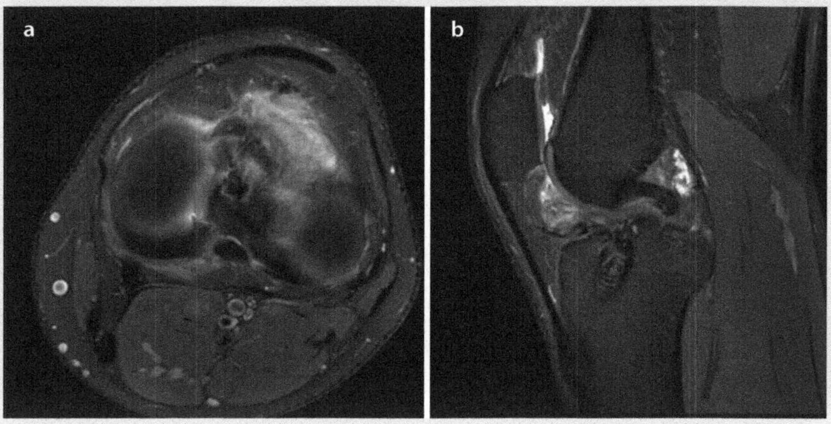

■ A 32-year-old male, post-ACL reconstruction, presented with restriction of joint movement, predominantly in extension

S. Saran et al., *101 Knee Imaging Case Series*, 101 MSK Imaging 1,
https://doi.org/10.1007/978-3-032-21567-3_75

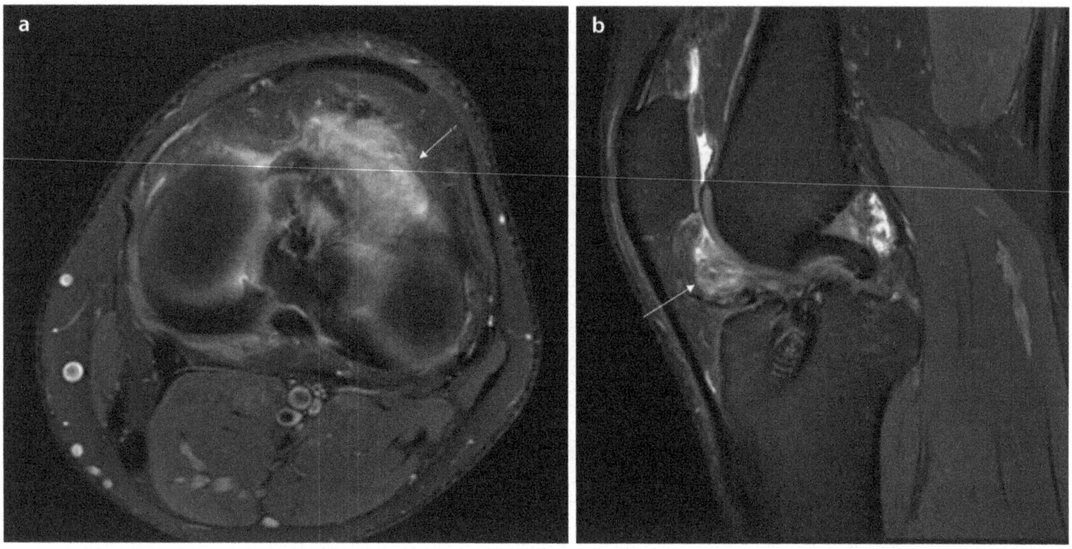

▪ MRI knee PDFS axial **a**, sagittal **b** shows the presence of a soft-tissue mass (arrows) anteriorly in the intercondylar notch near the tibial insertion of the reconstructed anterior cruciate ligament, showing mixed signal intensity on PDFS weighted sequences. MRI findings in the light of the clinical context favour the diagnosis of Cyclops lesion or localised anterior arthrofibrosis

Localised Anterior Arthrofibrosis (Cyclops Lesion)

Definition and Pathophysiology

- A Cyclops lesion is a specific type of localised anterior arthrofibrosis that occurs after Anterior Cruciate Ligament (ACL) reconstruction. It is a benign, nodular mass of fibrous tissue and granulation tissue that forms primarily at the anterolateral aspect of the tibial tunnel entrance, directly in front of the ACL graft.
- The lesion is named for its arthroscopic appearance, which resembles a "cyclops eye"—a reddish, nodular mass with a central pale spot (avascular core).

Clinical Presentation

- Typically presents 3–6 months after ACL reconstruction surgery.
- Symptom:
  - Painful, solid, "springy" block to terminal knee extension. The patient is unable to fully straighten the knee, often lacking the last 5–15 degrees of extension.

- Anterior knee pain, especially with attempts to force extension.
- Audible and palpable "clunk" during terminal extension as the nodule flips over the femoral condyle.
- Lack of instability (the graft itself is intact).

Imaging Findings

- MRI
  - The lesion has a characteristic location and appearance.
  - T1-weighted: The lesion appears as a well-defined, nodular mass of low to intermediate signal intensity located anterior to the ACL graft and posterior to the infrapatellar fat pad (Hoffa's fat pad).
  - T2-weighted/STIR (fat-saturated): The signal is heterogeneous but predominantly low to intermediate, reflecting its fibrous nature. There may be a central focus of a higher signal.
  - T1-weighted post-contrast: The lesion typically shows moderate to marked enhancement due to its vascularized granulation tissue component.

Differential Diagnosis

- Graft impingement: due to a malpositioned tibial tunnel (too anterior), causing the graft itself to abut the intercondylar roof during extension. The graft will appear thickened and bowed.
- Graft failure: presents with instability, not a mechanical block. MRI shows graft discontinuity.
- Hoffa's fat pad impingement/syndrome: causes anterior pain and possible loss of extension, but the pathology is within the fat pad itself, not a discrete nodule anterior to the graft.
- Post-operative infection: causes diffuse synovitis, effusion, and pain, not a discrete nodule.

Management

- The standard and highly effective treatment is arthroscopic excision.
- This procedure is extremely successful. Patients typically experience immediate restoration of full extension intraoperatively and have an excellent prognosis.

Suggested Reading

Kulczycka P, Larbi A, Malghem J, Thienpont E, Vande Berg B, Lecouvet F. Imaging ACL reconstructions and their complications. Diagn Interv Imaging. 2015;96(1):11–9.

Noailles T, Chalopin A, Boissard M, Lopes R, Bouguennec N, Hardy A. Incidence and risk factors for cyclops syndrome after anterior cruciate ligament reconstruction: a systematic literature review. Orthop Traumatol Surg Res. 2019;105(7):1401–5.

Case 76

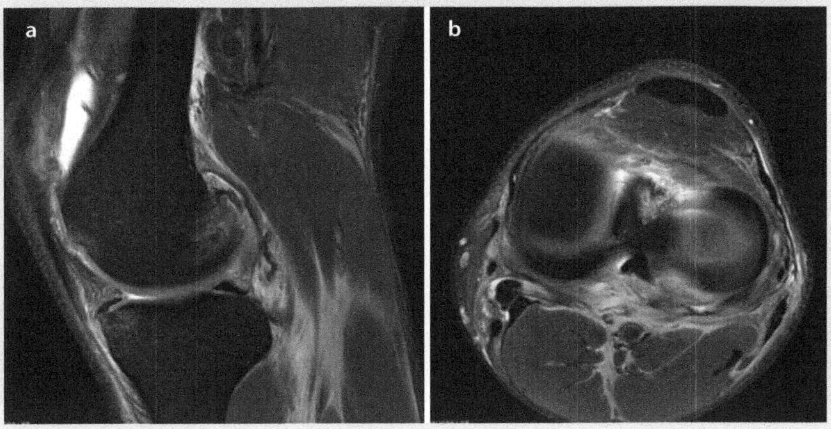

■ A 22-year-old football player presented with a severe twisting knee injury

S. Saran et al., *101 Knee Imaging Case Series*, 101 MSK Imaging 1,
https://doi.org/10.1007/978-3-032-21567-3_76

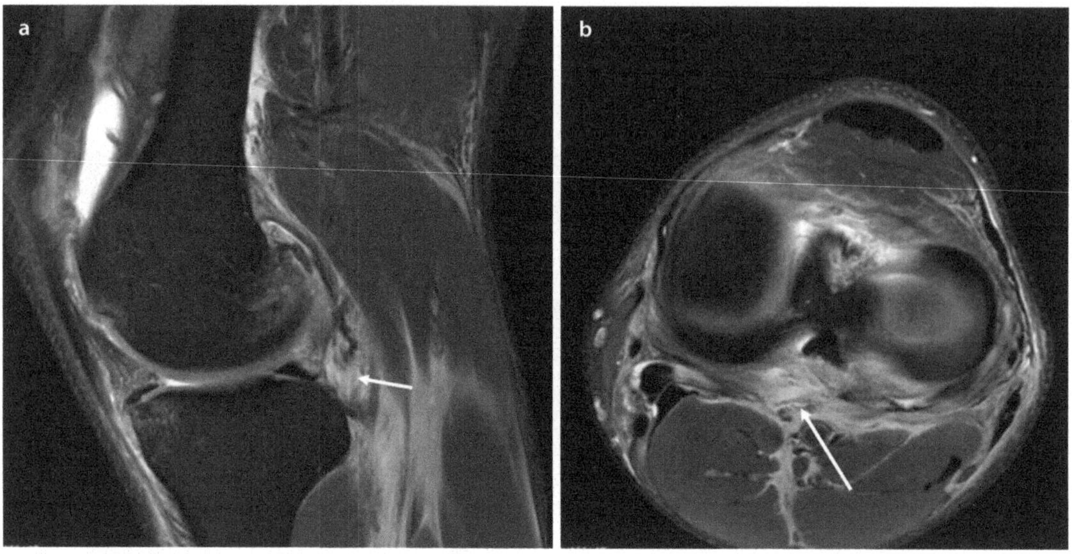

■ MRI knee **a**, **b** shows the presence of a breach in the posterior capsular ligament (arrows) with leakage of joint fluid in the popliteal soft tissue. Along with other ligament injuries, the patient also had the presence of posterior capsular ligament tear

Posterior Capsular Ligament Tear

Definition and Pathophysiology

- The posterior knee capsule is a taut, fibrous structure critical for stabilizing the knee against excessive translation and rotation. It is reinforced by two key ligaments—the posterior oblique ligament (POL) and the oblique popliteal ligament (OPL)—which are thickenings of the capsule itself and are prone to injury.
- Unlike the lax anterior capsule, the posterior capsule is taut to provide primary restraint against hyperextension and excessive tibio-femoral translation and rotation.
- Posterior oblique ligament (POL): Situated between the medial collateral ligament (MCL) and the semimembranosus tendon. Integrates with the semimembranosus tendon, the posteromedial capsule, and the OPL, forming a key part of the posteromedial corner.
- Oblique popliteal ligament (OPL): The largest posterior capsular ligament; it runs obliquely across the back of the knee. Serves as the primary restraint to knee hyperextension and a secondary restraint to axial rotation.
- Mechanism of injury: Usually caused by trauma involving hyperextension or intense rotational forces that strain the posterior structures.

- Clinical implication: Damage to these ligaments reduces knee stability against hyperextension and rotational forces, frequently happening alongside other ligament injuries such as PCL, ACL, or posterolateral corner injuries.

MRI Findings

- Injury is best appreciated on axial MRI images at the level of the knee joint.
- Since direct visualisation of a tear is uncommon, injury is inferred from the leakage of fluid and oedema and swelling within and around these specific capsular regions. This is distinguished from non-traumatic oedema by its location and association with a trauma history.
- Accurate diagnosis via MRI is crucial to understand the full extent of ligamentous damage, as these injuries rarely occur in isolation.

Management

- Management is directed at restoring stability to the posteromedial and posterolateral corners of the knee.
- Surgical Intervention: Severe sprains or tears, especially those that are part of a multi-ligament knee injury (like a knee dislocation), often require surgical repair or reconstruction to re-tension the posterior capsule and restore native knee kinematics.

Suggested Reading

Griffith JF. Five overlooked injuries on knee MRI. AJR Am J Roentgenol. 2021;217(5):1165–74.

Harris G, Kermanshah A, Patel N, Marmor WA, Rizzo MG Jr, Jose J. Characterization of posterior capsular injury for preoperative planning in closed knee injuries: a narrative review. J Orthop. 2025;15(68):323–30.

Case 77

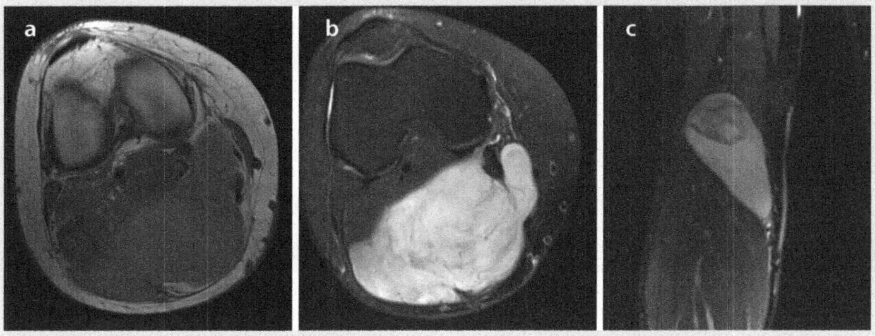

A 55-year-old male presented with a firm lump in the popliteal region

S. Saran et al., *101 Knee Imaging Case Series*, 101 MSK Imaging 1,
https://doi.org/10.1007/978-3-032-21567-3_77

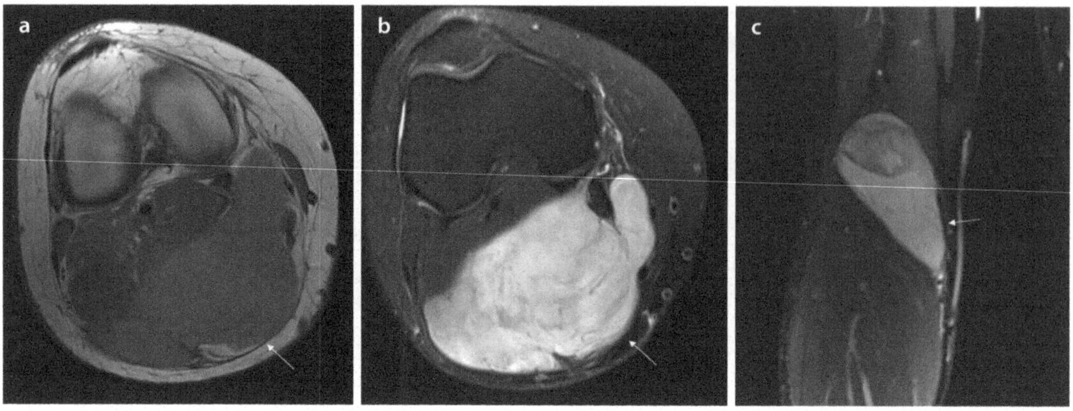

▪ MRI knee axial T1 **a**, T2FS **b** and coronal T2FS **c** shows the presence of a well-defined lesion (arrows) in the popliteal region in the intermuscular fascial plane, showing intermediate to high signal intensity on T1-weighted sequence **a** and very high signals ("light bulb") on T2FS sequences **b**, **c**. Though the lesion is insinuating between the medial head of gastrocnemius and semimembranosus tendons, it is not arising from the intervening bursa. The histopathological diagnosis was Myxoid liposarcoma. Differential diagnosis in this location will be Baker's cyst, myxoma and other soft tissue sarcomas

Myxoid Liposarcoma

Definition & Pathophysiology

- A myxoid liposarcoma (MLS) is a malignant soft tissue sarcoma that arises from primitive mesenchymal cells (not mature fat cells). It is the second most common subtype of liposarcoma and has a strong predilection for the deep soft tissues of the extremities, with the popliteal fossa being a common location.
- Pathology: Characterized by a unique genetic translocation, t(12;16) (q13;p11), which fuses the DDIT3 and FUS genes. This drives tumorigenesis.

Clinical Presentation

- Demographics: Most common in adults aged 30–50 years.
- Symptoms:
  - A slow-growing, painless mass.
  - The mass is typically deep-seated, firm, and fixed.
  - Myxoid liposarcoma has a high propensity for non-pulmonary metastases, spreading to other soft tissue sites (e.g., the retroperitoneum, opposite extremity) and bone.

Imaging Findings

- Imaging appearance varies significantly based on the tumour's cellularity and myxoid content.
- It is a "liposarcoma", but can be predominantly non-fatty on imaging. Its appearance is a spectrum, ranging from a cystic, water-like mass to a more solid, enhancing tumour with variable fat content.
- Ultrasound
  - Shows a hypoechoic, well-defined mass.
  - May show increased through-transmission, mimicking a cyst, but Doppler will reveal internal vascularity within the septations, confirming its solid nature.

MRI

- T1-weighted: The mass is typically iso to hyperintense to muscle. Small foci of fat may be seen as hyperintense strands or septa, a crucial diagnostic clue. If no fat is visible, it can mimic a cyst or other sarcoma.
- T2-weighted/STIR: The mass is markedly and homogeneously hyperintense, often described as "cyst-like" or "light-bulb bright" due to its high water content from the myxoid matrix. The internal fat foci will suppress on fat-sat sequences.
- T1-weighted post-contrast: Shows a characteristic "pseudocapsule" and "lace-like", "reticular", or "ring-and-arc" pattern of enhancement. The enhancement is often peripheral and septal rather than solid and homogeneous. This helps distinguish it from a simple cyst.

Differential Diagnosis

The "cyst-like" appearance on MRI creates a broad differential in the popliteal fossa:

- Baker's cyst: It follows a simple fluid signal on all MRI sequences (dark on T1, very bright on T2) and shows no internal enhancement. Characteristically located between the medial head of gastrocnemius and semi-membranosus tendons.
- Intramuscular myxoma: A benign lesion that is also T1 dark and T2 bright but typically occurs in older patients, shows minimal to no enhancement, and is almost always devoid of any internal fat.
- Haemangioma: A benign vascular tumour that may contain fat but often has characteristic phleboliths and a more heterogeneous, "bag of worms" appearance.

- Synovial sarcoma: Can be cystic but is often more solid and heterogeneous, frequently located close to a joint.
- Peripheral nerve sheath tumour (e.g., schwannoma): Typically associated with a nerve, shows the target sign on T2, and strong enhancement.

Management

- Management requires a multidisciplinary team at a specialist sarcoma centre.
- Pre-operative planning
  - Core needle biopsy: essential for diagnosis. Must be planned along the line of potential future excision.
  - Staging: whole body MRI, CT chest/abdomen/pelvis to evaluate for unusual metastatic sites.
- Surgical intervention (primary curative treatment).
  - Procedure: wide local excision.
  - The tumour must be removed en bloc with a margin of normal tissue (typically 1–2 cm) around it to minimise the risk of local recurrence.
- Radiation therapy
  - Neoadjuvant (pre-operative) or adjuvant (post-operative): often used for larger tumours (>5 cm) or high-grade lesions to reduce the risk of local recurrence.
  - Definitive radiotherapy: an option for surgically inoperable tumours.
- Systemic therapy
  - Chemotherapy: used for metastatic or unresectable disease. Myxoid liposarcoma is notably highly sensitive to radiotherapy and certain chemotherapy agents (e.g., trabectedin), which target the specific molecular translocation.

Suggested Reading

Encinas Tobajas VM, Almeida González C, Marcilla D, Vallejo M, Cano Rodríguez A, Reina Sánchez de Movellán JI, Morales Pérez JM. Myxoid liposarcoma: MRI features with histological correlation. Radiologia (Engl Ed). 2023;65(Suppl 2):S23–32.

Morán LM, Vega J, Gómez-León N, Royuela A. Myxomas and myxoid liposarcomas of the extremities: our preliminary findings in conventional, perfusion, and diffusion magnetic resonance. Acta Radiol Open. 2022;11(10):20584601221131481.

Shah A, James SL, Davies AM, Botchu R. A diagnostic approach to popliteal fossa masses. Clin Radiol. 2017;72(4):323–37.

Stevenson JD, Watson JJ, Cool P, Cribb GL, Jenkins JP, Leahy M, Gregory JJ. Whole-body magnetic resonance imaging in myxoid liposarcoma: a useful adjunct for the detection of extra-pulmonary metastatic disease. Eur J Surg Oncol. 2016;42(4):574–80.

Case 78

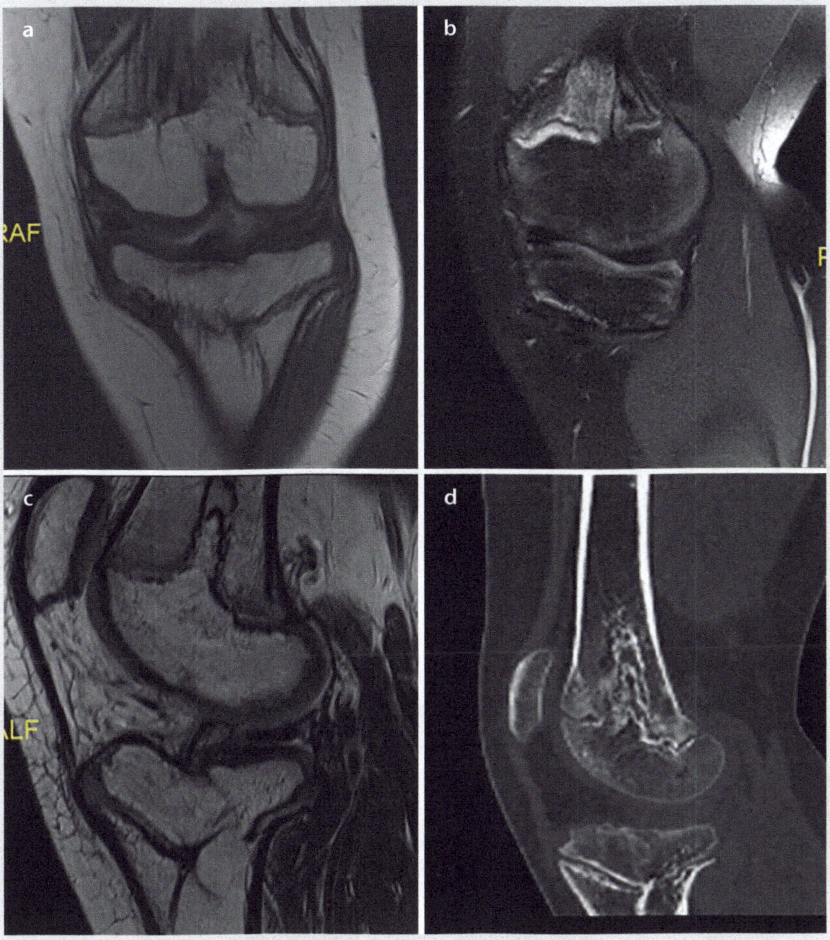

■ A 17-year-old male presented with limb length discrepancy. He had a history of trauma in the affected limb 2 years back

S. Saran et al., *101 Knee Imaging Case Series*, 101 MSK Imaging 1,
https://doi.org/10.1007/978-3-032-21567-3_78

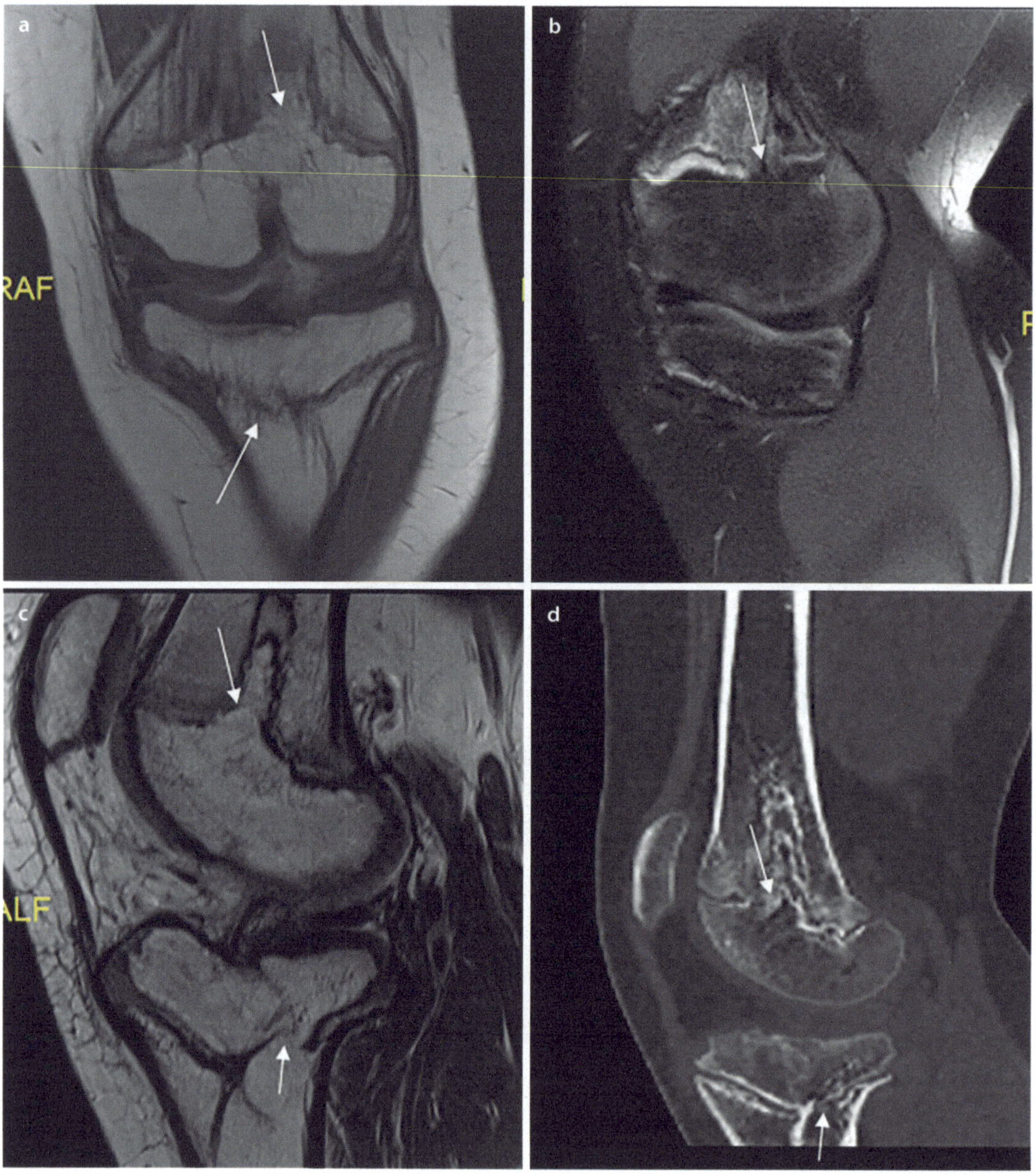

■ MRI knee, coronal T1 **a**, sagittal STIR **b**, and sagittal T1 **c** shows the presence of multiple regions of premature physeal fusion involving the distal femur and proximal tibia (arrows). Similar findings (arrows) can be seen on sagittal CT **d**. Imaging findings are suggestive of multiple physeal bars

Physeal Bars

Definition and Pathophysiology

- A physeal bar (or bridge) is a bony tether that forms across the growth plate (physis), connecting the epiphysis to the metaphysis. This abnormal bridge of bone disrupts the normal mechanism of longitudinal bone growth and is a common cause of growth disturbance in children.
- The most common cause is trauma, typically a Salter-Harris type III, IV, or V fracture that damages the germinal layer of cartilage-producing cells. Other causes include infection, ischemic injury, tumours, or metabolic disorders.
- The normal process of cartilage proliferation, maturation, and replacement by bone at the metaphysis is disrupted, which leads to bony bridge formation.
- The bony bar acts as a mechanical tether, preventing growth in that specific area of the physis. The uninjured portions of the physis continue to grow normally, leading to progressive angular deformity and/or limb shortening.

Clinical Features

- Limb length discrepancy: if the bar is central, it causes a symmetric growth arrest, leading to a shorter limb.
- Angular deformity: if the bar is peripheral, it causes asymmetric growth arrest, leading to a progressive angular deformity (e.g., genu varum or valgum in the knee).
- Loss of motion: possible if the deformity causes joint incongruity.
- The deformity progresses over time until the child reaches skeletal maturity.

Imaging Findings

- Radiography
  - Presence of a bony bridge across the physis with deformity.
- MRI
  - Loss of physeal cartilage: a focal interruption of the normal high T2 signal of the physis.
  - Bony bridge: a low signal intensity bony tract traversing the physis, connecting the epiphyseal and metaphyseal bone marrow.

Management

- The goal of treatment is to restore normal longitudinal growth and correct deformity.
- Prevention: Anatomic reduction of Salter-Harris fractures to minimise physeal damage is the primary preventive measure.
- Surgical resection (bar excision): the bony bar is surgically removed. The resulting defect is filled with an interposition material (e.g., fat, cranioplasty cement) to prevent the bar from re-forming. The goal is to untether the physis and allow for the resumption of normal growth.
- Osteotomy is performed to correct an established angular deformity. The bone is cut and realigned to correct the deformity.

Suggested Reading

Gauger EM, Casnovsky LL, Gauger EJ, Bohn DC, Van Heest AE. Acquired upper extremity growth arrest. Orthopedics. 2017;40(1):e95–e103.

Kim HHR, Menashe SJ, Ngo AV, Otjen JP, Maloney E, Iyer RS, Thapa M. Uniquely pediatric upper extremity injuries. Clin Imaging. 2021;80:249–61.

Samora JB. Distal radius Physeal Bar and ulnar overgrowth: indications for treatment. J Pediatr Orthop. 2021;41(Suppl 1):S6–S13.

Case 79

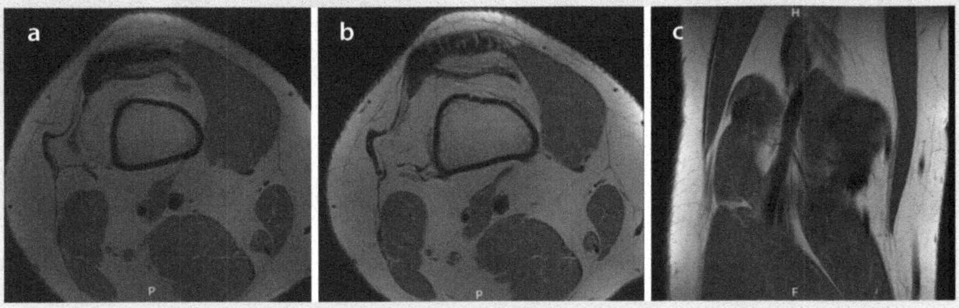

◘ A 22-year-old marathon runner presented with intermittent claudication in one leg following a period of activity

S. Saran et al., *101 Knee Imaging Case Series*, 101 MSK Imaging 1,
https://doi.org/10.1007/978-3-032-21567-3_79

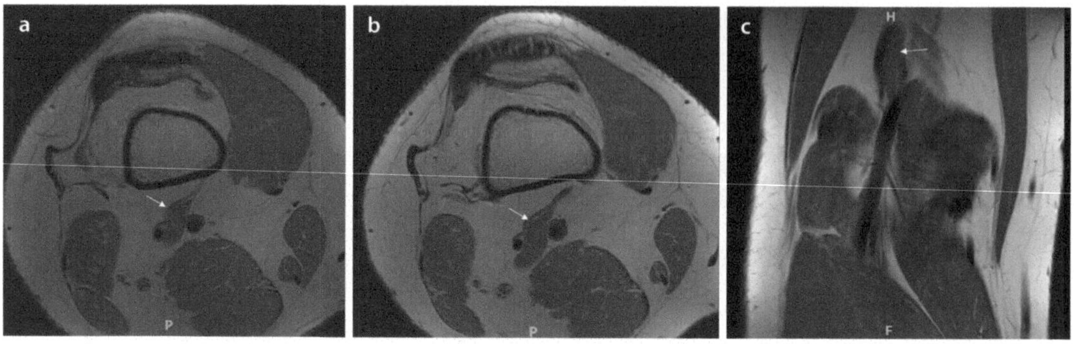

MRI knee PD axial **a**, **b** and PD coronal **c** shows the presence of an accessory slip of the gastrocnemius muscle (arrows), causing entrapment of the popliteal artery

Accessory Slip of the Gastrocnemius Muscle Causing Popliteal Artery Entrapment Syndrome (PAES)

Definition & Pathophysiology

- This condition is a specific anatomical variant classified as Popliteal Artery Entrapment Syndrome (PAES) Type III. It occurs when an aberrant or accessory muscle slip of the medial head of the gastrocnemius muscle compresses the popliteal artery during plantarflexion of the foot.
- Anatomy: Normally, the popliteal artery courses between the medial and lateral heads of the gastrocnemius, deep to the plantaris and soleus muscles. An accessory slip creates an abnormal fibrous band or muscle bundle that crosses the artery, acting as a "noose," causing intermittent ischemia.
- Chronic compression can lead to localised atherosclerosis, thrombosis, or the formation of a popliteal artery aneurysm.

Clinical Presentation

- Demographics: Typically affects young, healthy, athletic individuals (often <30 years old) with no cardiovascular risk factors.
- Symptoms:
  - Calf claudication: reproducible cramping, pain, or fatigue in the calf during exercise, relieved by rest. This is the hallmark symptom.
  - Paresthesia or numbness in the foot due to nerve ischemia.

  - Coolness or pallor of the foot after activity.
  - Absent or diminished pedal pulses after active plantarflexion against resistance.

Imaging Findings

- A multi-modality approach is essential for diagnosis, moving from rest to dynamic assessment.
- Duplex ultrasound
  - At rest: the popliteal artery may appear normal with triphasic flow.
  - During manoeuvre (active plantarflexion against resistance): colour Doppler shows turbulence, narrowing, or complete cessation of flow in the popliteal artery.
  - Spectral Doppler: demonstrates increased velocity at the site of compression or complete loss of flow signal.
  - Release of manoeuvre: shows a "burst" of high-velocity flow (reactive hyperaemia), confirming the dynamic nature of the entrapment.
- CT angiography (CTA) or MR angiography (MRA)
  - These are the gold standards for confirming the anatomical variant and planning surgery.
  - Shows the course of the popliteal artery and suggests the presence of an aberrant muscle slip.

Classification

- Anatomical types
  - Type I: The popliteal artery has an abnormal course, running medial to the normally positioned medial head of the gastrocnemius muscle.
  - Type II: The medial head of the gastrocnemius muscle is abnormally attached more laterally, causing it to compress the normally positioned popliteal artery.
  - Type III: The popliteal artery is compressed by an abnormal fibrous band or a slip of muscle from the medial or lateral condyle of the femur.
  - Type IV: The popliteal artery is compressed by the popliteus muscle or fibrous bands.
  - Type V: This involves the entrapment of both the popliteal artery and vein by any of the causes listed above.
- Functional Types
  - Type VI: This type is defined by functional compression of the popliteal artery and vein caused by hypertrophy (enlargement) of the gastrocnemius muscle. Unlike anatomical types, there is no structural anomaly; instead, the muscle itself is enlarged, causing compression.

Differential Diagnosis

- Atherosclerotic peripheral artery disease: uncommon in young athletes; presents with fixed stenoses, calcifications, and typically worse symptoms.
- Chronic exertional compartment syndrome: causes similar claudication but is due to increased pressure within a muscle compartment; pulses remain intact.

Management

- Surgical intervention is the definitive treatment to relieve the compression and prevent permanent arterial damage.

Suggested Reading

Abou-Ghaida J, Thapaliya D, Rua I. Differential diagnosis of popliteal artery entrapment syndrome in light of an atypical clinical manifestation. Cureus. 2023;15(2):e34889.

Al-Tayef TA, Rziki A, Rasras H, El Mahi O, Benzirar A. Popliteal artery entrapment syndrome: a case report with literature review. Pan Afr Med J. 2021;39:80.

Case 80

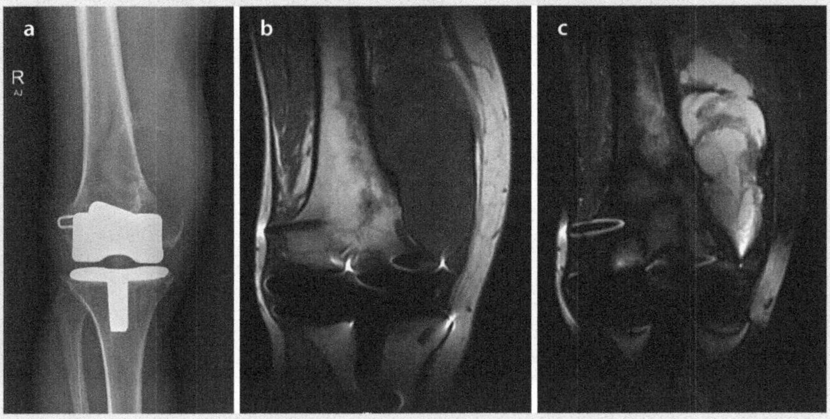

■ A 65-year-old female presented with swelling along the medial aspect of the knee joint, 2 years following total knee replacement (TKR)

S. Saran et al., *101 Knee Imaging Case Series*, 101 MSK Imaging 1,
https://doi.org/10.1007/978-3-032-21567-3_80

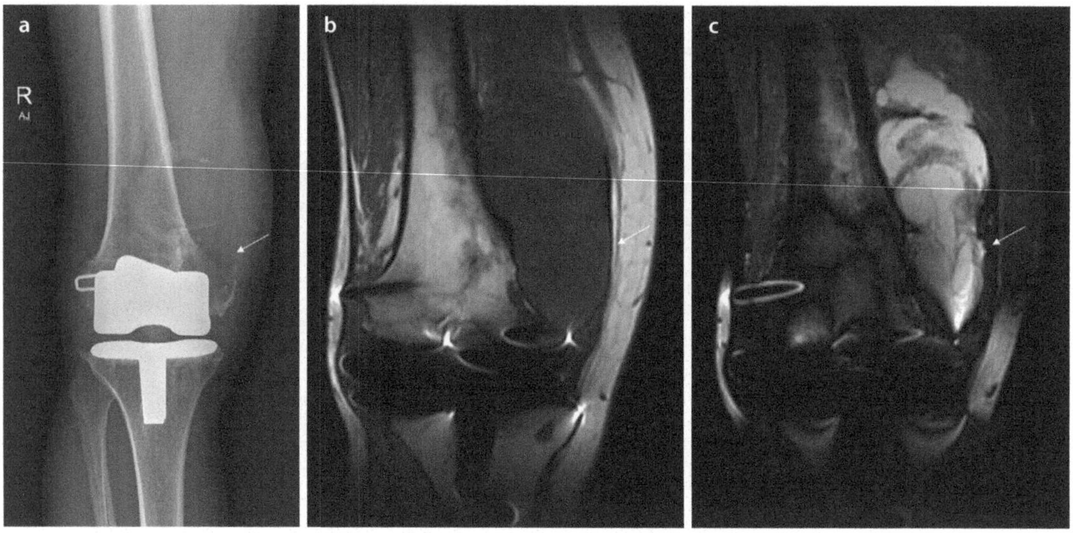

■ Anteroposterior radiograph **a** shows the presence of an aggressive lytic region (arrow) in the medial femoral condyle with cortical breach and periosteal reaction. MRI coronal T1 **b** and T2FS **c** shows the presence of a large soft tissue mass lesion (arrows) in the region showing low signals on T1 **b** and high signals on T2-weighted fat-suppressed **c** sequences. Findings are in favour of Particle disease

Particle Disease (Periprosthetic Osteolysis)

Definition & Pathophysiology

- Particle disease, formally known as aseptic lymphocytic-dominated vasculitis-associated lesion (ALVAL) or simply periprosthetic osteolysis, is a biologic response to wear debris from a total knee replacement. It is a non-infectious, inflammatory process that leads to progressive bone destruction around the implant, potentially resulting in component loosening, pain, and implant failure.
- Key feature: A cell-mediated, granulomatous foreign-body reaction that creates expansile, cystic lesions at the bone-implant interface.

Clinical Presentation

- Timeline: typically, a late complication, presenting 5–15 years after the surgery.
- Symptoms:
  - Progressive pain: often deep, aching, and worse with weight-bearing. The pain may be new after years of good function.
  - Swelling: effusion may be present.

- Instability or "giving way": as bone loss progresses, the implant can become loose.
- The patient is typically afebrile and has no systemic signs of infection, though the presentation can mimic low-grade infection.

Imaging Findings

- Radiography (initial and surveillance tool)
  - Serial radiographs are key to identifying progression.
  - Osteolysis occurs at the bone-prosthesis or bone-cement interface.
  - "ballooning" or expansile lytic lesions: well-defined, scalloped, cystic areas of bone loss.
  - Scalloped endosteal erosions.
  - Progressive radiolucent lines (>2 mm) at the implant interface.
  - Component migration or subsidence indicates loosening.
- CT (superior for defining bone stock loss)
  - Provides excellent 3D detail of the location, size, and extent of osteolytic lesions.
- MRI
  - Can visualize the soft tissue mass or "pseudomembrane" of the granulomatous reaction, which appears as an intermediate signal on T1 and T2.
  - Helps differentiate the fluid-filled cysts from solid tissue and can assess for alternative causes of pain.

Differential Diagnosis

- Periprosthetic joint infection: often presents with more acute pain, erythema, warmth, and systemic signs. Elevated serum ESR/CRP and a positive joint aspiration are diagnostic.
- Stress shielding: bone loss due to altered load transfer, typically in the anterior femur behind the flange of the femoral component. It is not expansile or cystic and is usually asymptomatic.

Management

- Surveillance
  - For small, asymptomatic lesions discovered incidentally, serial radiographs may be used to monitor for progression.

- Surgical intervention
  - Surgery is indicated for symptomatic lesions, progressive bone loss, or impending fracture/implant failure.
  - Procedure: revision arthroplasty.

Suggested Reading

Nawabi DH, Gold S, Lyman S, Fields K, Padgett DE, Potter HG. MRI predicts ALVAL and tissue damage in metal-on-metal hip arthroplasty. Clin Orthop Relat Res. 2014;472(2):471–81.

Sukur E, Akman YE, Ozturkmen Y, Kucukdurmaz F. Particle disease: a current review of the biological mechanisms in periprosthetic osteolysis after hip arthroplasty. Open Orthop J. 2016;15(10):241–51.

Case 81

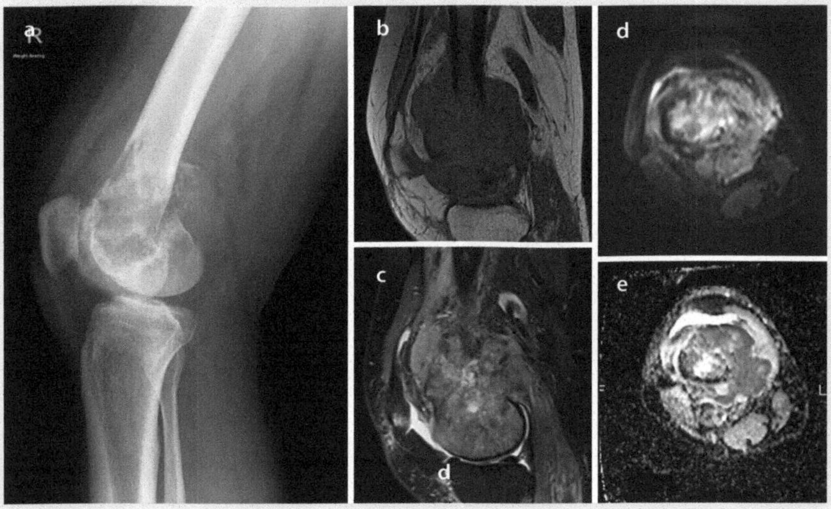

■ A 33-year-old female presented with a progressively increasing swelling around knee joint with limitation of joint movement

S. Saran et al., *101 Knee Imaging Case Series*, 101 MSK Imaging 1,
https://doi.org/10.1007/978-3-032-21567-3_81

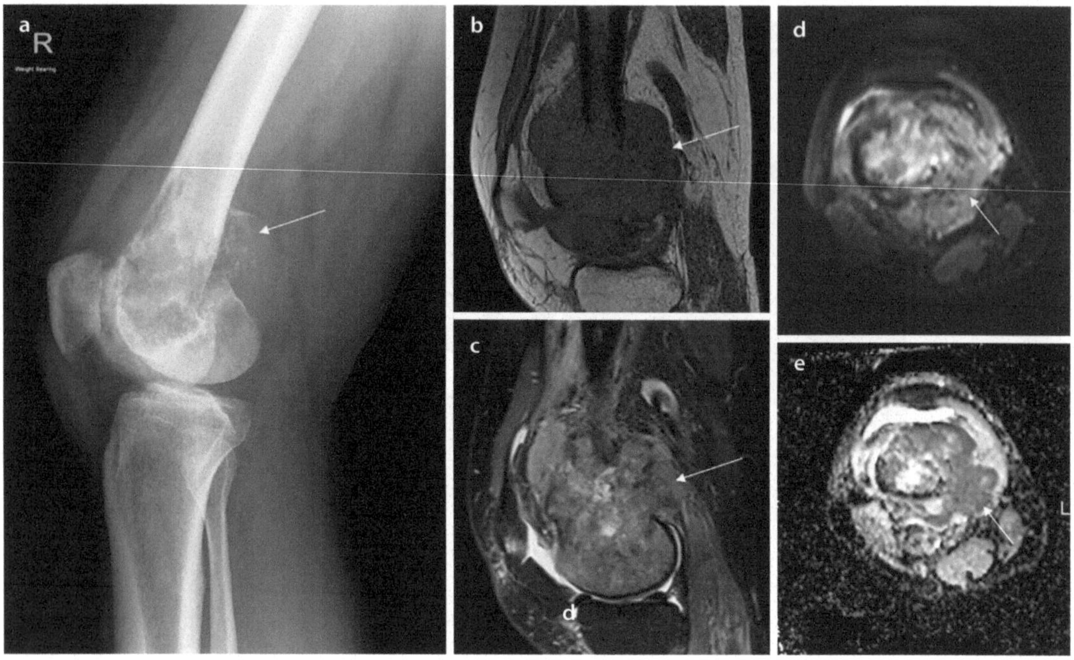

◘ Lateral radiograph **a** shows the presence of an ill-defined osteolytic lesion (arrow) in the distal femur with subarticular extension and cortical breach, and having extraosseous mass with calcification within. MRI sagittal T1 **b**, sagittal PDFS **b**, axial diffusion weighted imaging **d** and ADC **e** shows the lesion (arrows) as a heterogeneous destructive mass having hypointense signals on T1 **b**, hyperintense signals on PDFS **c**, and showing restriction of diffusion **d**, **e**, suggestive of malignant neoplasm. Differentials in this location and age will include malignant giant cell tumour and osteosarcoma. Histopathological diagnosis was malignant giant cell tumour

Malignant Giant Cell Tumour

Definition & Pathophysiology

- A malignant giant cell tumour (GCT) of bone is a rare, aggressive sarcomatous lesion. It can present in two primary forms:
  - Primary malignant GCT (de novo): A rare variant (<5% of GCTs) where high-grade sarcoma coexists with areas of conventional benign GCT from the outset.
  - Secondary malignant GCT: The more common form, arising at the site of a previously diagnosed and treated conventional benign GCT, typically following radiation therapy. The risk of malignant transformation post-radiation is estimated at 5–15%.
- Pathology: Histologically, it shows a dual population:
  - Areas resembling conventional benign GCT (osteoclast-like giant cells and mononuclear stromal cells).
  - Areas of high-grade sarcoma (typically osteosarcoma, fibrosarcoma, or undifferentiated pleomorphic sarcoma).

Clinical Presentation

- Demographics: Similar to conventional GCT, most common in adults aged 20–50 years.
- A history of a previously treated GCT (often with radiation) with a new onset of symptoms after a symptom-free interval.
- Symptoms:
  - Rapidly worsening pain, often more severe and progressive than with a benign GCT.
  - Rapidly enlarging mass or swelling.
  - Pathologic fracture due to aggressive bone destruction.

Imaging Findings

Imaging shows features of an aggressive, malignant bone tumour, often superimposed on changes from a previous benign GCT.

- Radiography
  - Location: Eccentric, metaphyseal, extending to the subchondral bone of the distal femur—the classic location for GCT.
  - Aggressive Features:
    - Permeative or moth-eaten bone destruction with a wide zone of transition (replacing the well-defined margin of a benign GCT).
    - Cortical destruction with a large soft tissue mass.
    - Aggressive periosteal reaction (e.g., sunburst pattern, Codman's triangle).
    - In secondary malignancy, these aggressive changes are seen at the site of a previously lytic, "soap-bubble" lesion.
- MRI
  - T1-weighted: The tumour is heterogeneously low to intermediate signal intensity, replacing the normal marrow fat. The soft tissue component is isointense to muscle.
  - T2-weighted/STIR: The tumour is heterogeneously hyperintense. Areas of necrosis, haemorrhage, and residual benign GCT contribute to the mixed signal.
  - T1-weighted post-contrast: Shows intense, heterogeneous enhancement of the viable tumour tissue and the soft tissue mass.

Differential Diagnosis

- Osteosarcoma: Typically, in a younger demographic (10–25 years). Shows cloud-like osteoid matrix mineralisation, which may also be present in malignant GCT with osteosarcomatous differentiation.
- Metastatic carcinoma: In older patients, a lytic metastasis can mimic this. A known primary cancer is the key.
- Lymphoma of bone: Can be purely lytic and permeative, often with a large soft tissue mass disproportionate to the bone destruction.
- Aneurysmal bone cyst (ABC): Can occur secondary to a GCT but appears as fluid-fluid levels on MRI and lacks the solid, enhancing tissue of a sarcoma.

Management

Management is aggressive and mirrors the protocol for other high-grade sarcomas, requiring a multidisciplinary team at a specialist sarcoma centre.

- Pre-operative (neoadjuvant) chemotherapy
  - Regimens: Similar to osteosarcoma, using multi-agent chemotherapy (e.g., Doxorubicin, Cisplatin, Methotrexate).
- Surgical intervention (definitive treatment)
  - Procedure: wide surgical resection.
  - The tumour must be removed en bloc with a margin of normal tissue to minimise the risk of local recurrence.
  - For distal femur lesions, this typically means a limb-salvage resection followed by reconstruction with a metal endoprosthesis (megaprosthesis) or sometimes an allograft.
  - Amputation is reserved for cases where the tumour involves critical neurovascular structures, making a safe margin impossible.
- Adjuvant chemotherapy: continues after surgery based on the tumour's response to neoadjuvant chemo.

Suggested Reading

Palmerini E, Picci P, Reichardt P, Downey G. Malignancy in giant cell tumor of bone: a review of the literature. Technol Cancer Res Treat. 2019;1(18):1533033819840000.

van Langevelde K, Cleven AHG, Navas Cañete A, van der Heijden L, van de Sande MAJ, Gelderblom H, Bovée JVMG. Malignant transformation of Giant cell tumor of bone and the association with Denosumab treatment: a radiology and pathology perspective. Sarcoma. 2022;17(2022):3425221.

Case 82

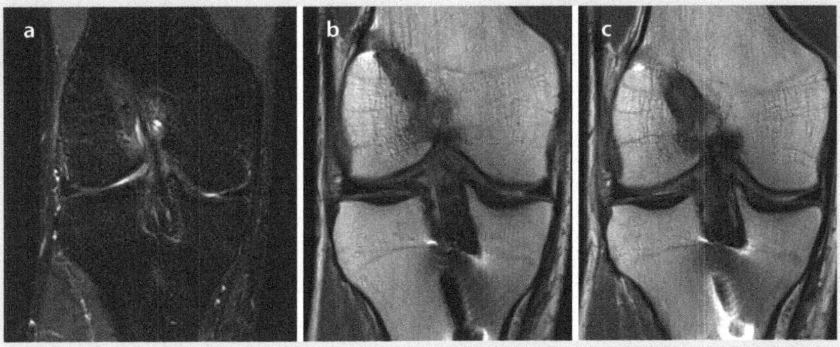

■ A 27-year-old male presented for an MRI post-ACL reconstruction. He complained of knee pain, instability, and a clicking sound on knee extension

S. Saran et al., *101 Knee Imaging Case Series*, 101 MSK Imaging 1,
https://doi.org/10.1007/978-3-032-21567-3_82

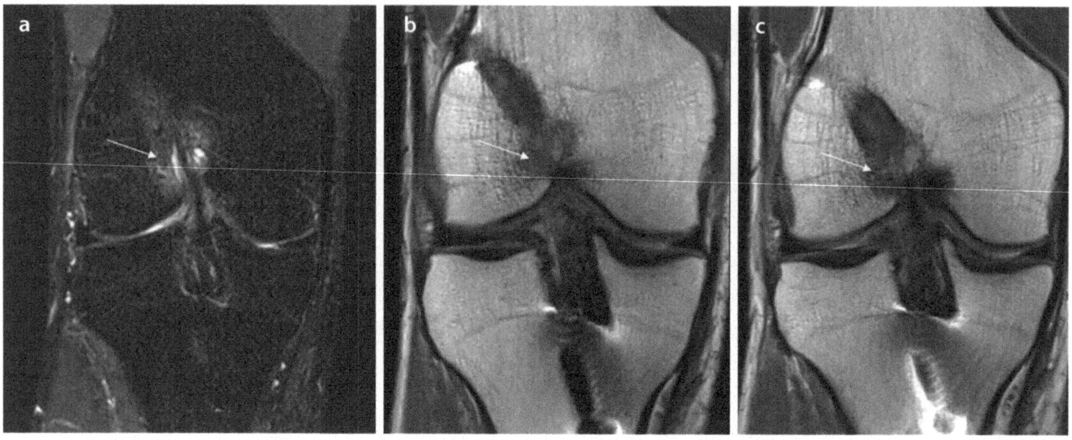

MRI knee, T2 FS weighted coronal **a** and T1 weighted coronal **b**, **c** sequences showing narrowing of the intercondylar notch with impingement of graft by the medial wall of the lateral femoral condyle (arrow), appearances are of ACL graft sidewall impingement

ACL Graft Sidewall Impingement

Definition & Pathophysiology

- ACL graft sidewall impingement occurs when the reconstructed graft path is improperly positioned, causing it to abut and rub against the lateral wall of the intercondylar notch. This is distinct from the more common roof impingement, which occurs in the sagittal plane.
- Mechanism: The primary cause is non-anatomic tunnel placement during surgery.
- Lateral Impingement: Can be caused by a femoral tunnel placed too anteriorly or a tibial tunnel placed too laterally, pushing the graft against the lateral condyle.
- Consequence: Chronic friction leads to:
  - Graft abrasion, fraying, and elongation.
  - Progressive graft failure and laxity.
  - Persistent pain, stiffness, and inflammation.
  - Cyclops lesion formation (from repetitive impingement and scar tissue).

Clinical Presentation

- Persistent anterior knee pain: deep, aching pain within the joint line, often worse with activity.
- Stiffness & loss of extension: a common finding, as the impinging graft acts as a mechanical block to full extension.
- Effusion: recurrent swelling after activity.

- Sense of instability: as the graft weakens and elongates from abrasion.
- Audible "clunk" or "catch": especially during terminal knee extension.

MRI Findings

- MRI is crucial for visualising the graft's position and signs of impingement.
  - Graft position:
  - "Vertical graft" sign: on coronal images, the graft appears nearly vertical instead of having a more oblique, anatomic orientation.
  - The graft is seen making direct contact with the lateral femoral condyle.
- Graft morphology:
  - Focal thinning or signal change: the portion of the graft contacting the wall may appear narrowed or show increased signal on T2/PD-weighted images (indicating degeneration/oedema).
- Secondary signs:
  - Bone marrow oedema: in the lateral femoral condyle at the site of impaction.
  - Synovitis: inflammation around the graft.
  - Cyclops lesion: a nodular mass of scar tissue anterior to the graft, a common sequela.

Management

- Prevention
  - Anatomic tunnel placement: The cornerstone of modern ACL reconstruction. Placing tunnels within the native ACL footprints avoids impingement.
  - Adequate notchplasty: ensuring the intercondylar notch is wide enough to accommodate the graft without friction.
- Surgical intervention
  - Arthroscopic debridement & revision notchplasty: involves arthroscopically removing scar tissue (e.g., cyclops lesion) and performing a targeted notchplasty to widen the space between the graft and the sidewall, eliminating the source of impingement.
  - Revision ACL reconstruction: indicated for failed grafts with significant laxity, extensive graft degeneration, or if the tunnel malposition is so severe that a simple notchplasty is insufficient.

Suggested Reading

Kim SG, Kobayashi K, Uchino S, Nozawa M. Radiographic assessment of the tibiofemoral relationship in anterior cruciate ligament deficient knees. J Orthop. 2021;9(23):256–8.

Udagawa K, Niki Y, Enomoto H, Toyama Y, Suda Y. Factors influencing graft impingement on the wall of the intercondylar notch after anatomic double-bundle anterior cruciate ligament reconstruction. Am J Sports Med. 2014;42(9):2219–25.

Wilson WT, Hopper GP, O'Boyle M, Henderson L, Blyth MJG. Quantifying graft impingement in anterior cruciate ligament reconstruction. Knee. 2022;34:270–8.

Case 83

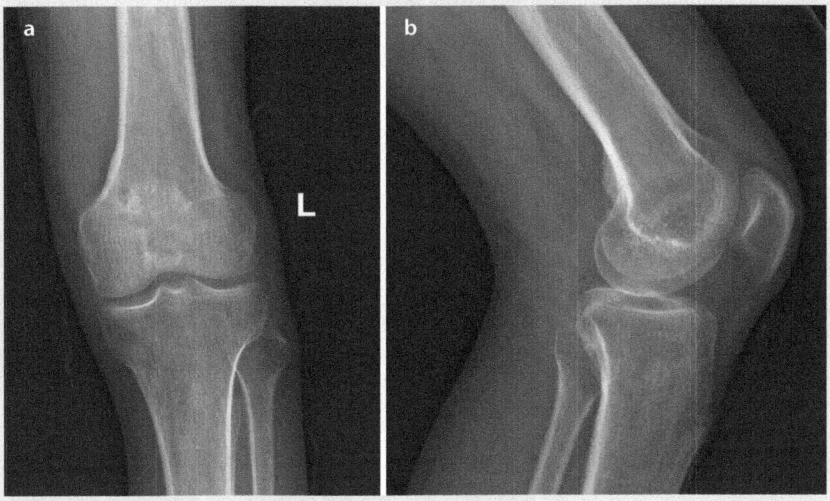

■ A 32-year-old female with knee pain

S. Saran et al., *101 Knee Imaging Case Series*, 101 MSK Imaging 1,
https://doi.org/10.1007/978-3-032-21567-3_83

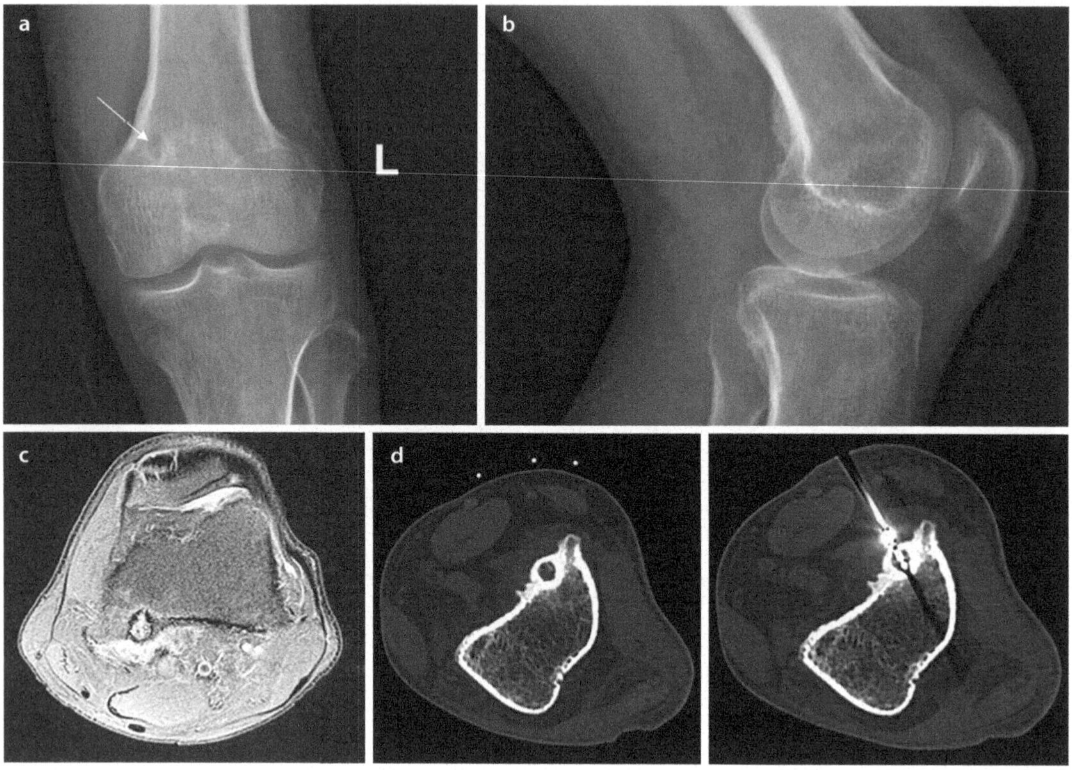

◘ Anteroposterior radiograph **a** and lateral radiograph **b** show a well-defined osteolytic lesion in the posterior cortex of the medial femoral condyle (arrow). A detailed history revealed typical nocturnal pain relieved by salicylates, suggesting osteoid osteoma. PDFS axial MRI **c** shows the lesion as a well-defined osteolytic cortical-based nidus with surrounding oedema. **d**. CT-guided Microwave ablation of the nidus was performed

Osteoid Osteoma

Osteoid osteoma is a benign, osteogenic bone tumour characterized by a small nidus (<2 cm) surrounded by reactive sclerosis. It commonly occurs in the femur and tibia.

Clinical Presentation

Classic symptom: Localised pain, typically worse at night and relieved by NSAIDs (especially aspirin).

Imaging Findings

1. Radiography (initial screening): may show focal sclerosis with a small radiolucent nidus (often subtle in early stages). Periosteal reaction is less common in intra-articular lesions.

2. CT: CT is considered the gold standard for diagnosis. It clearly visualises the radiolucent nidus with central calcification and surrounding sclerotic rim. The vascular groove sign is diagnostic.
3. MRI: Shows bone marrow oedema and synovitis, but may miss the nidus.
4. Bone scan: Intense focal uptake on triple-phase scintigraphy ("double-density" sign).

Differential Diagnosis

1. Stress fracture
2. Brodie's abscess (chronic osteomyelitis)

Management

1. Medical management: NSAIDs (first-line, providing dramatic pain relief in 50–75% of cases). May lead to spontaneous resolution over 3–5 years (but impractical for most patients).
2. Minimally invasive interventions (preferred): CT-guided radiofrequency ablation (RFA) or microwave ablation (MWA): 90–95% success rate, outpatient procedure. Avoids open surgery, preserves joint integrity. Cryoablation or laser ablation are equally useful alternatives.
3. Surgical excision (rarely needed): Indicated if RFA fails or the lesion is difficult to access.

Suggested Reading

Asayama Y, Nishie A, Ishigami K, Kakihara D, Ushijima Y, Takayama Y, et al. Ct-guided radiofrequency ablation of osteoid osteoma in the long bones of the lower extremity. World J Radiol. 2012;4:278.

Singh DK, Katyan A, Kumar N, Nigam K, Jaiswal B, Misra RN. CT-guided radiofrequency ablation of osteoid osteoma: established concepts and new ideas. Br J Radiol. 2020;93(1114):20200266.

Case 84

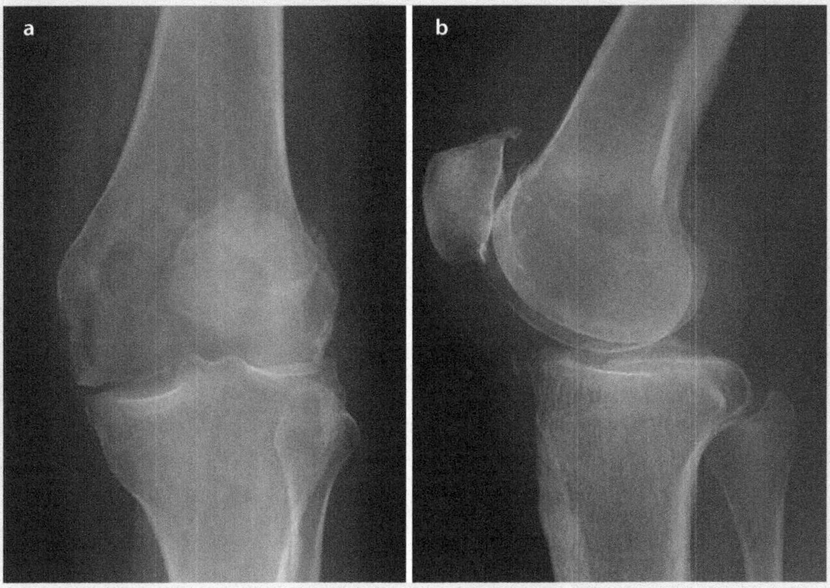

A 68-year-old male presents with a 3-week history of severe, progressive pain in his right knee. He reports significant unintentional weight loss of 7 kg over the past 4 months, along with generalised fatigue

S. Saran et al., *101 Knee Imaging Case Series*, 101 MSK Imaging 1,
https://doi.org/10.1007/978-3-032-21567-3_84

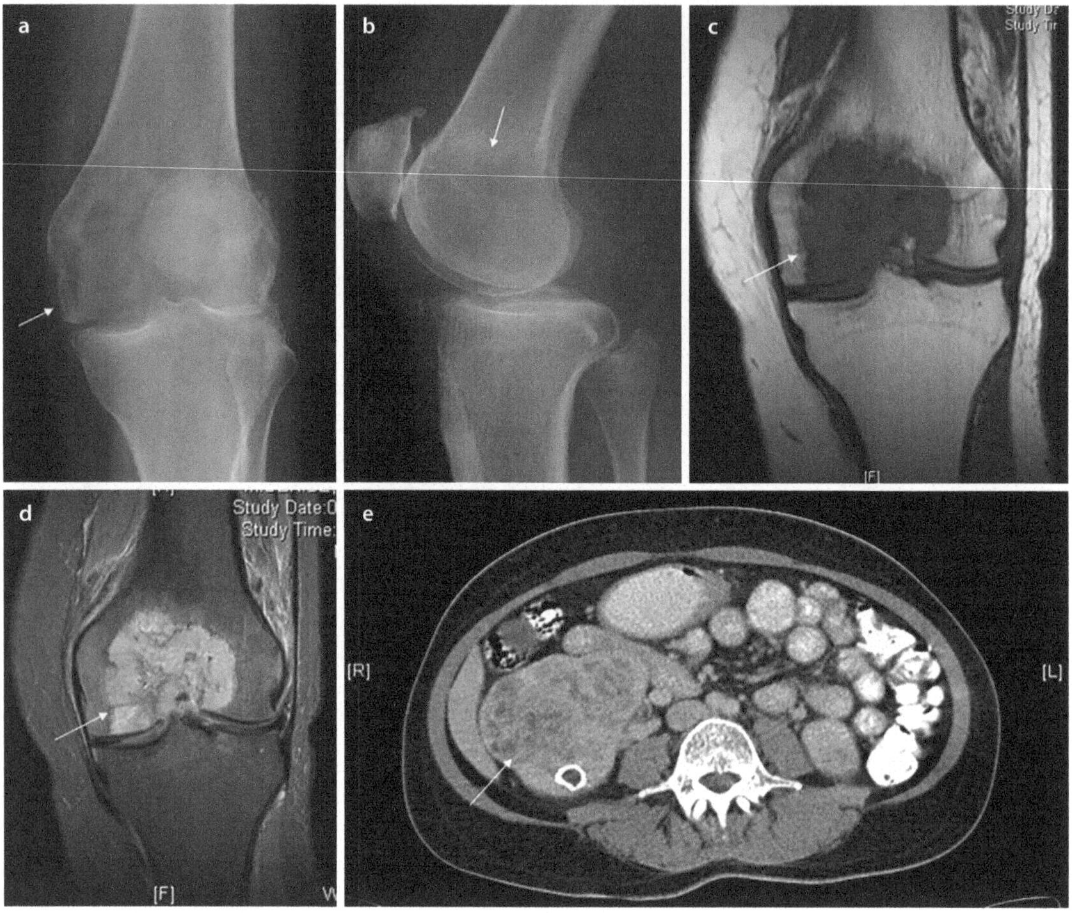

▪ Anteroposterior radiograph **a**, and lateral radiograph **b** show a permeative lytic lesion in the distal femoral metaphysis with subchondral extension (arrow) and no internal mineralisation. MRI shows a lytic lesion (arrows) appearing hypointense on the coronal T1-weighted sequence **c** and hyperintense on the coronal PDFS sequence **d** with no obvious soft tissue extension. Imaging differential in this case, considering the age of the patient, will be metastatic bone lesion, plasmacytoma, GCT, bone lymphoma and fibrosarcoma. On further probing, the patient revealed a history of hematuria. CECT abdomen axial **e** revealed a large heterogeneously enhancing lesion (arrow) in the right kidney, confirming the diagnosis of renal cell carcinoma with bone metastasis

Metastasis from Renal Cell Carcinoma (RCC)

Definition and Pathophysiology

- This is a lytic metastatic lesion in the distal femur, originating from a primary renal cell carcinoma (RCC). RCC is one of the most common primary cancers to metastasise to bone, and its metastases have several distinctive features.
- Mechanism: hematogenous spread and seeding of the highly vascular bone marrow.
- "Seed and soil" hypothesis: The bone marrow microenvironment provides a fertile "soil" for RCC cells (the "seeds") to grow.
- RCC-specific behaviour: RCC metastases are notoriously hypervascular, which influences their imaging appearance and poses a significant risk of severe bleeding during biopsy or surgery.

Clinical Presentation

- Often, a patient with a known history of RCC. However, the bone metastasis can be the first presenting sign of an otherwise silent kidney cancer in up to 30% of cases.
- Symptoms:
  - Deep, localised bone pain, often worse at night, may progress to constant, severe pain.
  - Pathologic fracture: A common and devastating complication due to progressive bone destruction. This can present as a sudden, severe pain after a minor trauma or even spontaneously.
  - Constitutional symptoms, such as weight loss, fatigue, and anaemia, may be present in advanced disease.

Imaging Findings

- Radiography
  - A "blown-out", "bubbly", or "moth-eaten" lytic lesion.
  - Margin: poorly defined, aggressive, with a wide zone of transition.
  - Cortex: marked cortical thinning, expansion, and often cortical breakthrough.
  - Lack of sclerosis: there is typically no reactive bone formation, making the lesion appear purely destructive.

- CT
  - Confirms the extensive bone destruction and soft tissue component.
  - Excellent for assessing the integrity of the cortex and risk of impending fracture.
  - Can detect the primary renal tumour if unknown.
- MRI: MRI is crucial for defining the true intramedullary and soft tissue extent.
  - T1-weighted: the metastasis appears as a heterogeneously low-signal intensity mass, replacing the normal bright fatty marrow.
  - T2-weighted/PDFS: typically, heterogeneously hyperintense. The high signal is due to the tumour's high fluid content and vascularity.
  - Post-contrast (T1 + C): Shows intense, vivid, and heterogeneous enhancement, a classic feature reflecting the lesion's hypervascular nature.
  - Soft tissue mass: Often, a large, enhancing soft tissue component is present.
- Angiography: May show a highly vascular "tumour blush" and is sometimes used pre-operatively for embolisation.

Differential Diagnosis

For a solitary, aggressive lytic lesion in the distal femur of an adult, consider

- Plasmacytoma/multiple myeloma
- Lytic osteosarcoma: Typically in a younger population (adolescents/young adults).
- Giant cell tumour (GCT): typically appears hypointense on T2 with internal cystic changes.
- Thyroid cancer metastasis.
- Lymphoma: It can be purely lytic and often exhibits a permeative pattern and a large, soft tissue mass.
- Brown tumour of hyperparathyroidism: Patients will have abnormal serum calcium and PTH levels.

Management

Management is multidisciplinary, involving oncology, orthopaedic surgery, and interventional radiology. The goals are to control the disease, relieve pain, and maintain structural integrity.

- Systemic therapy
  - Targeted therapy: the mainstay for advanced RCC. Includes Tyrosine Kinase Inhibitors (TKIs) like Sunitinib, Pazopanib, and Axitinib.
  - Immunotherapy: checkpoint inhibitors (e.g., Nivolumab, Ipilimumab) are now standard.
- Local control & surgical intervention
  - Pre-operative embolisation: performed 24–48 hours before surgery to devascularise the tumour, reducing intraoperative blood loss from a potential torrential haemorrhage.
  - Indications for surgery: pathologic fracture; impending pathologic fracture.
- Radiation therapy
  - Palliative Radiotherapy: Highly effective for pain relief and local control.
  - Pre-operative or Post-operative: May be used to reduce the risk of local recurrence.
- Minimally invasive techniques: Radiofrequency Ablation (RFA) or Cryoablation can be used for local tumour control in select patients, especially those who are poor surgical candidates.

Prognosis

- The presence of bone metastasis places RCC in Stage IV, which is incurable. However, with modern targeted therapies and immunotherapy, survival has significantly improved.
- The prognosis depends on factors like the number of metastases, response to systemic therapy, and the patient's overall performance status.
- Successful local control of the bone metastasis is critical for maintaining quality of life, mobility, and pain control.

Suggested Reading

Choudhury AK, Verma R, Dhyani A, Paul S, Goyal T. Late metastasis of renal cell carcinoma in distal femur treated with knee joint preservation: a case report. J Orthop Case Rep. 2022;12(1):1–5.

Mohakud S, Tripathy S, Bag ND, Mishra N. Multidisciplinary management of solitary hypervascular metastatic recurrence of renal cell carcinoma presenting with pathological femoral fracture. BMJ Case Rep. 2021;14(11):e245422.

Case 85

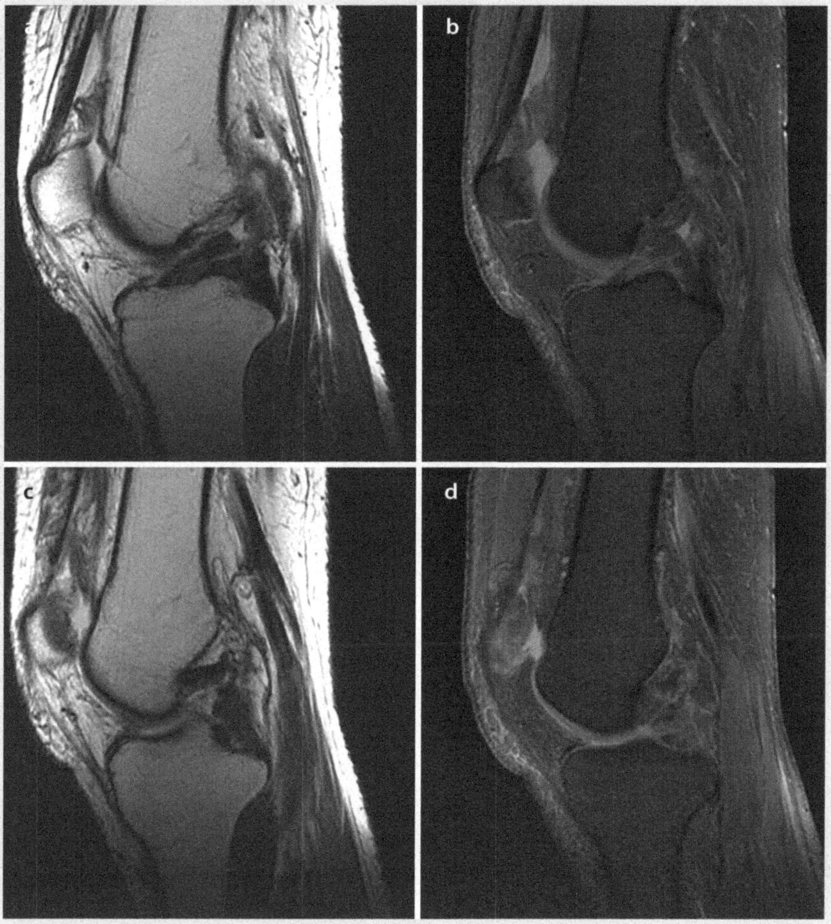

A 28-year-old male with significant trauma to the knee joint

S. Saran et al., *101 Knee Imaging Case Series*, 101 MSK Imaging 1,
https://doi.org/10.1007/978-3-032-21567-3_85

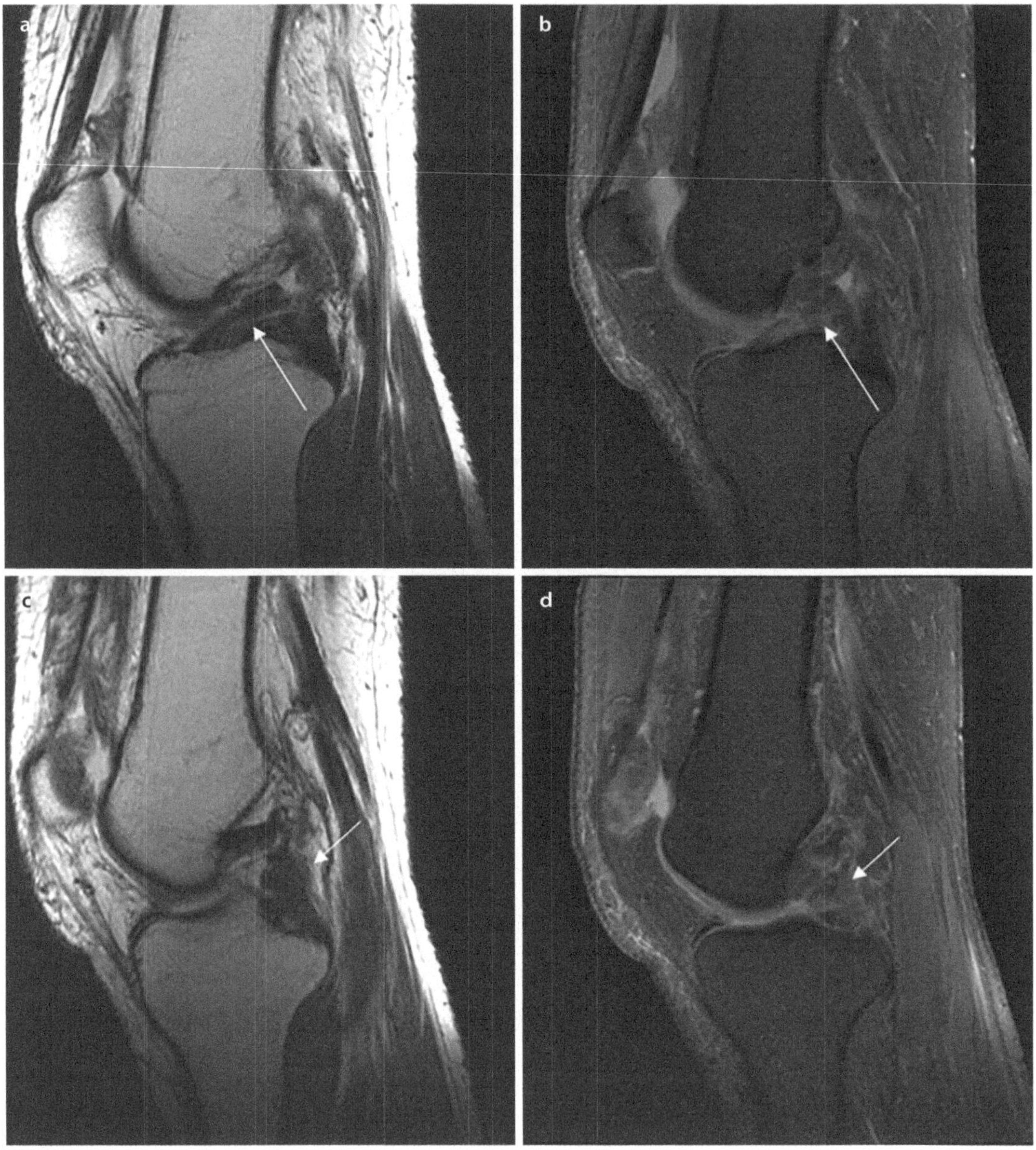

▪ MRI knee, T2 weighted sagittal **a**, **c** and PDFS weighted sagittal **b**, **d** sequences showing a full-thickness tear involving the Anterior cruciate ligament (ACL) (arrow in **a** and **b**) and the Posterior cruciate ligament (PCL) (arrow in **c** and **d**). This is a case of bicruciate injury

Bicruciate Ligament Injury

Definition & Pathophysiology

- A combined tear of the anterior cruciate ligament (ACL) and posterior cruciate ligament (PCL) is a severe, debilitating knee injury that results in global knee instability. It is often the result of high-energy trauma and is frequently part of a more complex injury pattern.
- The knee loses its two primary stabilisers against anterior-posterior translation and rotational stability, leading to a grossly unstable joint.

Mechanism of Injury

- Knee dislocation/hyperextension: the most common cause (e.g., dashboard injury in a car accident, fall from height. Hyperextension in sports).
- Severe rotational or dashboard injury: a posteriorly directed force on the proximal tibia with the knee flexed.

Clinical Presentation

- History: Significant high-energy trauma. The patient may report feeling a "pop" or the knee "going out of place"
- Symptoms:
  - Severe pain and immediate, massive swelling (hemarthrosis).
  - Instability: A profound sensation of the knee "giving way" or buckling in multiple directions.
  - Inability to bear weight.
- Physical exam:
  - Positive Lachman test & anterior drawer: suggests ACL tear.
  - Positive posterior drawer test & posterior sag sign: the tibia sags backwards relative to the femur, indicating a PCL tear.
  - Assessment of neurovascular status: the popliteal artery and peroneal nerve are at high risk with this injury pattern.

Associated Injuries

- A bicruciate injury is rarely isolated. It is often part of a knee dislocation (even if it reduces spontaneously) and is associated with:
  - Collateral ligament tears: (MCL, LCL, posterolateral corner (PLC)—most common combination is ACL/PCL/PLC).
  - Meniscal tears.
  - Neurovascular injury: Popliteal artery injury occurs in up to 40% of knee dislocations. This requires immediate vascular surgery consultation and often an angiogram.
  - Fractures (avulsion fractures, tibial plateau fractures).

Imaging Findings

- Radiography
  - Assess for fractures (avulsion fractures, tibial plateau).
  - Posterior sag sign: may be visible on a lateral view.
  - Check for knee dislocation: even if reduced, subtle incongruity may be present.
- MRI
  - Confirms complete tears of both the ACL and PCL.
  - Essential for evaluating all other injured structures: collateral ligaments, posterolateral corner, menisci, and cartilage.
  - Assesses the extent of the tears (mid-substance vs. avulsion).

Management

This is a severe injury requiring a structured, often surgical, approach.

- Acute phase & emergency care.
  - Address life-threatening injuries first.
  - Reduction: if the knee is dislocated, immediate closed reduction under sedation is required.
  - Neurovascular assessment: continuous monitoring. Vascular injury is limb-threatening.
  - Immobilisation: place the knee in a hinged knee brace or long-leg splint locked in extension to protect the reduced joint.
- Surgical management: Surgery is almost always required due to the profound instability.
  - Timing: Often performed 2–3 weeks post-injury to allow swelling to decrease and soft tissues to recover, but after any vascular issues are stabilised.
  - Procedure: multi-ligament knee reconstruction.

- Rehabilitation
  - Prolonged and phased: recovery takes 9–12 months or longer.

Complications

- Stiffness (arthrofibrosis) is very common.
- Persistent instability if reconstruction fails.
- Post-traumatic osteoarthritis.
- Chronic pain.

Prognosis

Good outcomes can be achieved with expert surgery and dedicated rehab, but the knee is unlikely to return to its pre-injury level, especially for high-impact sports.

Suggested Reading

Boutany M, Abdelnour D, Elnaggar A, Schweller E, Vaidya R. Sensitivity of MRI reports for ligamentous injuries in high-grade knee dislocations: a single-center retrospective analysis of radiology reports and operative findings. SICOT J. 2025;11:43.

Cruz JK, Al Habsi S, Ying Ren M, Lee YHD. Repair of posterior cruciate ligament femoral avulsion in multiligament knee injuries. Video J Sports Med. 2025;5(4):26350254251315498.

Hassebrock JD, Hartigan DE, Makovicka JL, et al. Anatomy and biomechanics of the cruciate ligaments and their surgical implications. In: Fanelli GC, editor. The multiple ligament injured knee: a practical guide to management. Cham: Springer International Publishing; 2019. p. 25–34.

Yang T, Li Y, Yang L, Liu Q. Magnetic resonance imaging of cruciate ligament disorders: current updates. EFORT Open Rev. 2025;10(7):475–86.

Case 86

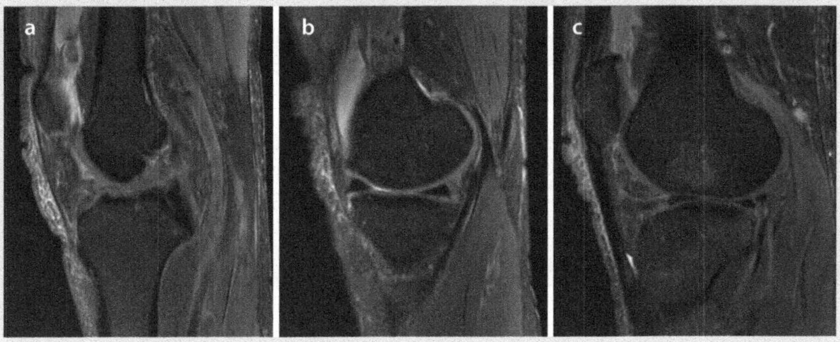

A 24-year-old football player presented with a twisting injury to the left knee joint followed by severe pain and swelling

S. Saran et al., *101 Knee Imaging Case Series*, 101 MSK Imaging 1,
https://doi.org/10.1007/978-3-032-21567-3_86

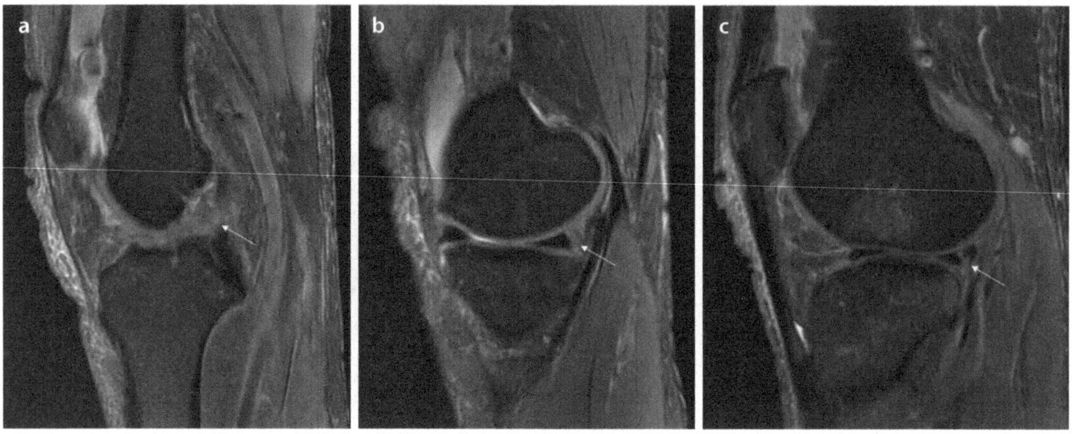

MRI knee sagittal PDFS weighted sagittal sequences **a**–**c** show the presence of a complete anterior cruciate ligament (ACL) tear (arrow in **a**) with joint effusion. The RAMP lesion (arrow in **b**) is also seen as a posterior medial meniscocapsular separation. Wrisberg rip (arrow in **c**), a longitudinal vertical meniscal tear at the junction of the ligament of Wrisberg and the posterior horn of the lateral meniscus is also seen

RAMP Lesion

Definition & Pathophysiology

- A RAMP lesion is a specific injury of the medial meniscus involving a tear of the peripheral capsular attachment of the posterior horn of the medial meniscus (PHMM). The term "RAMP" refers to the injury's location at the meniscocapsular junction and its extension superiorly along the meniscosynovial junction.
- Anatomy: The "ramp region" is the posteromedial corner of the knee, where the PHMM attaches to the joint capsule and the deep portion of the medial collateral ligament (MCL).
- Mechanism: It is highly associated with Anterior Cruciate Ligament (ACL) tears. The injury occurs during the pivoting event, where a combination of anterior tibial translation, valgus force, and external rotation of the tibia creates a shearing force that avulses the meniscus from its capsular attachment.
- Biomechanical Significance: A RAMP lesion creates anteroposterior and rotational instability of the medial meniscus, which can contribute to persistent knee instability even after a successful ACL reconstruction if left unrepaired.

Clinical Presentation

- The patient presents with a clinical picture of an ACL tear (pain, instability, effusion, positive Lachman/pivot shift test).
- Symptoms: There are no specific clinical signs that reliably diagnose a RAMP lesion in isolation. The symptoms are those of the concomitant ACL injury.

Imaging Findings

- MRI is the key to pre-operative diagnosis, but these lesions are often subtle and can be missed if not specifically looked for.
- The lesion is best visualised on PDFS sagittal sequences. The posteromedial corner must be carefully scrutinised in every ACL-deficient knee.
- Seen as a fluid signal intensity interposed between the medial meniscus and the joint capsule.

Greif's Classification

Type 1: Meniscocapsular ligament tear

Type 2: Partial superior peripheral posterior meniscal horn tear

Type 3A: Partial inferior peripheral posterior horn meniscal tear

Type 3B: Meniscotibial ligament tear

Type 4A: Complete peripheral posterior horn meniscal tear

Type 4B: Complete meniscocapsular junction tear

Type 4: Complete meniscocapsular disruption (a full-thickness RAMP lesion)

Type 5: Peripheral posterior horn meniscal double tear

Management

The decision to repair a RAMP lesion is based on its size, chronicity, and the patient's profile.

- Surgical repair (recommended in most cases)
- Indications
  - All RAMP lesions identified during ACL reconstruction in young, active patients.
  - Lesions causing significant meniscal hypermobility or instability.

- Rationale: Repairing the RAMP lesion restores the "sling" function of the medial meniscus, improving rotational stability and protecting the ACL graft.
- Procedure: Arthroscopic Repair. Using a portal placed in the posteromedial corner, specialised suturing devices are used to place sutures through the meniscus and the capsule, pulling them together to heal.

Wrisberg Rip (Wrisberg-Type Lateral Meniscal Tear)

Definition & Pathophysiology

- A "Wrisberg rip" is a specific and uncommon injury involving the posterior horn of the lateral meniscus. It is characterised by a vertical, longitudinal tear that destabilises the meniscus by disrupting its key stabilising attachments, particularly the meniscofemoral ligaments (Wrisberg).
- Mechanism: In case of the ACL tear, anterior tibial translation occurs, resulting in traction of the ligament of Wrisberg against the PCL and tearing a longitudinal fragment of the lateral meniscus.

Imaging Findings

- MRI is the primary diagnostic tool, but the findings can be subtle.
- MRI characteristics.
- A vertical, longitudinal tear in the posterior horn of the lateral meniscus, appearing as a cleft extending anteriorly from the posterior root of the lateral meniscus on several consecutive slices.

Pitfall

- The pitfall in diagnosing this type of tear is that normally there is a cleft at the attachment site of the ligament of Wrisberg to the posterior horn of the lateral meniscus, which can be mistaken for a tear.

- Due to variability in the ligament attachment site, this cleft can extend variably far, and as a result, the discrimination between a true tear and a "pseudo-tear" may pose a challenge.

Management

- Due to the inherent instability of this tear pattern, surgical intervention is almost always required.
- Arthroscopic suture repair is usually performed.

Suggested Reading

Gupta S, Dwivedi A, Chavan SK, Gupta P. Lateral meniscus zip lesion of knee: classification and repair methods. Arthrosc Tech. 2024;13(4):102911.

Kumar N, Ghimire P, Shukla S, Meena PK, Saxena S, Saran S. Is trochlear dysplasia associated with a high prevalence of repaired anterior medial portal lesions in anterior cruciate ligament-deficient knees? Indian J Radiol Imag. 2025;35(02):272–9.

Tomsan H, Gorbachova T, Fritz RC, Abrams GD, Sherman SL, Shea KG, Boutin RD. Knee MRI: meniscus roots, ramps, repairs, and repercussions. Radiographics. 2023;43(7):e220208.

Case 87

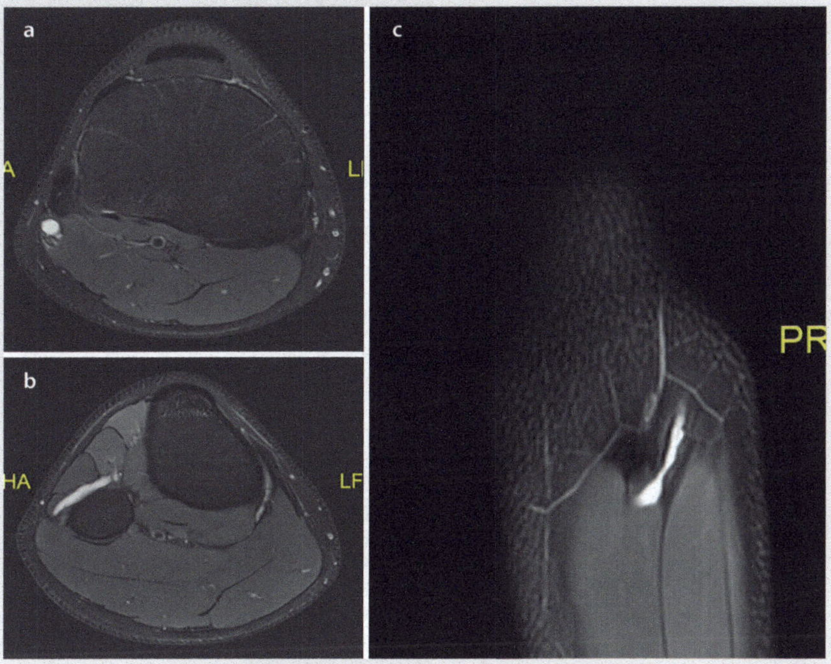

▪ A 34-year-old female presented with weakness in dorsiflexion and eversion of the foot

S. Saran et al., *101 Knee Imaging Case Series*, 101 MSK Imaging 1,
https://doi.org/10.1007/978-3-032-21567-3_87

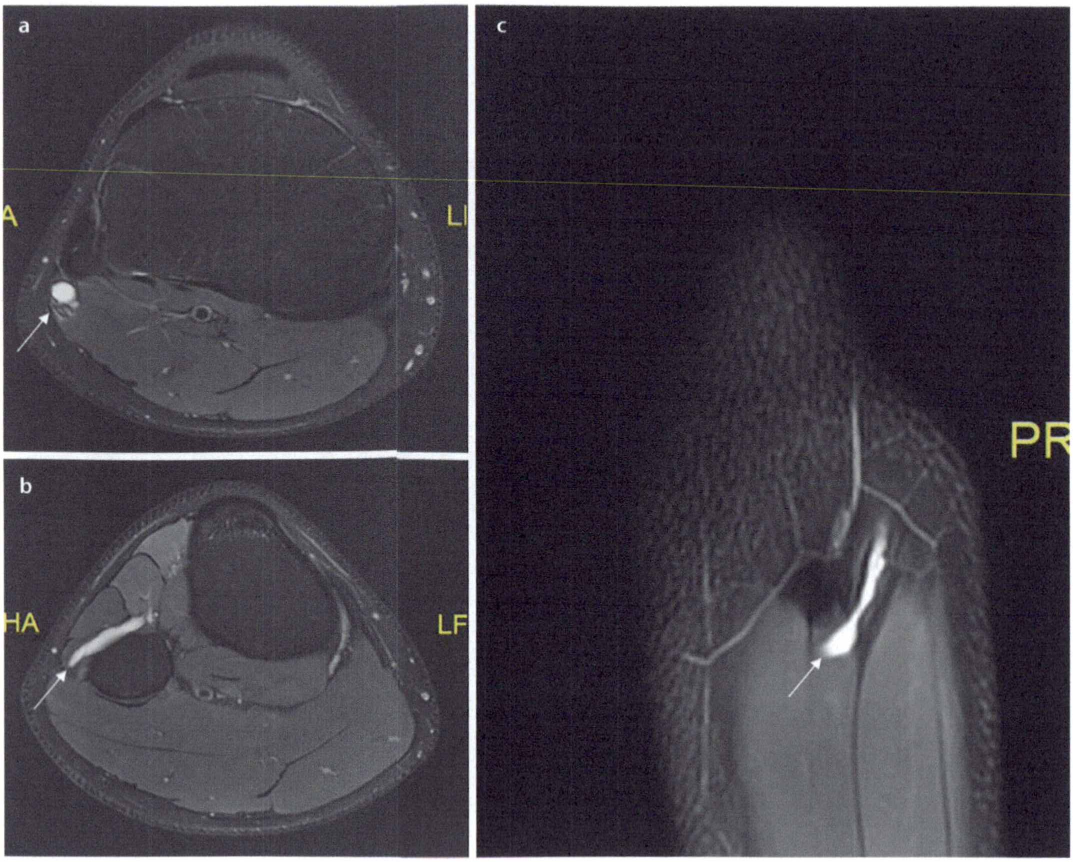

■ MRI knee PDFS weighted axial **a**, **b** and sagittal **c** sequences show a linear hyperintense lesion tracking along the course of the common peroneal nerve (arrow), appearances are of a common peroneal intraneural ganglion cyst

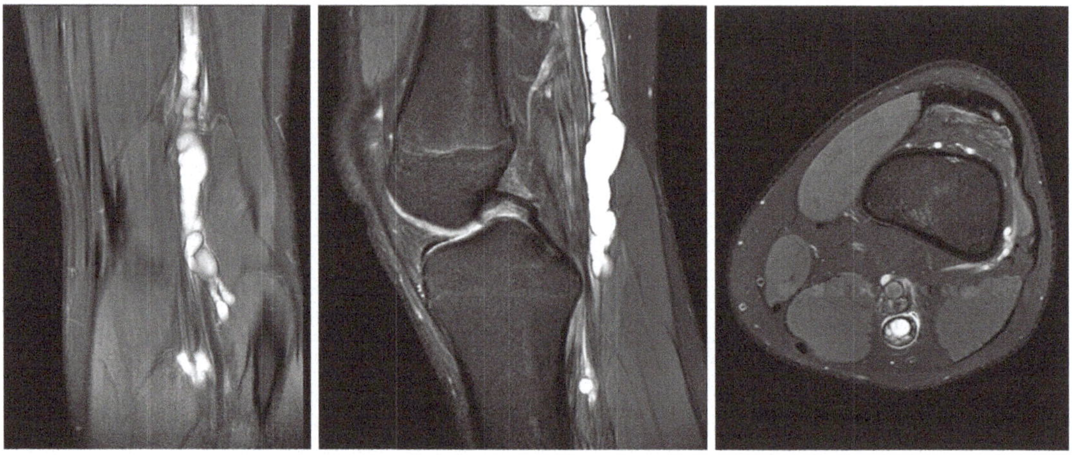

■ Companion case: Intraneural ganglion cyst in the sciatic nerve extending into tibial nerve

Common Peroneal Intraneural Ganglion Cyst

Definition and Pathophysiology

- A common peroneal intraneural ganglion cyst is a non-neoplastic, mucinous cyst that forms within the epineurium of the common peroneal nerve. It is a cause of progressive mononeuropathy and represents a longitudinal dissection of synovial fluid from a neighbouring joint, not a degenerative cyst.
- Articular (synovial) theory: A capsular defect in the superior tibiofibular joint (STFJ) allows synovial fluid to track along the articular branch of the common peroneal nerve. Under pressure, this fluid dissects within the epineurium, travelling proximally and distally along the path of least resistance within the nerve.
- The cyst is intraneural (within the nerve sheath) but extrafascicular (between the nerve fascicles), which explains why neurological function can sometimes be preserved until late stages.

Clinical Presentation

- Progressive foot drop: the hallmark symptom, due to compression of the deep peroneal nerve fibres. This manifests as weakness in ankle and toe dorsiflexion.
- Weakness in ankle eversion: due to involvement of the superficial peroneal nerve fibres.
- Sensory deficits: numbness, tingling, or pain in the anterolateral leg and dorsum of the foot.
- Palpable mass: a firm, non-tender, or slightly tender mass may be palpable near the fibular head.
- Tinel's sign: tapping over the cyst at the fibular head may elicit a tingling sensation radiating into the leg/foot.

Imaging Findings

- Ultrasound
- Can show a well-defined, anechoic, cystic mass within the common peroneal nerve.
- Useful for guiding diagnostic or therapeutic aspiration.
- MRI
- Location: cystic lesion centred at the fibular neck/head, intimately associated with the common peroneal nerve.

- T1-weighted: well-defined, homogeneously low signal intensity mass.
- T2-weighted/STIR: markedly hyperintense, fluid-signal mass with a characteristic "tail sign"—a thin tract of fluid signal tracking back to the superior tibiofibular joint (STFJ). This is a pathognomonic finding.
- Morphology: often has a multilobulated or "bunch of grapes" appearance as it ascends and descends within the nerve sheath.
- Mass effect: the cyst causes fusiform enlargement and splaying of the common peroneal nerve fascicles.

Differential Diagnosis

- Extraneural ganglion cyst: a cyst adjacent to, but not within, the nerve. It may cause mass effect but lacks the classic intraneural "tail sign"
- Peroneal nerve schwannoma/neurofibroma: a solid, enhancing nerve sheath tumour. It typically shows contrast enhancement, unlike the non-enhancing cyst fluid.
- Traumatic neuroma: a disorganised proliferation of nerve fibres and scar tissue following trauma, usually with a history of injury.

Management

- Image-guided aspiration (temporary/palliative)
- Ultrasound-guided aspiration of the cyst can provide temporary symptomatic relief.
- Recurrence is nearly universal because the connection to the joint remains patent, and the cyst rapidly refills.
- Surgical intervention (definitive treatment)
- The goal is to disconnect the cyst from its articular source at the superior tibiofibular joint.
- Articular branch disconnection and cyst decompression: this is the key step. The articular branch leading from the STFJ to the common peroneal nerve is identified and ligated or cauterised.
- Cyst decompression: The cyst is then incised and decompressed. A complete resection of the cyst wall is not necessary and risks damaging the nerve fascicles.

Suggested Reading

Panwar J, Mathew A, Thomas BP. Cystic lesions of peripheral nerves: are we missing the diagnosis of the intraneural ganglion cyst? World J Radiol. 2017;9(5):230–44.

Pemmari A, Mäkelä K, Niemi J, Kiekara T, Himanen SL. Large Intraneural ganglion cyst in the peroneal nerve. Case Rep Neurol. 2022;14(1):44–50.

Case 88

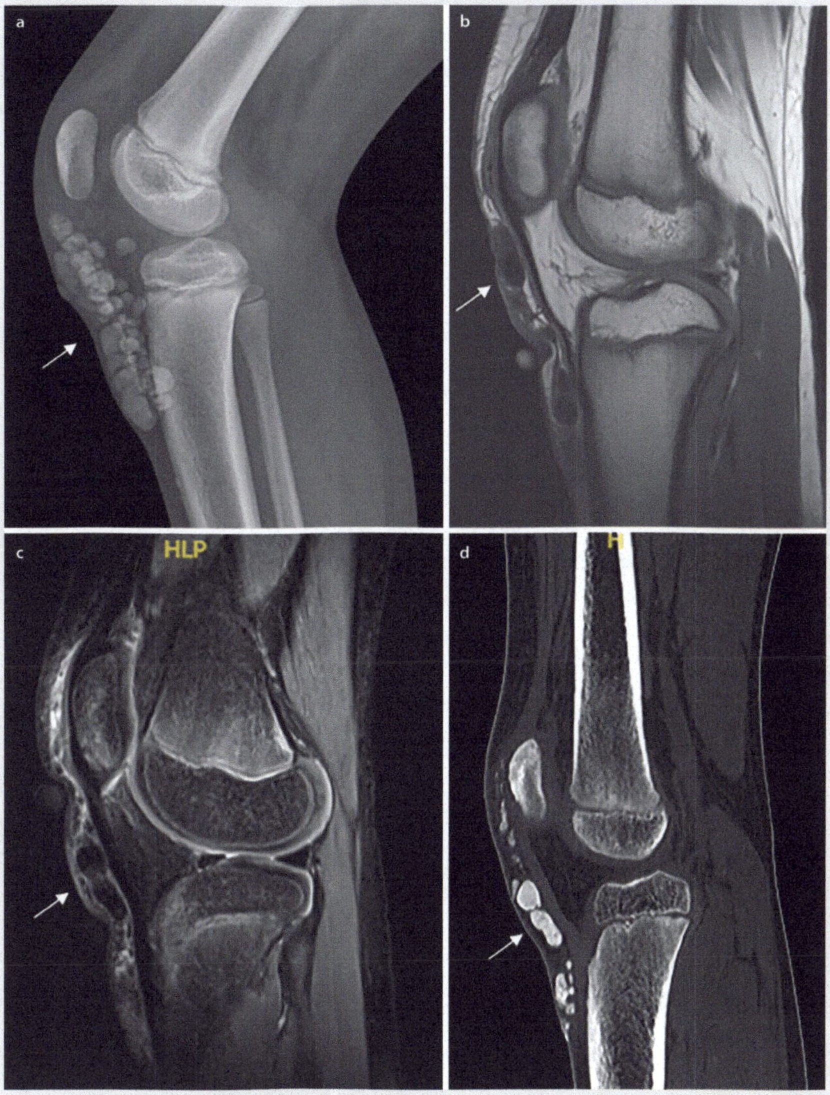

◘ A 16-year-old male presented with a 9-month history of a slowly enlarging, painless mass in the front of his right knee

S. Saran et al., *101 Knee Imaging Case Series*, 101 MSK Imaging 1,
https://doi.org/10.1007/978-3-032-21567-3_88

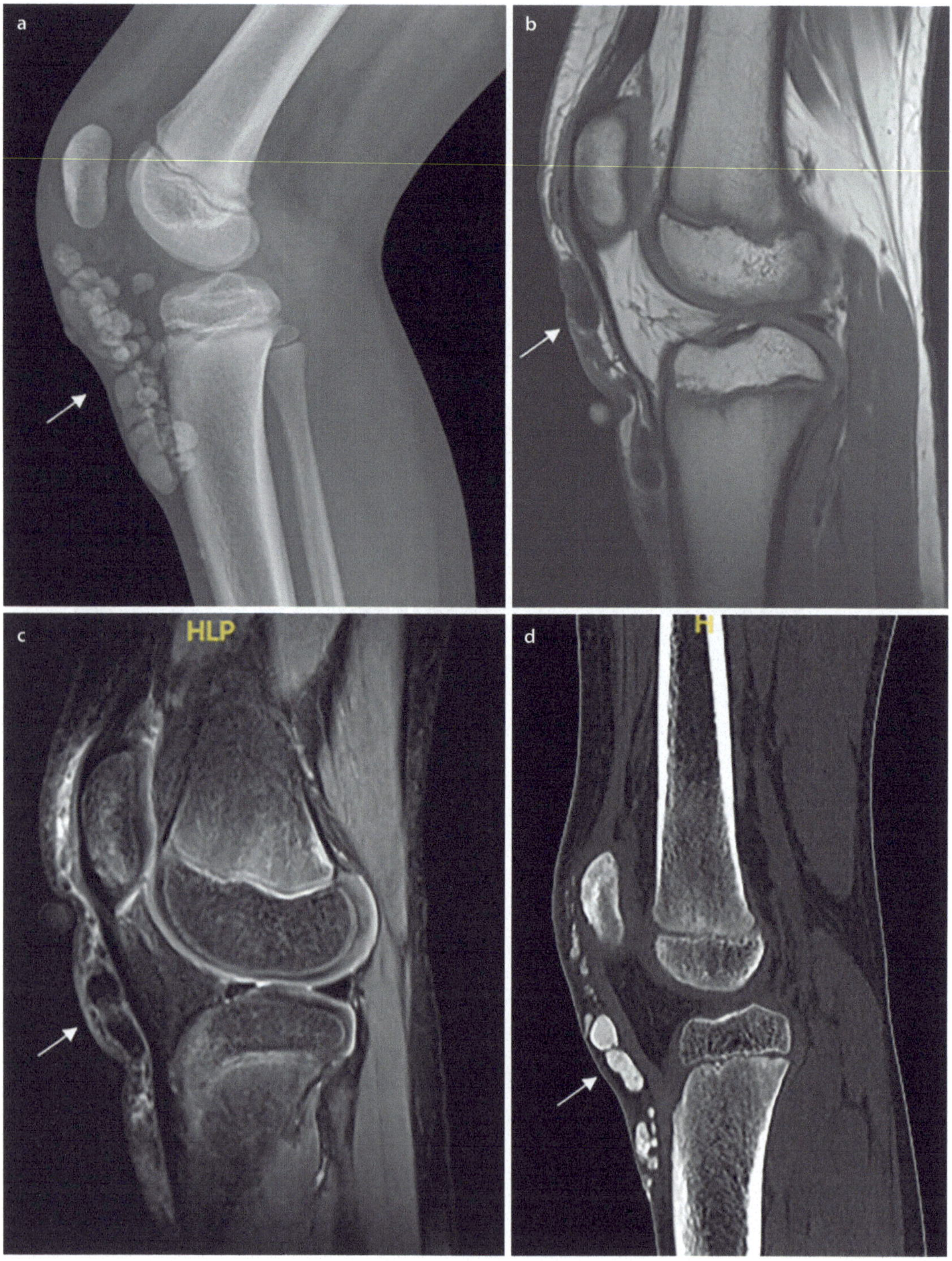

■ Lateral radiograph **a** shows multiple small, amorphous, cloud-like, and densely calcified masses (arrow) in the extensor aspect of the knee. MRI knee sagittal T1 **b**, and PDFS **c** sequences show the masses (arrows) as hypointense areas. The underlying patellar tendon is normal. Sagittal CT **d** confirms the masses (arrow) as densely calcified areas. The appearances are of tumoral calcinosis

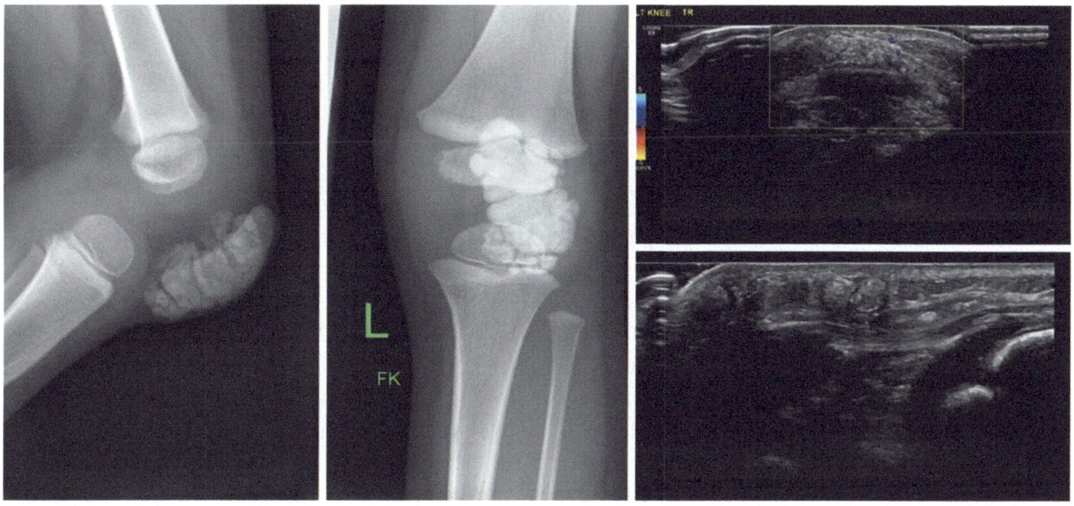

Companion case: Another case of tumoral calcinosis in the pre-patellar region shown on radiography and Ultrasound

Tumoral Calcinosis in the Extensor Aspect of the Knee

Definition & Pathophysiology

- Tumoral calcinosis is a rare condition characterised by the progressive, periarticular deposition of calcium hydroxyapatite crystals, forming large, calcified, tumour-like masses. When it occurs around the knee, it typically affects the extensor mechanism (quadriceps tendon, prepatellar bursa, patellar tendon).
- Pathogenesis: The exact mechanism is unclear, but involves a combination of:
  - Repetitive microtrauma: chronic stress to the extensor mechanism (e.g., from kneeling, strenuous activity).
  - Local tissue ischemia & necrosis: followed by calcium deposition.
  - Connective tissue disease: strongly associated with scleroderma, dermatomyositis, and SLE.
  - Chronic renal failure can cause secondary tumoral calcinosis due to hyperphosphatemia.

Clinical Presentation

- A slowly growing, firm, painless mass over the anterior knee. It may become painful if it impinges on surrounding structures, becomes inflamed, or reaches a large size.
- Restricted range of motion.

- The overlying skin can be tense, shiny, or even ulcerate, discharging a chalky, white paste.
- The mass is typically rock-hard, fixed to deep structures, and non-tender unless secondarily inflamed.

Imaging Findings

- Radiography
  - "Cobblestone" or "mass-like" calcification: shows multi-lobulated, dense calcific masses with a fluid-calcium level (a.k.a. "sedimentation sign") within the lobules. This is due to the layering of calcific sediment in a semi-liquid suspension.
  - The underlying bones are typically normal, which helps distinguish it from a bone-forming tumour.
- CT: confirms the radiographic findings with exquisite detail. Clearly demonstrates the multi-loculated cysts with fluid-calcium levels and the absence of bone destruction.
- Ultrasound
  - Shows hyperechoic masses with posterior acoustic shadowing.
  - Can visualise the lobulated architecture and may show the fluid-debris levels.
- MRI
  - While not a first-line approach, MRI is useful for assessing the relationship to critical structures, such as tendons and neurovascular bundles.
  - T1 & T2-weighted: The calcific components appear as signal voids.
  - Surrounding inflammation: may show oedema in the adjacent soft tissues.

Differential Diagnosis

- Calcific tendinitis/bursitis: acute, painful inflammation with smaller, more amorphous calcifications, often resolving spontaneously.
- Synovial sarcoma: a malignant tumour that may contain calcifications (30%), but they are typically more peripheral and stippled. The mass is more aggressive and painful.
- Myositis ossificans: heterotopic bone formation within muscle, showing a characteristic "zonal pattern" with mature bone at the periphery and immature tissue in the centre.
- Gout (tophaceous): tophi can be firm but are not as densely calcified.

- Chronic infection (e.g., TB): Can cause dystrophic calcification but usually has a more systemic and destructive presentation.

Management

Management is challenging due to high recurrence rates. It must address the underlying cause.

- Medical management
  - Treat the underlying disease: crucial in cases associated with renal failure or connective tissue disease (e.g., phosphate binders for hyperphosphatemia).
  - Phosphate-lowering diet: for primary and secondary forms.
  - Medications: acetazolamide or phosphate-lowering agents (e.g., sevelamer) have been used with variable success to reduce the calcium-phosphate product.
  - Probenecid: can increase urinary phosphate excretion in the hereditary form.
- Image-guided intervention
  - Aspiration & lavage: rarely successful due to the thick, pasty nature of the content, but can provide temporary relief for symptomatic cysts.
- Surgical intervention
  - Indications: pain, functional impairment, nerve compression, ulceration, or cosmesis.
  - Procedure: the goal is complete surgical excision. This can be technically difficult due to the mass's adherence to tendons and neurovascular structures.
  - Recurrence: the recurrence rate is high (up to 50%) if the underlying metabolic cause is not controlled. Incomplete excision almost guarantees recurrence.

Suggested Reading

Ayoub E, Youssef B, Badr B, Meriem OI, Najate CIE. Tumoral calcinosis producing peripheral nerve compression of the suprascapular nerve: a case report. Radiol Case Rep. 2024;20(1):670–3.

Kumar M, Sai RL, Mandal T, Keshav K, Kishan H, P TK. Pre-patellar Tumoral calcinosis of knee with intra-articular extension: an index case study. J Orthop Case Rep. 2025;15(1):73–8.

Sha Y, Hong K, Liew MKM, Lum JL, Wong RCW. Juxta-articular tumoral calcinosis associated with the temporomandibular joint: a case report and concise review. BMC Oral Health. 2019;19(1):138.

Case 89

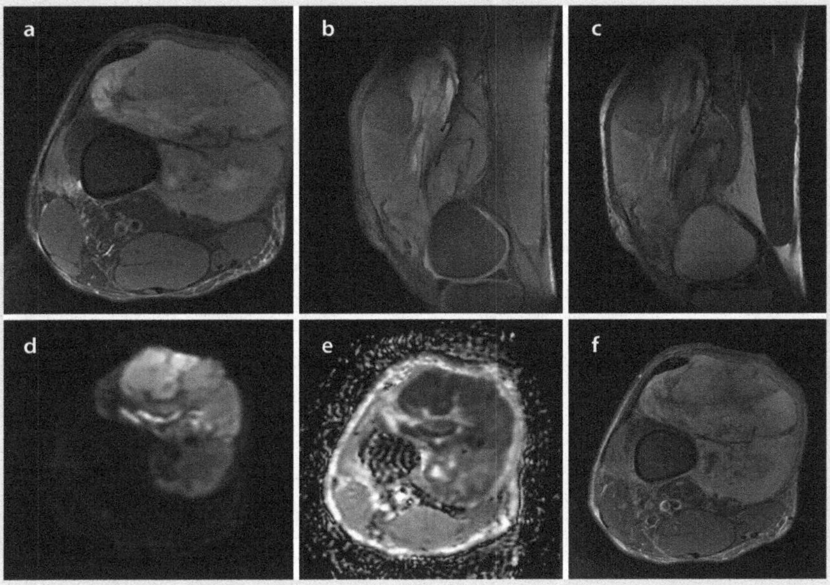

◘ A 34-year-old male presented with progressively increasing swelling in the anteromedial aspect of the knee joint, accompanied by restriction of joint movement

S. Saran et al., *101 Knee Imaging Case Series*, 101 MSK Imaging 1,
https://doi.org/10.1007/978-3-032-21567-3_89

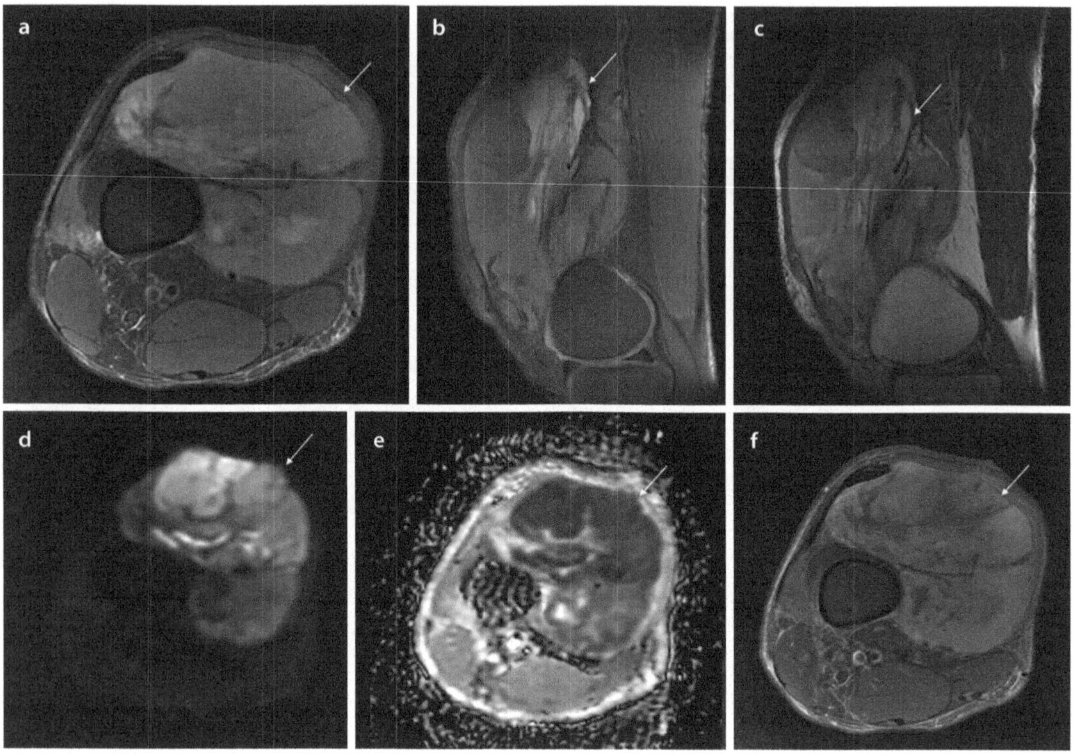

■ MRI knee **a**–**f** (PDFS axial **a**, sagittal **b**, T2 sagittal **c**, diffusion weighted imaging **d**, ADC **e** and post-contrast axial **f**) shows the presence of a large mass lesion in the anteromedial aspect of the knee joint (arrows), predominantly in the suprapatellar region with heterogeneous signal intensities (combination of hypo, iso and hyperintense signals) on PDFS weighted axial **a**, PDFS weighted sagittal **b** and T2 weighted sagittal **c** sequences. The lesion shows restriction of diffusion with a corresponding drop in signals on apparent diffusion coefficient maps **d**, **e**. The lesion shows heterogeneous enhancement **f** on post-contrast T1-weighted images. The histopathological diagnosis was Synovial sarcoma

Synovial Sarcoma

Definition & Pathophysiology

- Synovial sarcoma is a malignant, high-grade soft tissue tumour of mesenchymal origin. Despite its name, it does not typically arise from pre-existing synovial tissue but from pluripotent mesenchymal cells that differentiate to resemble synovial tissue. It is one of the most common soft tissue sarcomas to occur in the vicinity of large joints, with the knee being a predominant site.
- The tumour originates from primitive mesenchymal (stem) cells in the periarticular soft tissues, not from the synovial lining itself. This is why it is often found near, but not within, the joint capsule.
- Characteristic genetic abnormality: Over 90% of cases harbour a specific chromosomal translocation, t(X;18)

(p11.2;q11.2). This fusion creates an abnormal fusion oncogene (most commonly *SS18-SSX1* or *SS18-SSX2*) that drives tumorigenesis.
- It has significant potential for local invasion and distant metastasis (most commonly to the lungs).
- Biphasic & monophasic histology:
  - Biphasic: contains both epithelial cells (forming gland-like structures) and spindle cells.
  - Monophasic: composed almost entirely of spindle cells, which is more common and can be difficult to diagnose.

Clinical Features

- Demographics: most common in adolescents and young adults (15–40 years old).
- Symptoms: presents as a slow-growing, deep-seated mass. Pain is a frequent feature, unlike many other soft tissue masses, which are painless. Symptoms can be present for months to years before diagnosis, leading to a large tumour size at presentation.

MRI Findings

- MRI is the primary imaging modality for characterising the mass and its relationship to surrounding structures.
- "Triple Sign" (classic finding): A heterogeneous mass with a mixture of three signal intensities on T2-weighted images, representing:
  - Hyperintense: cystic/necrotic areas.
  - Intermediate-to-high intensity: solid tumour components.
  - Hypointense: fibrous tissue or calcifications.
- "Bowl of Grapes" Sign: describing multi-lobulated cystic components separated by internal septa.
- The solid components of the tumour show prominent, heterogeneous enhancement after gadolinium contrast administration.
- Intratumoral calcifications are seen in up to 30% of cases, best seen on CT or as focal low signal on MRI.

Management

- Management requires a multidisciplinary team at a specialised sarcoma centre.

- Core needle biopsy: performed to obtain a tissue sample for histopathological diagnosis and genetic testing for the t(X;18) translocation, which is diagnostic.
- Wide surgical resection: the cornerstone of treatment.
- Adjuvant therapies:
  - Radiation therapy: almost always used, either pre-operatively (to shrink the tumour and sterilise the margins) or post-operatively (to eradicate any residual microscopic disease).
  - Chemotherapy: the role is debated but is often used for large (>5 cm), high-grade tumours or those with metastatic disease.

Prognosis

- Dependent on tumour size, stage, and the ability to achieve a complete surgical resection.
- The 5-year survival rate ranges from 50% to 80%. Long-term follow-up is essential due to the risk of late recurrence and metastasis.

Suggested Reading

Kuruvilla N, Dang BTD, Dobtsis J. Synovial sarcoma: a radiologic case report. Radiol Case Rep. 2024;20(3):1569–73.

Singh C, Gharde P, Shah R, Nagtode T, Sapkale B. Synovial sarcoma in the right thigh of a 25-year-old male: a case report. Cureus. 2024;16(6):e62526.

Case 90

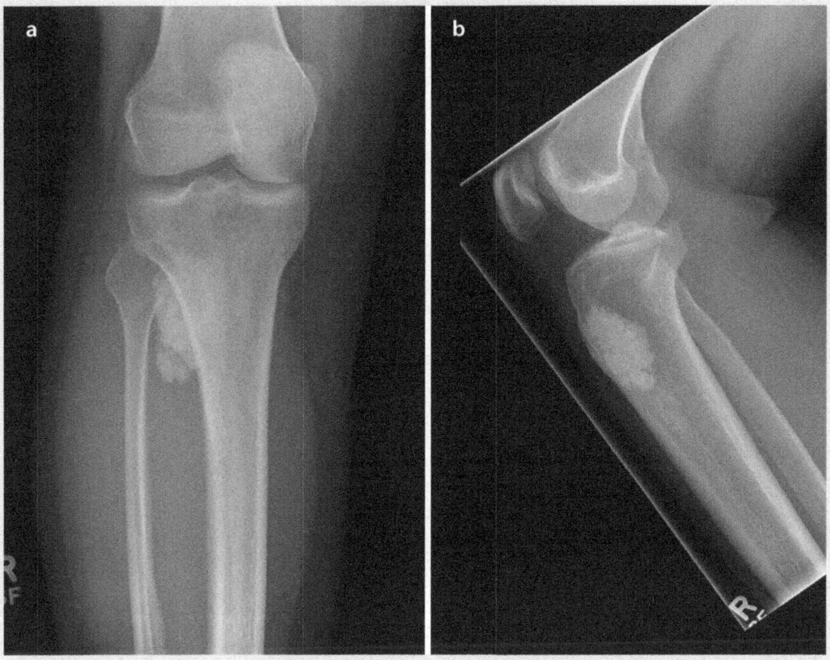

A 27-year-old female presented with a hard swelling in the proximal leg

S. Saran et al., *101 Knee Imaging Case Series*, 101 MSK Imaging 1,
https://doi.org/10.1007/978-3-032-21567-3_90

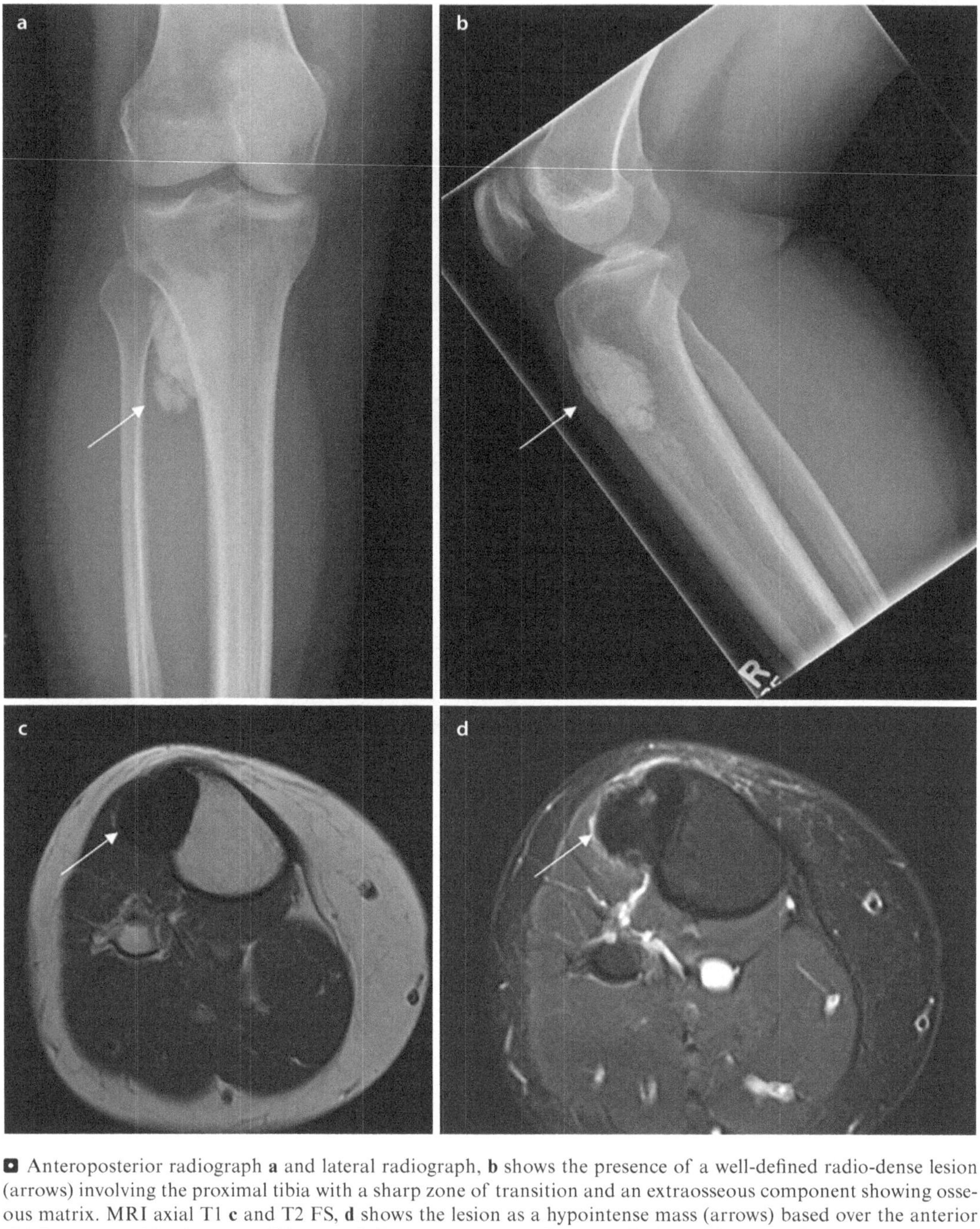

■ Anteroposterior radiograph **a** and lateral radiograph, **b** shows the presence of a well-defined radio-dense lesion (arrows) involving the proximal tibia with a sharp zone of transition and an extraosseous component showing osseous matrix. MRI axial T1 **c** and T2 FS, **d** shows the lesion as a hypointense mass (arrows) based over the anterior tibial cortex and having a small intramedullary component. The constellation of imaging findings supports the diagnosis of Parosteal osteosarcoma

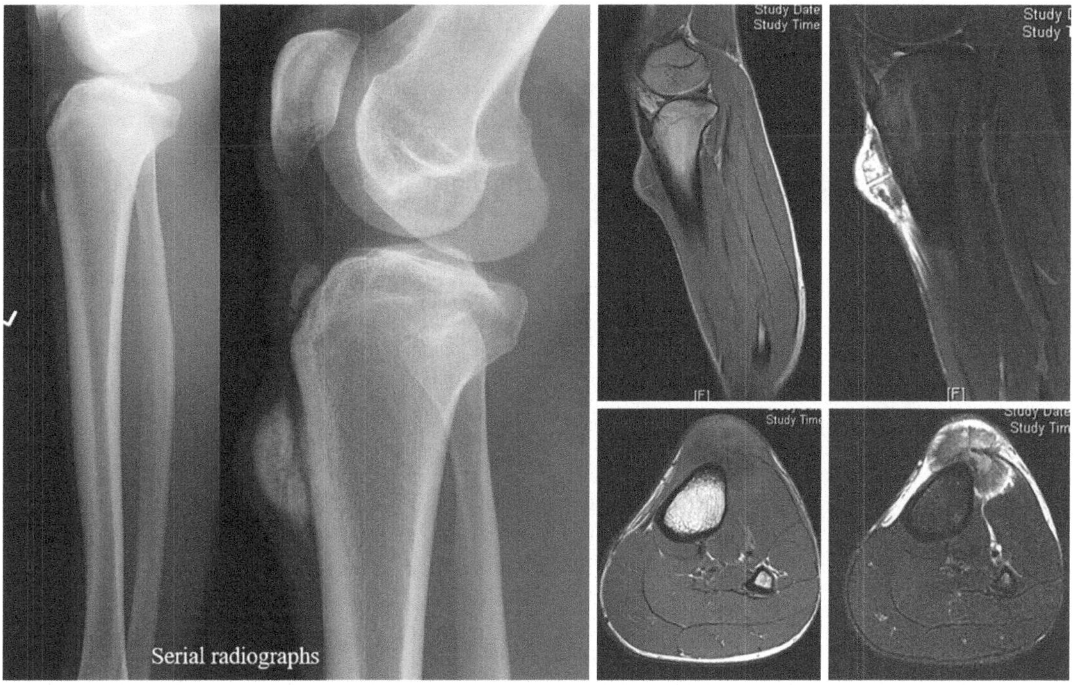

Companion case: Surface osteosarcoma of the proximal tibia

Parosteal Osteosarcoma

Definition & Pathophysiology

- Parosteal osteosarcoma is a low-grade, malignant bone-forming tumour that arises from the periosteum of the bone. It is the most common type of surface osteosarcoma and is characterised by its slow growth and excellent prognosis when treated appropriately.
- Origin: Arises from the cortical surface of the bone, most commonly in the posterior distal femur (~70% of cases). The proximal tibia is a less common but well-documented site.
- Pathology: It is a well-differentiated (low-grade) tumour that produces abundant osteoid and woven bone. Its key histological feature is the presence of bony trabeculae with a parallel arrangement, often showing a "mosaic" pattern.
- The tumour typically encases the underlying bone but initially does not invade the medullary canal. However, long-standing or recurrent lesions can eventually invade the medulla.

Clinical Presentation

- Demographics: Most common in young adults (second to fourth decades), with a slight female predominance.
- Symptoms:
  - Slow-growing, hard, fixed mass on the bone surface. The mass is often present for months to years before diagnosis.
  - Dull, aching pain is common, but the mass may be painless.
  - Limited range of motion if located near a joint.

Imaging Findings

- Radiography
  - Juxtacortical dense, heavily ossified mass attached to the external bone surface, typically in the metaphysis.
  - The classic finding is a radiolucent cleavage plane between the tumour and the underlying cortex at its periphery, best seen on tangential views. The base of the tumour is broadly attached to the cortex.
  - Underlying cortex usually appears intact and thickened, but may show saucerization or erosion in advanced cases.
- MRI
  - MRI best defines the full extent of the tumour, including its relationship to neurovascular structures and the medullary canal.
  - The ossified components appear as low signal intensity on all the sequences.
  - The non-mineralised, cellular components may appear hyperintense on T2/STIR and show moderate to marked enhancement.
  - The tumour appears as a lobulated, juxtacortical mass that "hugs" the bone without a significant soft tissue component (unless dedifferentiated).

Differential Diagnosis

- Myositis ossificans (heterotopic ossification): the most important mimic. It shows a zonal phenomenon with mature, organised bone at the periphery and immature tissue in the centre. It typically has a clear cleavage plane with the underlying bone.
- Osteochondroma: has cortical and medullary continuity with the underlying bone.
- Periosteal chondroma: a lucent, cartilaginous lesion with scalloping of the underlying cortex and periosteal reaction.

- High-grade surface osteosarcoma: a more aggressive tumour with a permeative growth pattern and poorly defined margins.

Management

- Surgical intervention
  - The standard of care is wide surgical excision with a margin of normal tissue to prevent local recurrence.
  - A cadaveric bone graft can be used to reconstruct the defect.
  - Endoprosthesis: a custom metal implant may be used for large defects.
- Role of chemotherapy: for classic low-grade parosteal osteosarcoma, chemotherapy is not indicated due to its low-grade nature and excellent prognosis with surgery alone. If a high-grade (dedifferentiated) component is identified on histology, neoadjuvant and adjuvant chemotherapy is administered, as for conventional osteosarcoma.

Suggested Reading

Hang J-F, Chen PC-H. Parosteal osteosarcoma. Arch Pathol Lab Med. 2014;138(5):694–9.

Prabowo Y, Kamal AF, Kodrat E, Prasetyo M, Maruanaya S, Efar TS. Parosteal osteosarcoma: a benign-looking tumour, amenable to a variety of surgical reconstruction. Int J Surg Oncol. 2020;2020:4807612.

Case 91

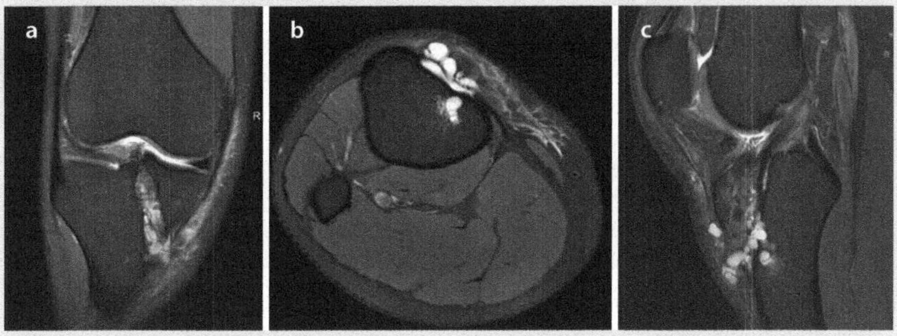

■ A 33-year-old female presented with palpable, painful masses along the anterior surface of the proximal tibia 3 years post ACL reconstruction

S. Saran et al., *101 Knee Imaging Case Series*, 101 MSK Imaging 1,
https://doi.org/10.1007/978-3-032-21567-3_91

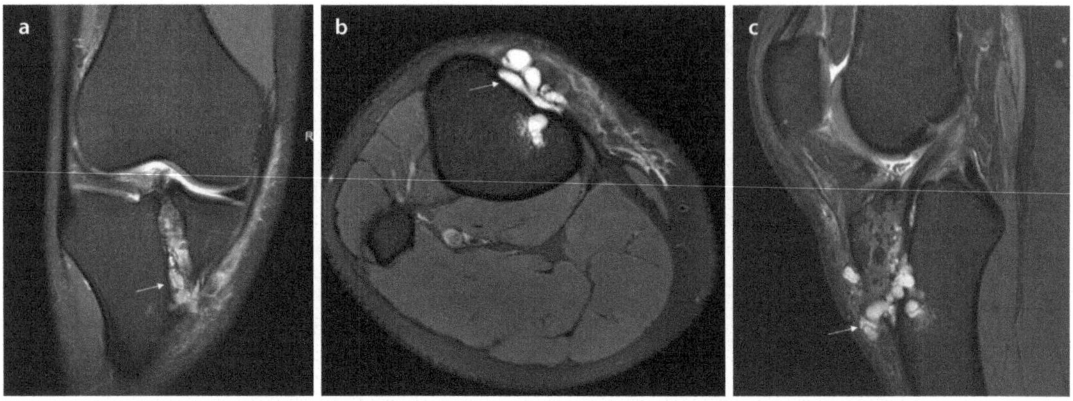

■ MRI PDFS coronal **a**, axial **b** and sagittal **c** shows the presence of multiloculated cystic lesions, typically appearing hyperintense on PDFS sequences in or around the osseous tibial tunnel (arrows), appearances are of Tibial tunnel cysts

Tibial Tunnel Cysts Post-ACL Reconstruction

Definition & Pathophysiology

- A tibial tunnel cyst is a ganglion cyst of the tibial tunnel, a fluid-filled collection that forms within or around the tibial bone tunnel following Anterior Cruciate Ligament (ACL) reconstruction. It is a late, non-infectious complication.
- Mechanism: The leading theory is a "check-valve" mechanism. Synovial fluid from the knee joint is forced into the tibial tunnel through a communication (often a gap between the graft and the tunnel wall or a fissure in the graft) during weight-bearing and knee motion. The fluid becomes trapped, unable to flow back into the joint, leading to cyst formation and expansion.

Clinical Presentation

- Timeline: Typically presents months to years after ACL reconstruction surgery.
- Symptoms:
  - Anterior knee pain: deep, aching pain localised to the proximal tibia, often worse with activity.
  - Palpable mass: a firm, tender mass may be palpable over the anteromedial aspect of the proximal tibia, near the tibial tunnel incision site.
  - Loss of extension: a cyst located at the intra-articular tunnel aperture can cause a mechanical block to full knee extension, mimicking a classic cyclops lesion.
  - Sense of instability: rarely, if the cyst compromises graft fixation or integrity.

Imaging Findings

- MRI
  - MRI clearly depicts the cystic nature of the lesion and its extent. Cystic mass centred on and expanding the tibial tunnel.
  - T1-weighted: The cyst appears as a well-defined, homogeneously low signal intensity mass within the tibial tunnel.
  - T2-weighted/STIR (fat-saturated): The cyst is markedly hyperintense, confirming its fluid content. It often appears multiloculated.
  - T1-weighted post-contrast: The fibrous cyst wall enhances, but the central fluid content does not. There is typically no surrounding bone marrow oedema unless there is significant pressure erosion.
  - Often shows a "tail sign"—a thin tract of fluid connecting the cyst to the joint space.
  - Assessment of the ACL graft is crucial; the graft may appear normal or show signs of mucoid degeneration.

Differential Diagnosis

- Graft failure/tear: presents with instability, not a palpable mass. MRI shows discontinuity of graft fibres.
- Hardware failure/screw loosening: pain around the hardware, often with lucency around the screw on X-ray.
- Deep infection (septic tunnel osteitis): Presents with constant pain, warmth, erythema, and systemic signs. MRI shows intense bone marrow oedema, soft tissue inflammation, and a thick, enhancing cyst wall.

Management

- Treatment is indicated for symptomatic cysts causing pain or mechanical symptoms.
- Ultrasound-guided aspiration and corticosteroid injection: The cyst is drained, and a corticosteroid is injected to reduce inflammation and sclerose the cyst lining.
- Surgical intervention: arthroscopic debridement and cyst excision.
  - Failed aspiration/injection.
  - Large, symptomatic, or recurrent cysts.

Suggested Reading

Ghazikhanian V, Beltran J, Nikac V, Feldman M, Bencardino JT. Tibial tunnel and pretibial cysts following ACL graft reconstruction: MR imaging diagnosis. Skeletal Radiol. 2012;41(11):1375–9.

Zappia M, Capasso R, Berritto D, Maggialetti N, Varelli C, D'Agosto G, Martino MT, Carbone M, Brunese L. Anterior cruciate ligament reconstruction: MR imaging findings. Musculoskelet Surg. 2017;101(Suppl 1):23–35.

Case 92

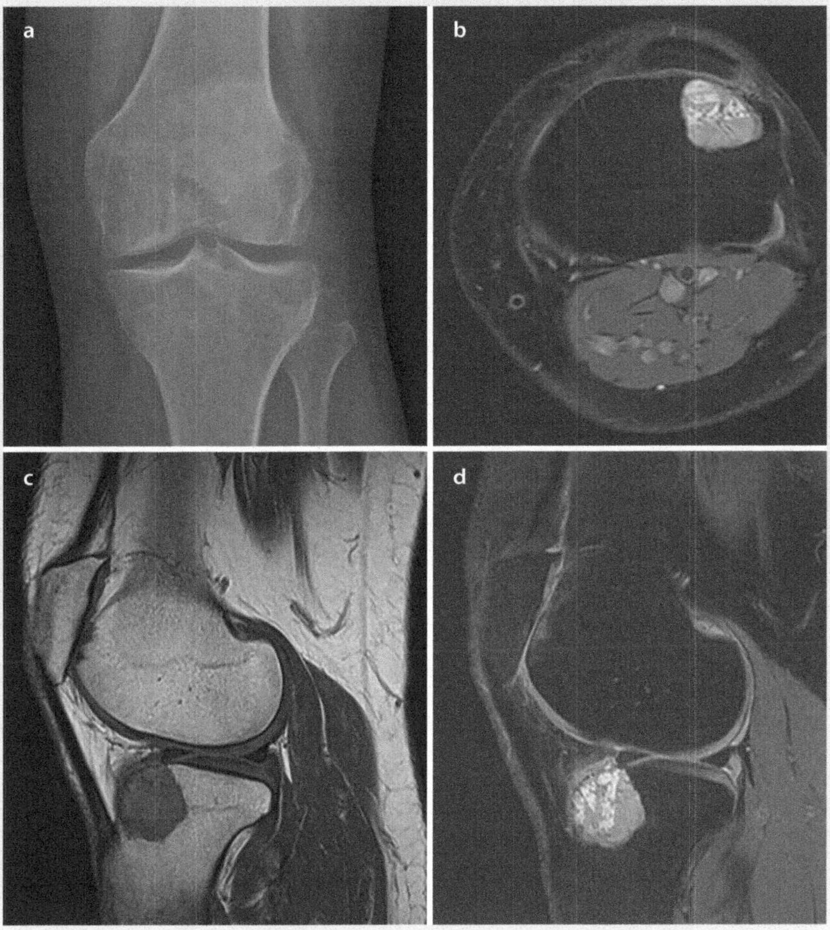

■ A 27-year-old female presented with mild knee pain

S. Saran et al., *101 Knee Imaging Case Series*, 101 MSK Imaging 1,
https://doi.org/10.1007/978-3-032-21567-3_92

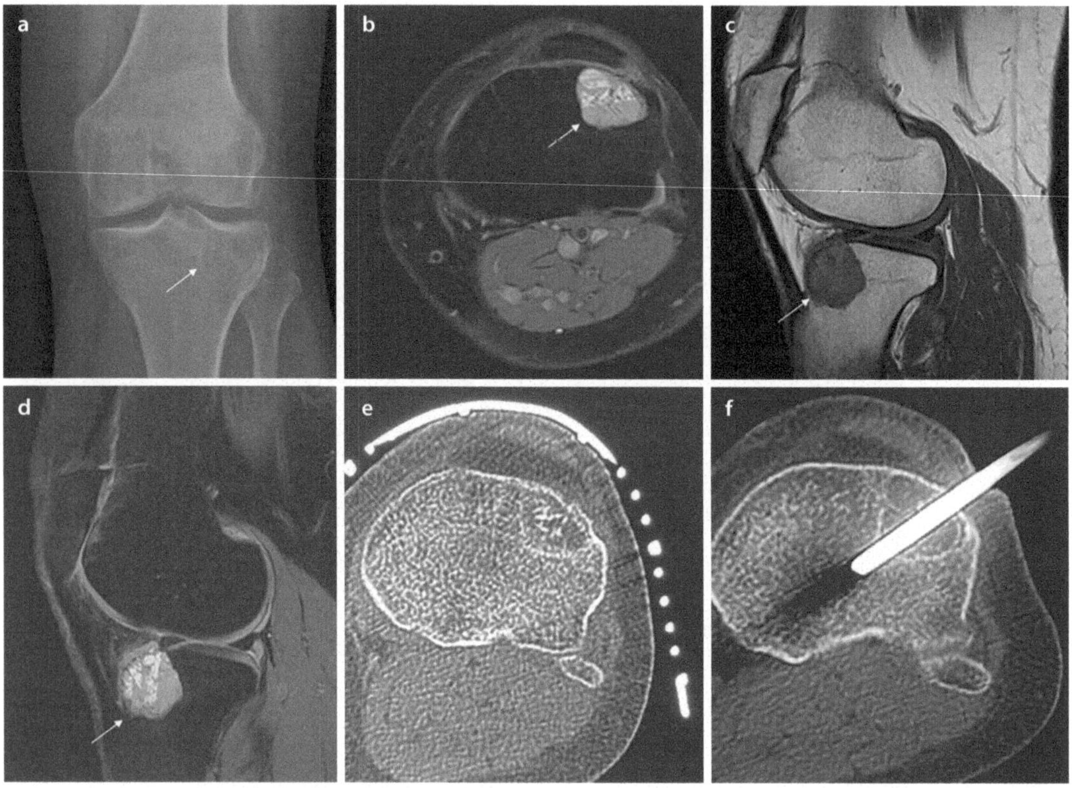

Radiograph **a** of the knee joint shows a well-defined osteolytic lesion (arrow) with a narrow zone of transition and thin sclerotic margins, absence of cortical breach and internal mineralisation. MRI PDFS axial **b** sagittal T1 **c**, PDFS **d** shows the lesion (arrow) appearing hypointense on the T1-weighted sequence **c** and hyperintense on PDFS sequences **b**, **d**. Internal cystic areas with fluid-fluid levels can also be observed, along with tiny hypointense dots that suggest flow voids. The possibility of a Giant cell tumour can be considered on radiograph and MRI. Planning CT **e** shows the lesion as an osteolytic area with prominent internal bony trabeculae, raising the suspicion of hemangioma. The biopsy **f** revealed the diagnosis of intraosseous haemangioma

Intraosseous Haemangioma

Definition & Pathophysiology

- An intraosseous hemangioma is a benign, slow-growing vascular tumour composed of newly formed blood vessels within the bone. It is a hamartoma rather than a true neoplasm.
- Location: While most common in the skull and vertebral bodies, they are rare in long bones.
- Histologically, they are classified as capillary or cavernous (the latter being more common in bone). They consist of thin-walled, blood-filled vessels lined by a single layer of endothelium.

Clinical Presentation

- The vast majority are asymptomatic and discovered incidentally on imaging for unrelated reasons (e.g., knee pain, trauma).
- Symptomatic cases can present with:
  - Dull, localised ache that may worsen at night or with activity.
  - Palpable swelling or deformity if the lesion expands the bone.
  - Pathologic fracture is rare due to the non-aggressive and non-destructive nature of the lesion.

Imaging Findings

- Radiography
  - Classic "corduroy cloth" or "honeycomb" appearance: A coarsened, vertically oriented trabecular pattern within a well-defined, geographic lytic area.
  - "Sunburst" pattern: rarely in long bones; more typical in the skull, showing radiating spicules from the centre of the lesion.
  - Margin: usually well-defined with a sclerotic rim.
  - Cortex: typically, intact but may be slightly expanded and thinned.
- CT
  - Shows the "polka-dot" appearance on axial images, created by the thickened, sclerotic vertical trabeculae seen in cross-section.
  - Excellent for confirming the intact cortex and lack of soft tissue extension.
- MRI
  - T1-weighted: intermediate to low signal intensity.
  - T2-weighted/PDFS: markedly hyperintense, often described as a "light bulb" sign, due to the slow-flowing blood and water content within the vascular spaces. The thickened trabeculae appear as low-signal striations, and arterial channels can be seen as black dots.
  - T1-weighted post-contrast: shows intense, homogeneous enhancement due to the highly vascular nature of the tumour.

Differential Diagnosis

For a lytic lesion in the proximal tibia, consider

- Giant cell tumour of bone (GCT): typically, subchondral, eccentric, and purely lytic without sclerotic margins. "Soap-bubble" appearance.
- Plasmacytoma/myeloma: a "punched-out" lytic lesion without a sclerotic rim, usually in older patients.

Management

- Asymptomatic lesion: no treatment is necessary. Reassurance is the standard of care. It is a "leave-me-alone" lesion.
- Symptomatic lesion (persistent pain, risk of fracture):
  - Pre-operative embolisation: to reduce vascularity and intraoperative bleeding.
  - Curettage.
  - Bone grafting: the resulting cavity is often filled with bone graft or bone cement.
  - Radiotherapy: an option for lesions that are inoperable or recur.

Suggested Reading

Cha JG, Yoo JH, Kim HK, Park JM, Paik SH, Park SJ. PET/CT and MRI of intra-osseous haemangioma of the tibia. Br J Radiol. 2012;85(1012):e94–8.

Zhou Q, Lu L, Yang Z, Su S, Hong G. Hemangioma of long tubular bone: imaging characteristics with emphasis on magnetic resonance imaging. Skeletal Radiol. 2020;49(12):2029–38.

Case 93

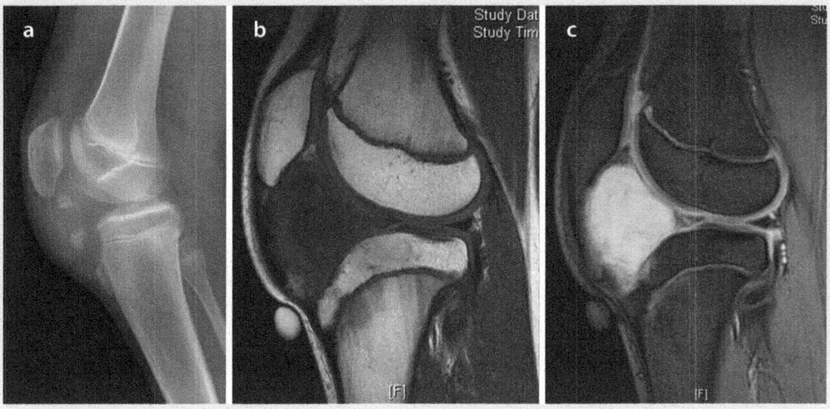

A 15-year-old male presented with anterior knee pain and intermittent locking

S. Saran et al., *101 Knee Imaging Case Series*, 101 MSK Imaging 1,
https://doi.org/10.1007/978-3-032-21567-3_93

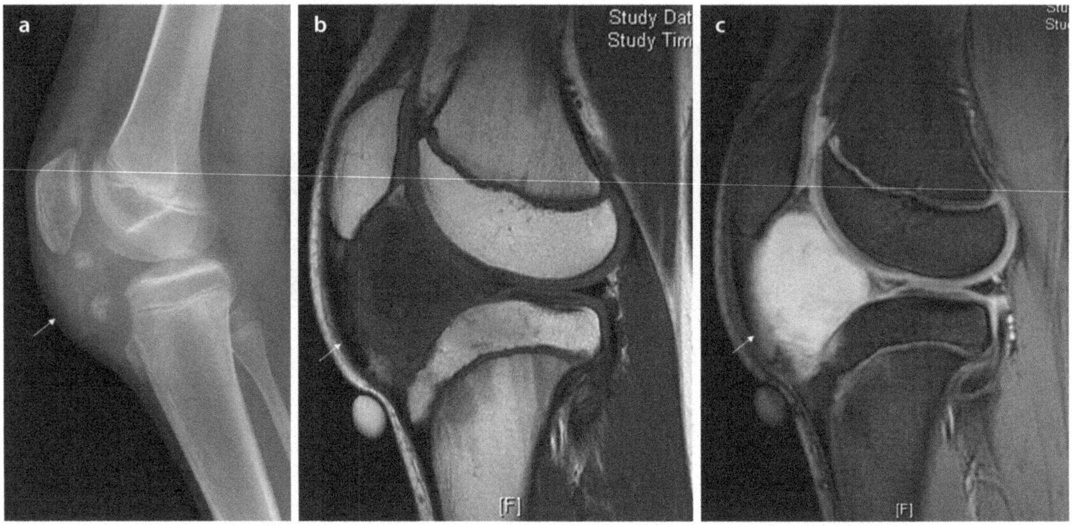

■ Lateral radiograph **a** shows the presence of soft tissue opacity in the Hoffa fat pad with stippled calcification (arrow). MRI sagittal T1 **b**, and PDFS **c** shows a well-circumscribed mass (arrows) within Hoffa's fat pad, appearing isointense to the muscles on T1 weighted **b** and hyperintense on PDFS weighted sequence **c**. Imaging findings are suggestive of an intracapsular chondroma/soft tissue chondroma of Hoffa's fat pad

Intracapsular Chondroma/Soft Tissue Chondroma of Hoffa's Fat Pad

Definition & Pathophysiology

- An intracapsular chondroma is a rare benign tumour composed of cartilage that develops in soft tissues. When it occurs within the knee, Hoffa's fat pad is the most common location.
- Arises from metaplastic synovial tissue. The synovial cells undergo transformation into cartilage-forming cells.
- It is a well-circumscribed, lobulated cartilaginous mass that is entirely contained within the intracapsular, extrasynovial space of Hoffa's fat pad.

Clinical Presentation

- Demographics: Most common in adults aged 30–60 years.
- Symptoms:
  - Often presents as chronic, dull anterior knee pain or a sensation of fullness.

- Mechanical symptoms: locking, catching, or limited range of motion can occur if the lesion becomes large enough to impinge between the femur and tibia.
- A palpable mass is rare due to the deep location within the fat pad.

Imaging Findings

- Radiography
  - Often normal if the chondroma is not calcified.
  - May show a soft tissue density in the anterior knee.
  - In 30–70% of cases, it shows characteristic "ring-and-arc", "popcorn", or stippled calcifications within the mass, which are pathognomonic for a cartilaginous tumour.
- MRI
  - T1-weighted: The lesion is typically isointense or hypointense to muscle. It appears as a well-defined, lobulated mass that replaces the normal bright signal of the fat pad.
  - T2-weighted / STIR (Fat-Saturated): Markedly hyperintense due to the high water content of cartilage. The classic "lobulated" or "septated" appearance is clearly visible. Low-signal fibrous septa may be seen between the lobules.
  - T1-weighted post-contrast: Shows a characteristic "ring-and-arc" or peripheral/septal enhancement pattern, reflecting the enhancement of the fibrovascular tissue surrounding the cartilaginous lobules. The central chondroid matrix does not enhance.

Differential Diagnosis

- Localised nodular synovitis/tenosynovial giant cell tumour: Typically shows low T2 signal due to hemosiderin, the opposite of the bright T2 signal of a chondroma.
- Synovial haemangioma: serpiginous, T2-bright lesion that shows strong, diffuse enhancement and often contains phleboliths.
- Ganglion cyst: a pure cyst that follows fluid signal and typically has a thin, non-enhancing wall.
- Hoffa's fat pad impingement syndrome: presents as diffuse oedema and fibrosis of the fat pad, not a discrete, lobulated mass.
- Synovial sarcoma: a malignant tumour that can contain calcifications but is typically more heterogeneous, invasive, and shows more solid enhancement.

Management and Prognosis

- Complete surgical excision is the standard of care due to the potential for local recurrence and mechanical symptoms.
- Arthroscopic excision is the preferred, minimally invasive approach for most lesions.
- The prognosis is excellent after complete excision.
- Recurrence rate is reported to be 10–20%, typically due to incomplete initial removal.
- Malignant transformation is extremely rare for soft tissue chondromas.

Suggested Reading

Albergo J, Gaston C, Davies M, et al. Hoffa's fat pad tumours: what do we know about them? International Orthopaedics (SICOT). 2013;37(11):2225–9.

O'Connell L, Memon AR, Foran P, Leen E, Kenny PJ. Synovial chondroma in Hoffa's fat pad: case report and literature review of a rare disorder. Int J Surg Case Rep. 2017;32:80–2.

Case 94

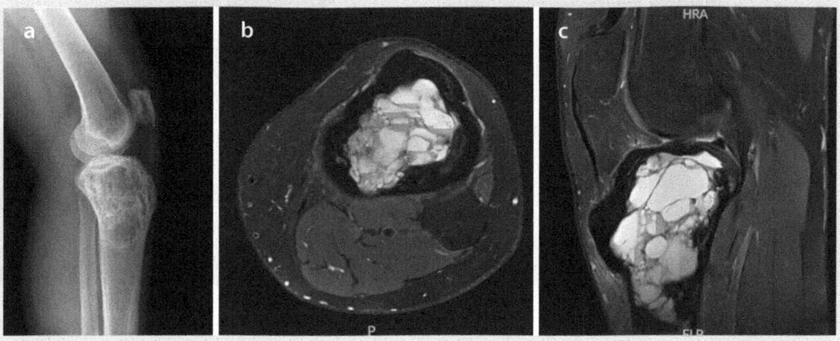

■ A 32-year-old female presented with a 4-month history of progressive pain and swelling in her right knee

S. Saran et al., *101 Knee Imaging Case Series*, 101 MSK Imaging 1,
https://doi.org/10.1007/978-3-032-21567-3_94

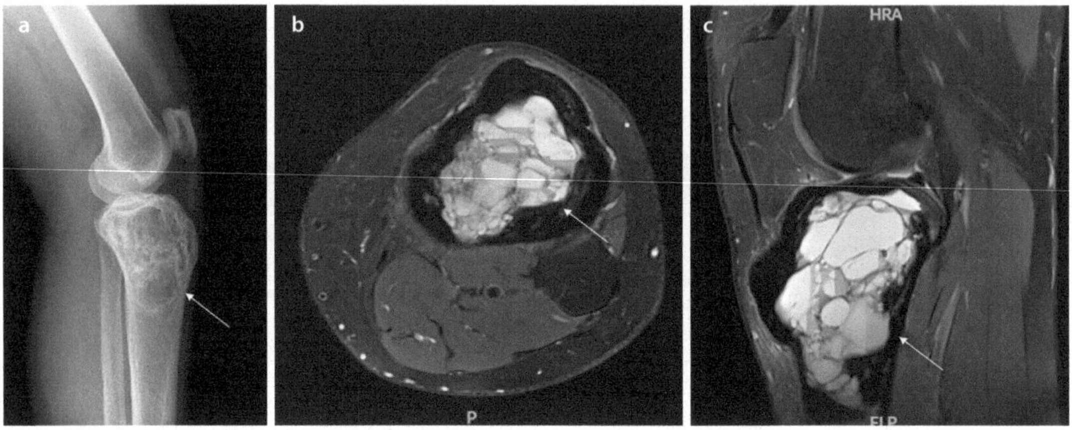

Lateral radiograph **a** shows a well-defined lytic sclerotic lesion (arrow) in the proximal tibia involving the metaphysis and epiphysis with subarticular extension, with a narrow zone of transition and no cortical breach. MRI PDFS weighted sequences axial **b**, and sagittal **c** show an expansile lesion (arrows) with endosteal scalloping in the epiphyseal-metaphyseal location with characteristic "fluid-fluid levels" indicative of secondary ABC changes. Provisional diagnosis was Giant cell tumour (GCT) with secondary ABC. Other differentials can be Brown tumour of hyperparathyroidism with secondary ABC. The biopsy came out to be GCT

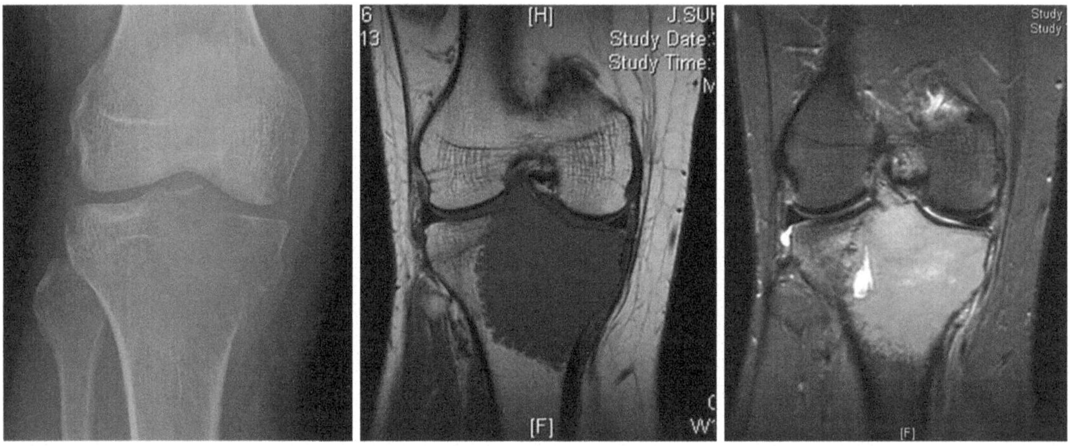

Companion case: GCT in proximal tibia

Giant Cell Tumour (GCT) with Secondary Aneurysmal Bone Cyst (ABC) Changes

Definition & Pathophysiology

- Giant cell tumour of bone is a locally aggressive, benign tumour composed of mononuclear stromal cells and numerous scattered, multinucleated osteoclast-like giant cells. The rapidly growing GCT is thought to cause an alteration in local haemodynamics (blood flow), leading to the formation of the secondary ABC components.
- ABC Changes: These are secondary, reactive changes within the primary tumour. They are characterised by blood-filled, cystic cavities separated by fibrous septae containing osteoclast-type giant cells and reactive bone.

Clinical Presentation

- Demographics: Typically occurs in skeletally mature adults aged 20–45 years. It is rare before the closure of the growth plate.
- Location: The proximal tibia is the second most common site after the distal femur. The tumour is almost always eccentric and subchondral, extending to the articular surface.
- Symptoms:
  - Progressive pain: often worse at night and with activity.
  - Swelling & tenderness: over the proximal, medial aspect of the tibia.
  - Limited range of motion: due to pain and proximity to the joint.
  - Pathologic fracture: a common presenting complication due to the bone's weakening.

Imaging Findings

The imaging appearance is a combination of features from both GCT and ABC.

- Radiography
  - A purely lytic, "soap-bubble" or multiloculated lesion.
  - Eccentric location in the metaphysis, extending to the subchondral bone.
  - Geographic bone destruction with a narrow zone of transition (well-defined, non-sclerotic margin).
  - ABC Changes: Can cause more rapid expansion and a more "blown-out" or "ballooned" appearance of the cortex.
- MRI
  - MRI is essential for visualising the "dual" nature of the lesion and its soft tissue extent.
  - Solid GCT component: T1-weighted: Intermediate to low signal intensity; T2-weighted/STIR: Heterogeneously low to intermediate signal is a key feature, as most tumours are bright on T2. This is due to the hemosiderin and collagen content.
  - Secondary ABC: fluid-fluid levels; a classic finding, seen within the cysts due to the layering of blood products of different densities. Best seen on T2-weighted images.
  - Post-contrast (T1 + C): The solid GCT components and septae enhance vividly, while the cystic ABC components do not enhance. This creates a characteristic "honeycomb" or "sponge-like" enhancement pattern.

Differential Diagnosis

- Brown tumour of hyperparathyroidism: Biochemically identical on histology, but patients have abnormal serum calcium and PTH levels.
- Telangiectatic osteosarcoma: A malignant tumour that can also have fluid-fluid levels. It typically has a more aggressive, permeative pattern of bone destruction.
- Chondroblastoma: Occurs in the epiphysis of skeletally immature patients and often has chondroid matrix calcification.

Management

- Primary treatment: Surgery is the mainstay of treatment for resectable GCT. The goal is to completely remove the tumour while preserving as much limb function as possible.
  - Intralesional curettage (with local adjuvants): This is the preferred and most common surgical procedure for GCT in the proximal tibia, especially when the joint can be preserved. Local adjuvants include phenol, liquid nitrogen and argon beam coagulation. The resulting cavity is then filled with bone graft, bone cement, or a synthetic bone substitute to restore strength and facilitate healing.
  - En bloc resection: This is reserved for very large, destructive tumours where curettage is not feasible, tumours with a pathological fracture that have compromised the joint surface and recurrent tumours that have failed previous curettage.
- The role of denosumab.
  - Denosumab is a monoclonal antibody that has revolutionised the management of GCT. It is not a cure, but a powerful tool used in specific scenarios.
  - Mechanism of action: GCT cells overexpress a protein called RANK Ligand (RANKL), which stimulates bone-destroying cells called osteoclasts. Denosumab binds to RANKL, inhibiting osteoclast activity, halting bone destruction, and even allowing for re-ossification.
  - It is used to reduce tumour size before surgery. It induces re-ossification of the bony shell, making the tumor less fragile. This can convert an unresectable tumour to a resectable one or allow for a less morbid curettage instead of a resection.
  - For tumours that are inoperable due to location, size, or patient comorbidities, denosumab can be used as a long-term control therapy to suppress tumour growth and prevent complications.
  - It is also the standard treatment for metastatic GCT.
- Other applicable drug therapies: While denosumab is the primary systemic drug for GCT, other options exist, typically used when denosumab is not suitable or has failed.
  - Bisphosphonates (e.g., zoledronic acid): These are anti-resorptive drugs that also inhibit osteoclasts, but through a different pathway than denosumab.
  - Interferon-alpha: An immunomodulatory agent that was historically used for advanced or metastatic GCT.

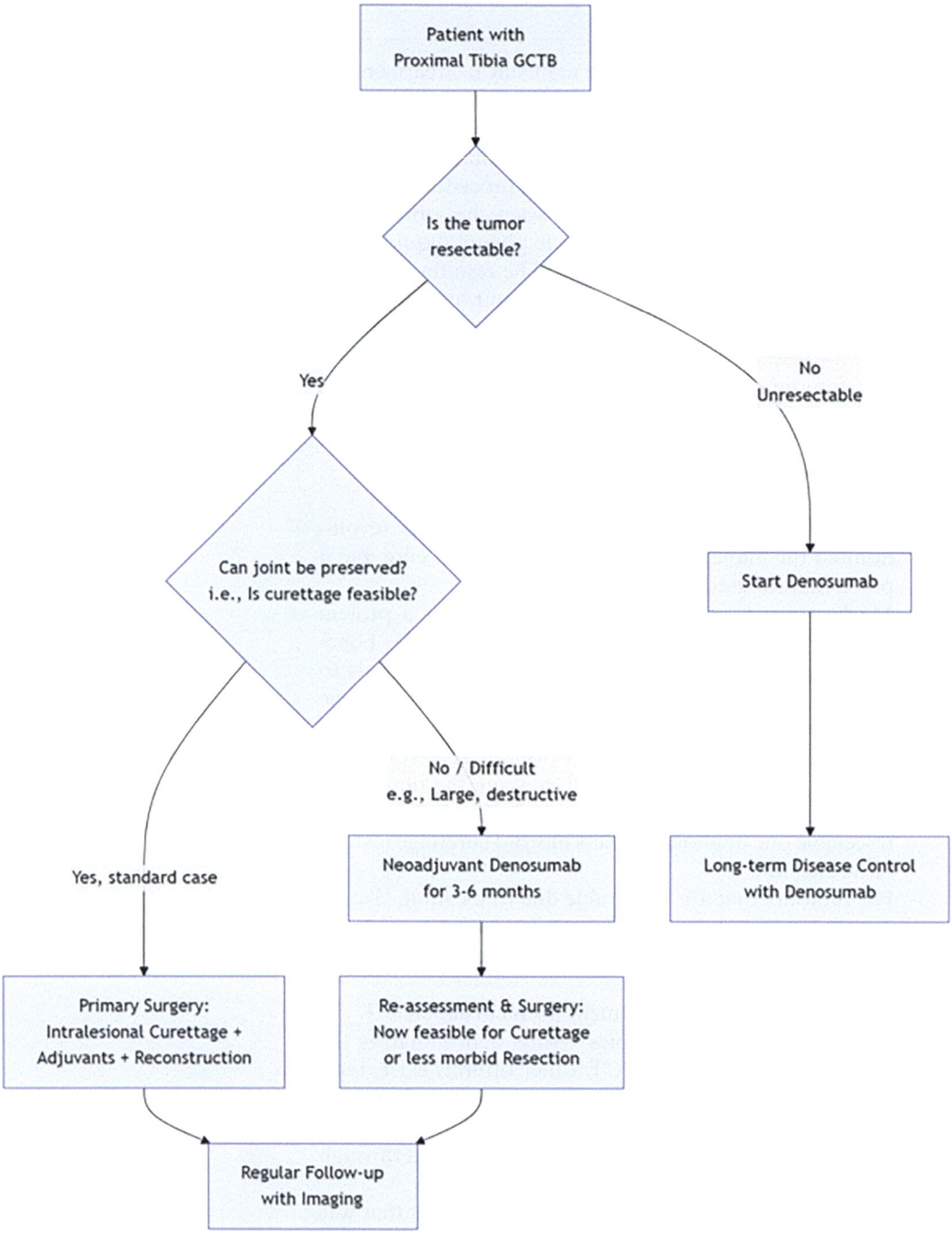
Patient with
Proximal Tibia GCTB
Is the tumor
resectable?
Yes
No
Unresectable
Can joint be preserved?
i.e., Is curettage feasible?
Start Denosumab
No / Difficult
e.g., Large, destructive
Yes, standard case
Neoadjuvant Denosumab
for 3-6 months
Long-term Disease Control
with Denosumab
Primary Surgery:
Intralesional Curettage +
Adjuvants + Reconstruction
Re-assessment & Surgery:
Now feasible for Curettage
or less morbid Resection
Regular Follow-up
with Imaging

Suggested Reading

Alhulaimi Y, AlAbbasi KK, AlShaya OS, Alrawaf TN, Aldosari NH, Zogel B. Giant cell tumor with secondary aneurysmal bone cyst in the left distal humerus: a case report. Cureus. 2024;16(7):e65507.

Guhan TVR, Raghav RV, Kumar MM, Vanchi PK. Giant cell tumor of intermediate cuneiform evolving into aneurysmal bone cyst: a rare case report. J Orthop Case Rep. 2021;11(9):12–5.

Case 95

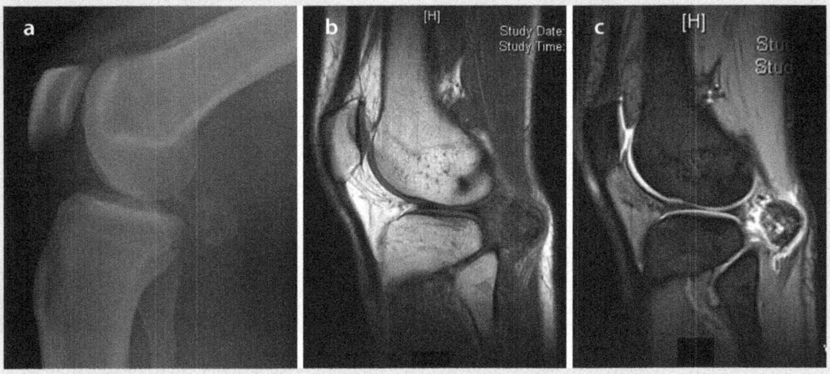

■ A 22-year-old football player presented with a 5-week history of a painful, firm mass in the back of his right knee. The pain and stiffness are now limiting his ability to run and fully flex his knee

S. Saran et al., *101 Knee Imaging Case Series*, 101 MSK Imaging 1,
https://doi.org/10.1007/978-3-032-21567-3_95

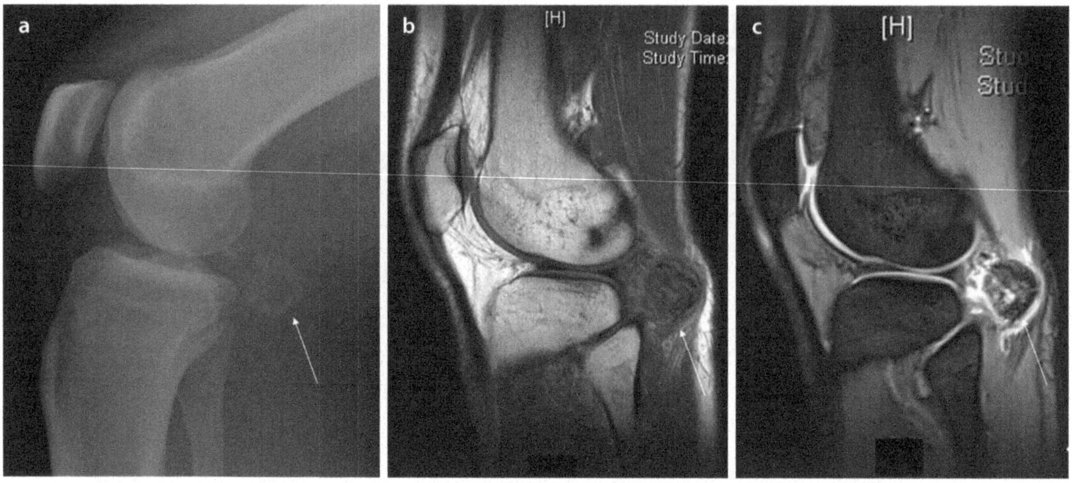

■ Lateral radiograph **a** shows fluffy, cloud-like density (arrow) with poorly defined margins in the popliteal fossa, separate from the femur and tibia with a characteristic "zonal phenomenon" beginning to form (more mature, dense periphery and a less dense, immature centre). MRI sagittal T1 **b**, T2 gradient echo **c** shows the lesion appearing heterogeneously hypointense on the T1-weighted sequence **b** and showing blooming on the GRE **c** sequence. Clinical differentials with the provided clinical history are: (1) Myositis ossificans. (2) Soft tissue sarcoma (e.g., synovial sarcoma, extraskeletal osteosarcoma). (3) Popliteal (baker's) cyst. (4) Post-traumatic hematoma with organisation and calcification. The diagnosis based on the imaging shown will be myositis ossificans

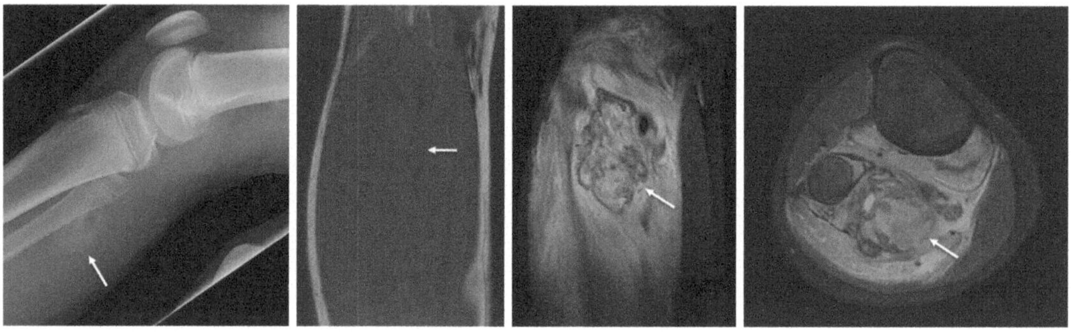

■ Companion case: Myositis ossificans in the proximal aspect of the posterior compartment of the leg

Myositis Ossificans

Definition & Pathophysiology

- Myositis ossificans (MO), now more accurately termed heterotopic ossification, is a benign, self-limiting process characterised by the formation of mature bone in soft tissue (typically muscle) outside the skeletal periosteum. When it occurs in the popliteal fossa, it can cause significant symptoms due to the confined neurovascular anatomy.
- Mechanism: Typically triggered by trauma (single significant injury or repetitive microtrauma) or, less commonly, occurs spontaneously. The process involves a reactive, inflammatory proliferation of fibroblasts and osteoblasts within the muscle.
  - Key feature: zonal phenomenon; the lesion matures in a distinct pattern:
  - Central zone: immature, highly cellular fibroblastic tissue.
  - Intermediate zone: osteoid formation (immature bone).
  - Peripheral zone: mature, lamellar bone with a well-defined cortical rim.
  - This "outside-in" maturation is a critical diagnostic clue.

Clinical Presentation

- A history of trauma is common, though not always recalled. Symptoms develop over weeks.
- Deep, aching pain in the back of the knee.
- A firm, often tender palpable mass.
- Progressive and painful loss of joint movement.
- Neurological symptoms.

Imaging Findings

Imaging evolution is pathognomonic and crucial for avoiding misdiagnosis as a sarcoma.

- Radiography
  - Weeks 2–4: May be normal or show a faint, fluffy soft tissue density.
  - Weeks 4–6: Peripheral "eggshell" calcification appears, forming a well-defined rim around the lesion. This is the classic sign.
  - Months 3–6: The calcification matures into trabecular bone with a clear, radiolucent centre, maintaining a clear cleavage plane from the underlying femur.

- CT
  - Clearly demonstrates the zonal architecture before it is visible on X-ray.
  - Shows the peripheral rim of mineralisation with a central non-mineralised, low-attenuation core.
  - Confirms the lesion is separate from the bone cortex, a key feature distinguishing it from a parosteal osteosarcoma.
- MRI
  - While its appearance can be confusing and mimic a sarcoma in the early stages, the key is to correlate with the clinical timeline.
  - Early Stage (0–4 weeks):
    - T1-weighted: isointense to muscle.
    - T2-weighted/PDFS: Diffuse, intense hyperintensity with surrounding muscle inflammation. May show a "fluid-fluid level" from haemorrhage.
    - T1 + C: Intense, heterogeneous enhancement.
    - This early appearance is highly aggressive and can be mistaken for a soft tissue sarcoma.
  - Mature stage (>6–8 weeks):
    - The peripheral rim becomes a low-signal intensity border on all sequences (representing the mature bony rim).
    - The central zone remains heterogeneous but becomes more defined.

Differential Diagnosis

- Extraskeletal osteosarcoma: A malignant tumour that calcifies in a reverse zonal pattern—most mature, organised bone is in the centre, with disorganised, immature tissue at the periphery. It lacks a clear cleavage plane from the bone.
- Parosteal osteosarcoma: Attached to the underlying cortex without a clear cleavage plane and has a heavily ossified base.
- Synovial Sarcoma: Often calcified (30% of cases), but calcifications are more central or peripheral in a stippled pattern, not in a mature rim.
- Popliteal artery aneurysm: A pulsatile mass that can calcify. Ultrasound or CT angiography is diagnostic.
- Pigmented villonodular synovitis (PVNS): Can extend posteriorly but does not calcify; it shows a low T2 signal due to hemosiderin.

Management

- Conservative management
  - Observation: The natural history is spontaneous maturation and often gradual regression. Many lesions become asymptomatic.
  - Rest & NSAIDs.
  - Physical therapy: Gentle, passive range of motion is encouraged, but aggressive manipulation is avoided as it can worsen inflammation and ossification.
- Medical management
  - Bisphosphonates (e.g., Etidronate) can be used in the early phase to block mineralisation, but they do not prevent the initial osteoblastic proliferation.
- Surgical intervention indicated in:
  - Persistent, significant pain unresponsive to conservative care.
  - Neurovascular compression.
  - Crucial timing: Surgery must be delayed until the lesion is radiographically mature (indicated by a well-defined bony rim on CT and decreased activity on a bone scan). Excision during the active phase carries a very high risk of recurrence.

Suggested Reading

Wang H, Nie P, Li Y, Hou F, Dong C, Huang Y, Hao D. MRI findings of early myositis ossificans without calcification or ossification. Biomed Res Int. 2018;2018:4186324.

Werenski JO, Hung YP, Chang CY, Nielsen GP, Lozano-Calderón SA. Myositis ossificans mimicking bone surface osteosarcoma: case report with literature review. APMIS. 2024;132(8):535–43.

Case 96

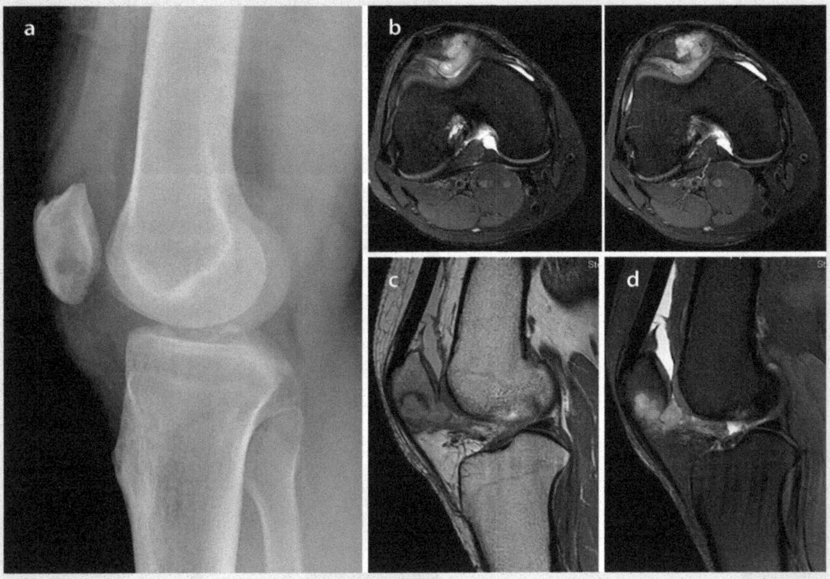

A 33-year-old female presented with pain and swelling in the lower pole of the patella

S. Saran et al., *101 Knee Imaging Case Series*, 101 MSK Imaging 1,
https://doi.org/10.1007/978-3-032-21567-3_96

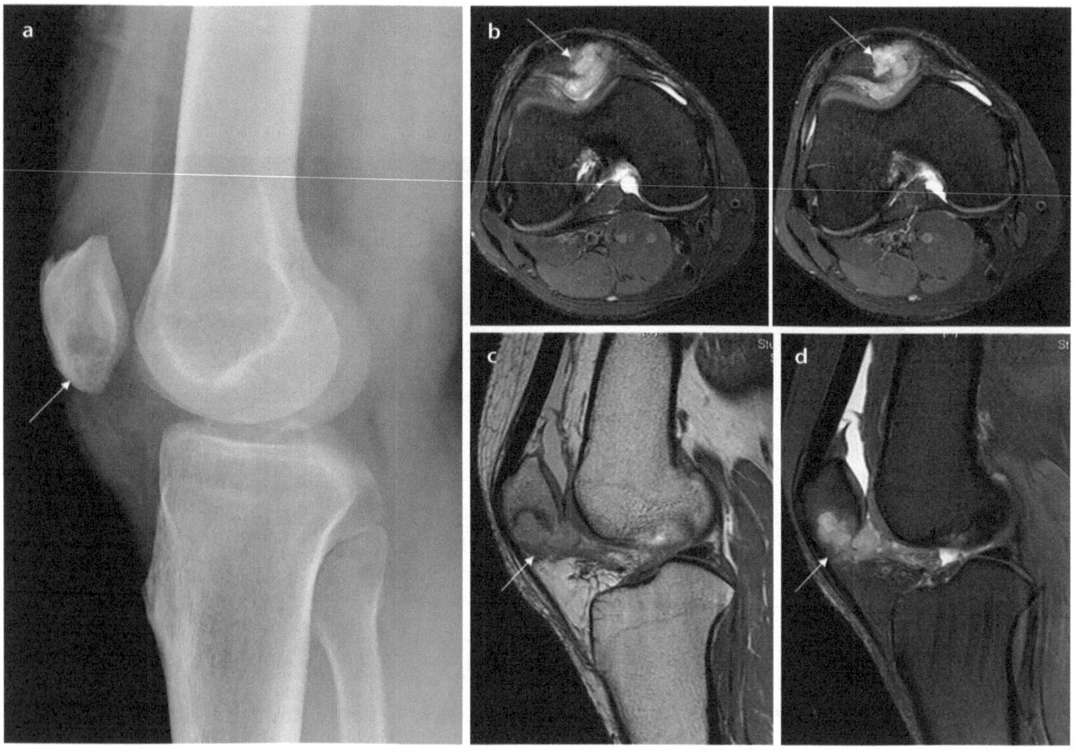

Lateral radiograph of knee **a** shows the presence of an ill-defined osteolytic area affecting the lower pole of the patella (arrow) with soft tissue opacity in Hoffa's fat pad. MRI **b**–**d** shows the lesion (arrows) as a hyperintense area on PDFS axial **b** and sagittal **d** sequences, and iso to hyperintense on T2-weighted sagittal sequence **c**. Aspiration analysis revealed Mycobacterium tuberculosis

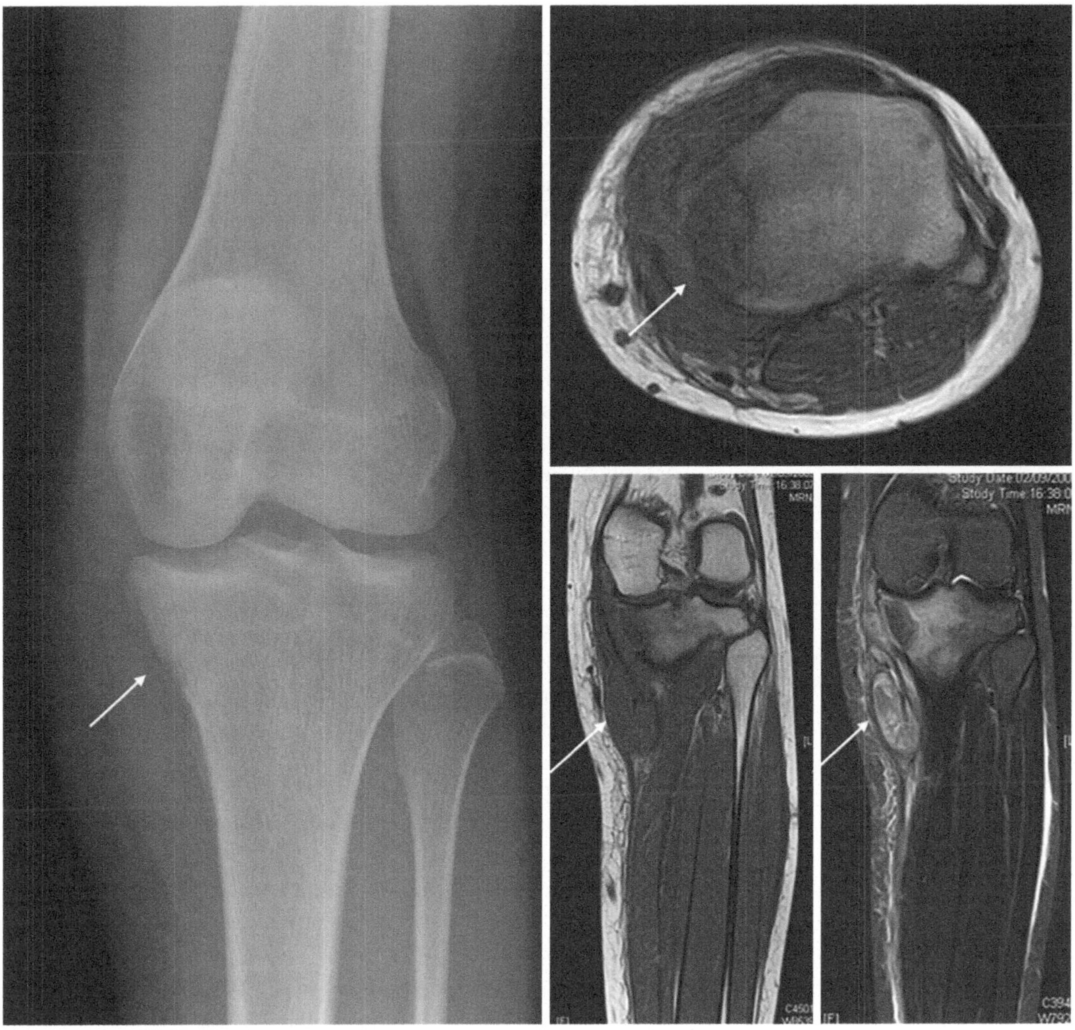

Companion case: Tuberculosis of the medial tibial condyle with extra-osseous abscess (arrows)

Tuberculosis of the Patella

Definition & Pathophysiology

- Tuberculosis (TB) of the patella, also known as tuberculous osteomyelitis, is a rare form of skeletal TB caused by hematogenous spread of mycobacterium tuberculosis from a primary focus (often pulmonary). The patella is an uncommon site, accounting for <1% of all skeletal TB cases.
- Pathogenesis: The bacilli lodge in the highly vascular cancellous bone of the patella. This triggers a cell-mediated immune response, leading to the formation of caseating granulomas. Enzymes released by the granulomas cause osteolysis and can spread to the adjacent joint, causing tuberculous arthritis.

Clinical Presentation

- Demographics: More common in children and young adults in endemic areas. Can occur in immunocompromised individuals.
- Symptoms (insidious onset):
  - Chronic anterior knee pain and swelling, developing over weeks to months.
  - Local warmth and tenderness over the patella.
  - Joint effusion: if the TB has spread to the knee joint.
  - Limited range of motion due to pain and swelling.
  - "Cold abscess": a painless fluctuant swelling without signs of acute inflammation may be present. A sinus tract can form if it drains to the skin.

Imaging Findings

- Imaging reveals a destructive process, but findings are often non-specific and can mimic a tumour.
- Radiography
  - Early stage: may be normal or show osteopenia.
  - Established disease: shows a lytic lesion with ill-defined, "geographic" margins.
  - Multiple, small, interconnected lytic areas creating a "woven" or "spongy" appearance.
  - Periosteal reaction is minimal or absent.
  - Sequestrum: a small, dead piece of bone may be seen within the lytic area.
  - Late stage: can show near-total destruction of the patella.

- MRI
  - MRI is superior for evaluating the bone marrow, soft tissue, and joint involvement.
  - Bone marrow oedema and destruction in the patella.
  - Soft tissue involvement: a cold abscess appears as a fluid collection with a thick, enhancing wall.
  - Synovitis: thickened, enhancing synovium if there is associated tuberculous arthritis of the knee joint.

Differential Diagnosis

- Chronic pyogenic osteomyelitis: can appear identical. History and culture are key differentiators.
- Brodie's abscess: a localised subacute pyogenic infection that is well-circumscribed with a sclerotic rim.
- Giant cell tumour of bone: a lytic, expansile lesion in a skeletally mature patient, but it is typically not painful and lacks systemic features.
- Metastasis: rare in the patella; usually in older patients with a known primary cancer.

Diagnosis

Aspiration/biopsy: definitive diagnosis requires identification of the bacilli. Cartridge-Based Nucleic Acid Amplification Test (CBNAAT/GeneXpert) is used for rapid diagnosis and detection of rifampicin resistance.

Management

Treatment involves a combination of anti-tubercular chemotherapy and, in some cases, surgery.

Suggested Reading

Khan A, Amedu OS, Kumar P, Chukwurah A, Kolawole OA, Unedu OR. Tuberculosis of patella complicated by synovitis of knee joint: a case report. Cureus. 2022;14(4):e24618.

Khezami K, Bennour MA, Basssalah E, Lahssini W, Brahim NB, Annabi H. Primary patella tuberculosis mimicking pre-patellar bursitis: a case report and review of the literature. Int J Surg Case Rep. 2021;86:106367.

Case 97

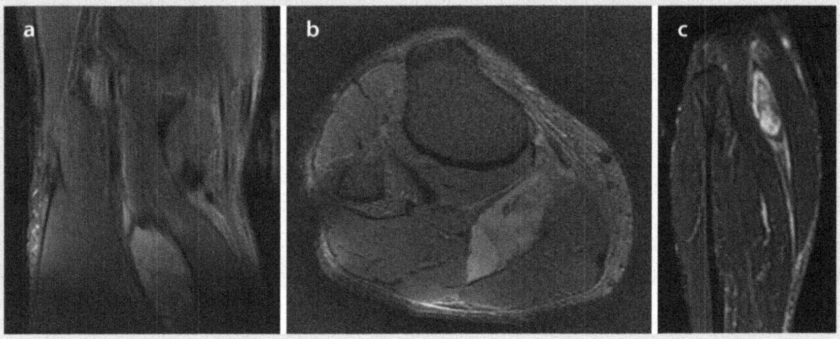

A 62-year-old presented with pain and swelling around the posteromedial leg region

S. Saran et al., *101 Knee Imaging Case Series*, 101 MSK Imaging 1,
https://doi.org/10.1007/978-3-032-21567-3_97

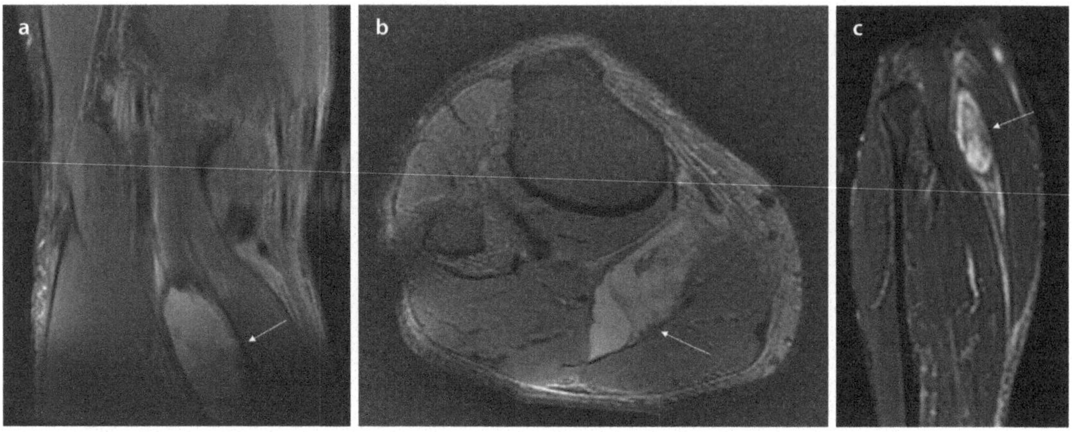

■ MRI knee STIR coronal **a**, and axial **b** sequences show the presence of a well-defined hyperintense area between the medial head of gastrocnemius and soleus muscle (arrow). MRI leg STIR coronal **c** shows the collection as a hyperintense area (arrow) with cranio-caudal extension

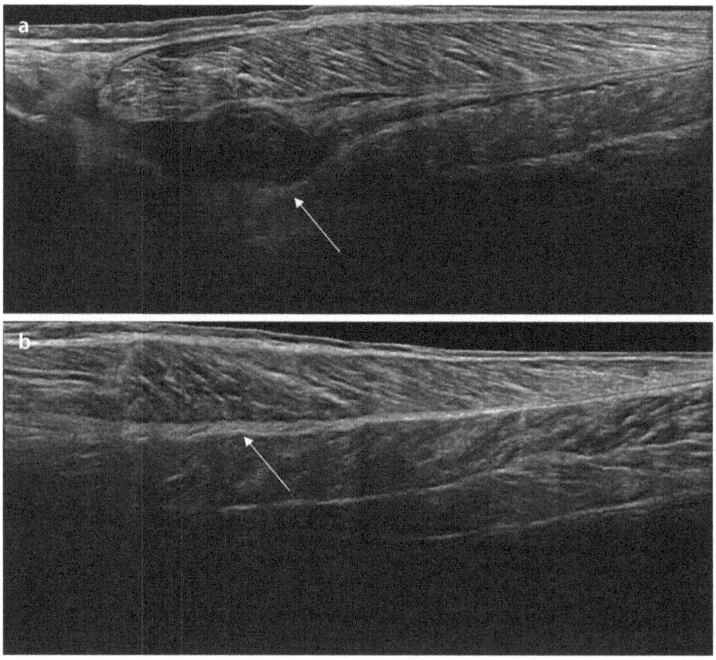

■ Ultrasound leg in the same patient demonstrates the presence of an organised collection between the medial head of gastrocnemius and soleus muscle **a**. **b** The normal contralateral leg shows a normal myotendinous junction of the medial head of gastrocnemius (arrow). Imaging findings are highly suggestive of Tennis leg

Tennis Leg

Definition & Pathophysiology

- Tennis Leg is a clinical diagnosis referring to an acute, painful injury at the musculotendinous junction of the medial head of the gastrocnemius, often involving a partial tear.
- Classically, it was thought to represent a rupture of the plantaris tendon, but modern imaging has shown this to be rare; the primary pathology is tearing of the medial gastrocnemius muscle fibres.
- Mechanism: A sudden, forceful eccentric contraction of the gastrocnemius muscle with the knee extended and the ankle dorsiflexed. This commonly occurs during a sudden push-off, a lunge, or jumping.

Clinical Presentation

- Classic history: a middle-aged "weekend warrior" who feels a sudden, sharp pain or a "pop" in the mid-calf during a sporting activity (e.g., tennis, racquetball, basketball).
- Can also occur in old age from sudden movements, even during daily activities.
- Symptoms: immediate pain and difficulty bearing weight.
- Physical exam:
  - Tenderness localised to the medial aspect of the mid-calf, at the gastrocnemius muscle belly.
  - Swelling and ecchymosis that may track down into the ankle and foot over several days.

Imaging Findings

- Imaging is not always necessary, but it is used to confirm the diagnosis, assess the extent of injury, and rule out more serious conditions like a deep vein thrombosis (DVT).
- Ultrasound
  - Can visualise the tear in real-time and assess muscle retraction with movement.
  - A fluid-filled gap (hematoma) between the medial gastrocnemius and the underlying soleus muscle.
  - Architectural disruption and hypoechoic oedema within the medial gastrocnemius fibres.

- MRI
  - MRI provides exquisite detail of the muscle injury and is crucial for excluding other pathologies.
  - T2-weighted/STIR: Pathognomonic finding is the presence of fluid signal (high intensity) interposed between the medial head of the gastrocnemius and the soleus muscle.

Differential Diagnosis

- Baker's cyst rupture: presents with posterior knee and proximal calf pain. Anatomic location on imaging is different from the tennis leg.
- Achilles tendon rupture.
- Deep vein thrombosis (DVT).
- Plantaris tendon rupture.

Management

- Acute phase (first 48–72 hours)
  - Optimal loading with ice and compression.
- Rehabilitation phase (subacute to recovery)
  - Physical therapy: the cornerstone of treatment.
  - Stretching: gradual, gentle stretching of the gastrocnemius-soleus complex.
  - Strengthening: progressive exercises, starting with isometrics, then concentric, and finally eccentric strengthening.
  - Gait training: to restore a normal walking pattern.
  - Gradual return to activity: typically, over 4–8 weeks, depending on severity.

Suggested Reading

Dai M, Liu X, Liu X, Yang L, Duan D. Diagnosis and follow-up MRI evaluation of tennis leg:New understanding of the pathogenesis and imaging. Injury. 2021;52(11):3355–61.

Shah JR, Shah BR, Shah AB. Pictorial essay: ultrasonography in 'tennis leg'. Indian J Radiol Imaging. 2010;20(4):269–73.

Case 98

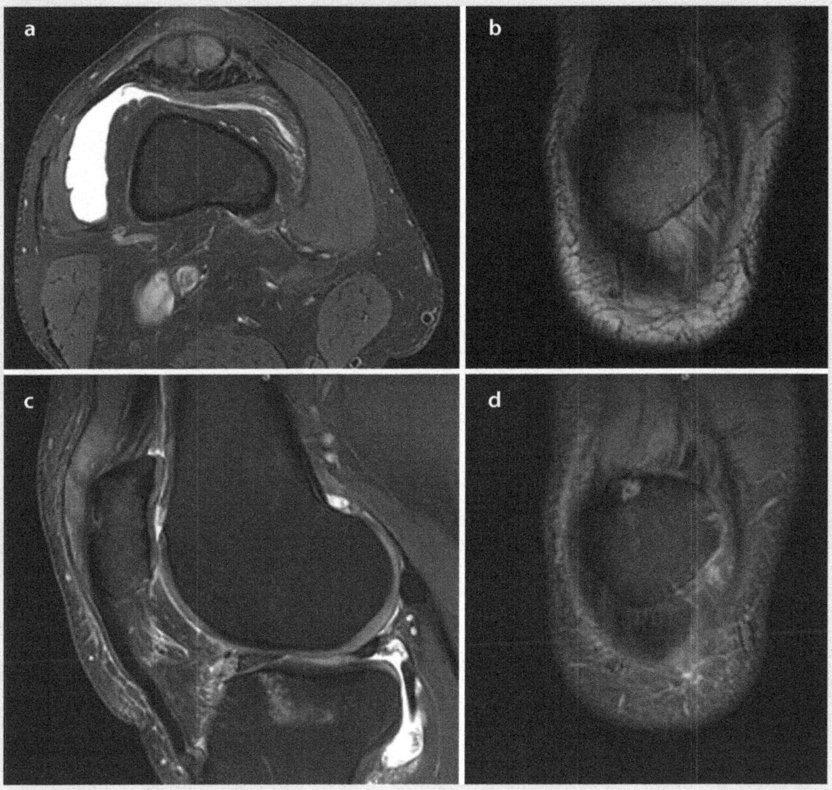

■ A 51-year-old male presented with a slightly painful soft tissue lump at the superior pole of the patella and limited range of motion in the joint. The patient has been admitted with alcohol overconsumption for many years and has had previous arthritic attacks in the feet

S. Saran et al., *101 Knee Imaging Case Series*, 101 MSK Imaging 1,
https://doi.org/10.1007/978-3-032-21567-3_98

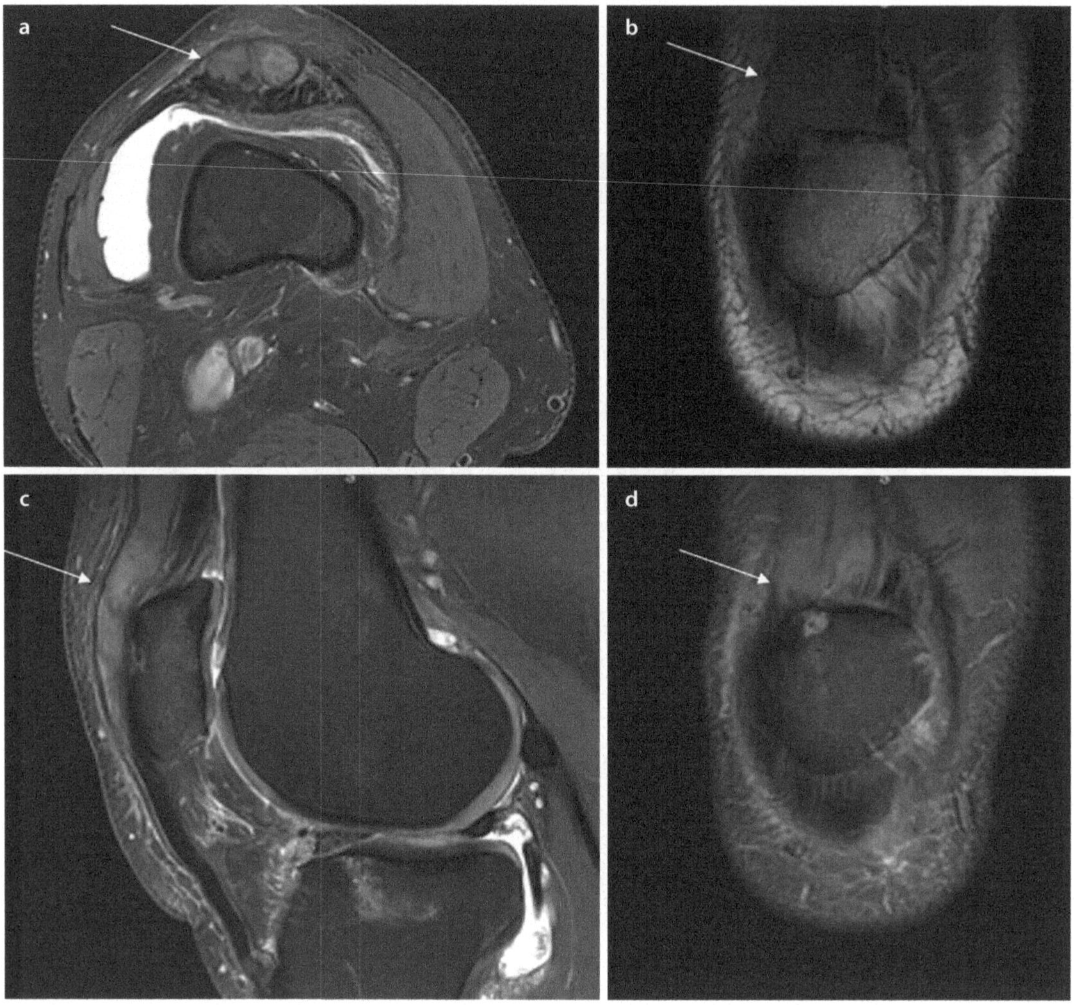

■ MRI of the left knee (PDFS axial **a**, T1 coronal **b**, PDFS sagittal **c** and coronal **d** shows a soft tissue mass (arrow) within the distal quadriceps extending anteriorly and inferiorly into the superior aspect of the patella. The mass is heterogeneously hypointense on PDFS weighted sequences **a**, **c**, **d** and hypointense on the T1-weighted sequence **b**. The clinical and imaging findings suggested tophaceous gout, which was confirmed by biopsy showing monosodium urate crystals

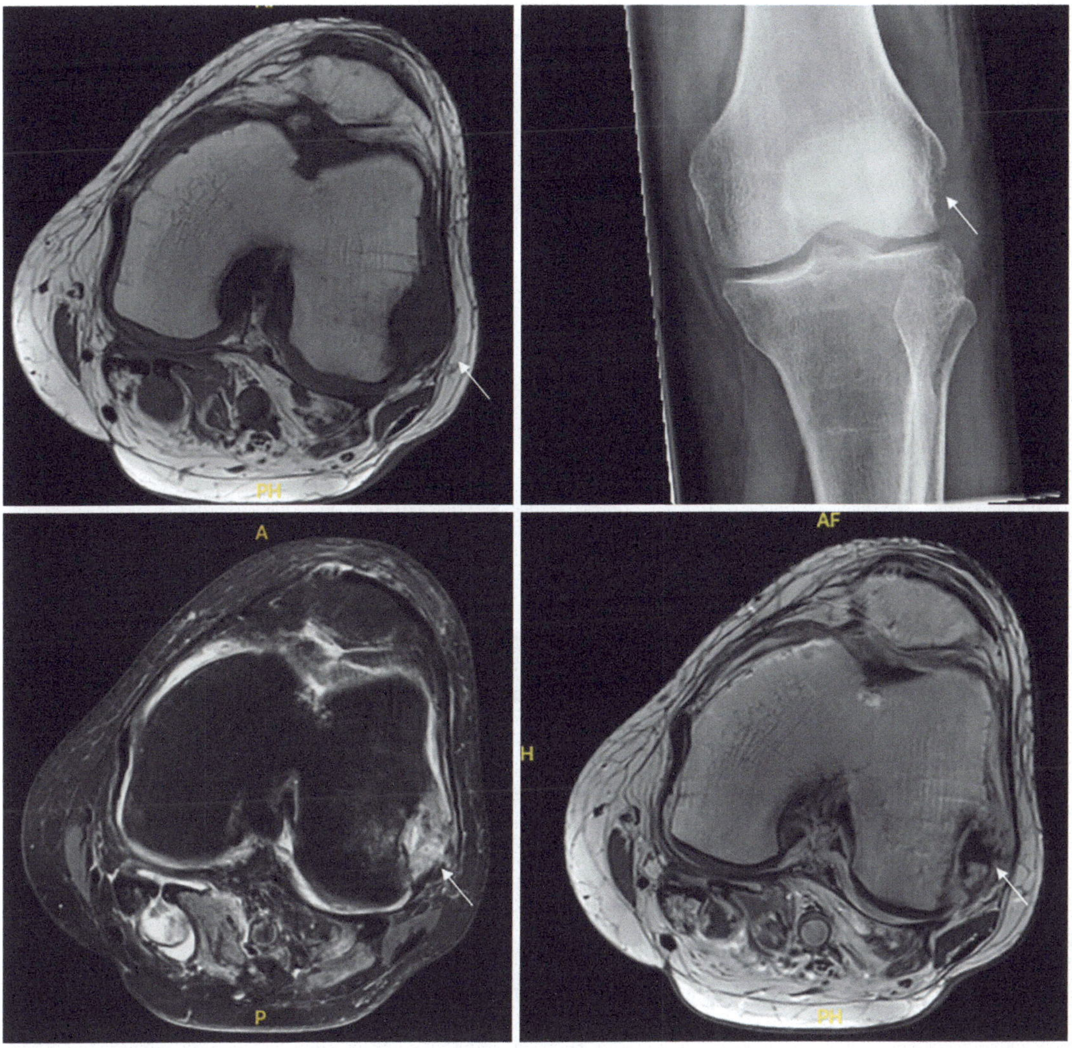

Companion case: Gouty tophus involving popliteal hiatus (arrows)

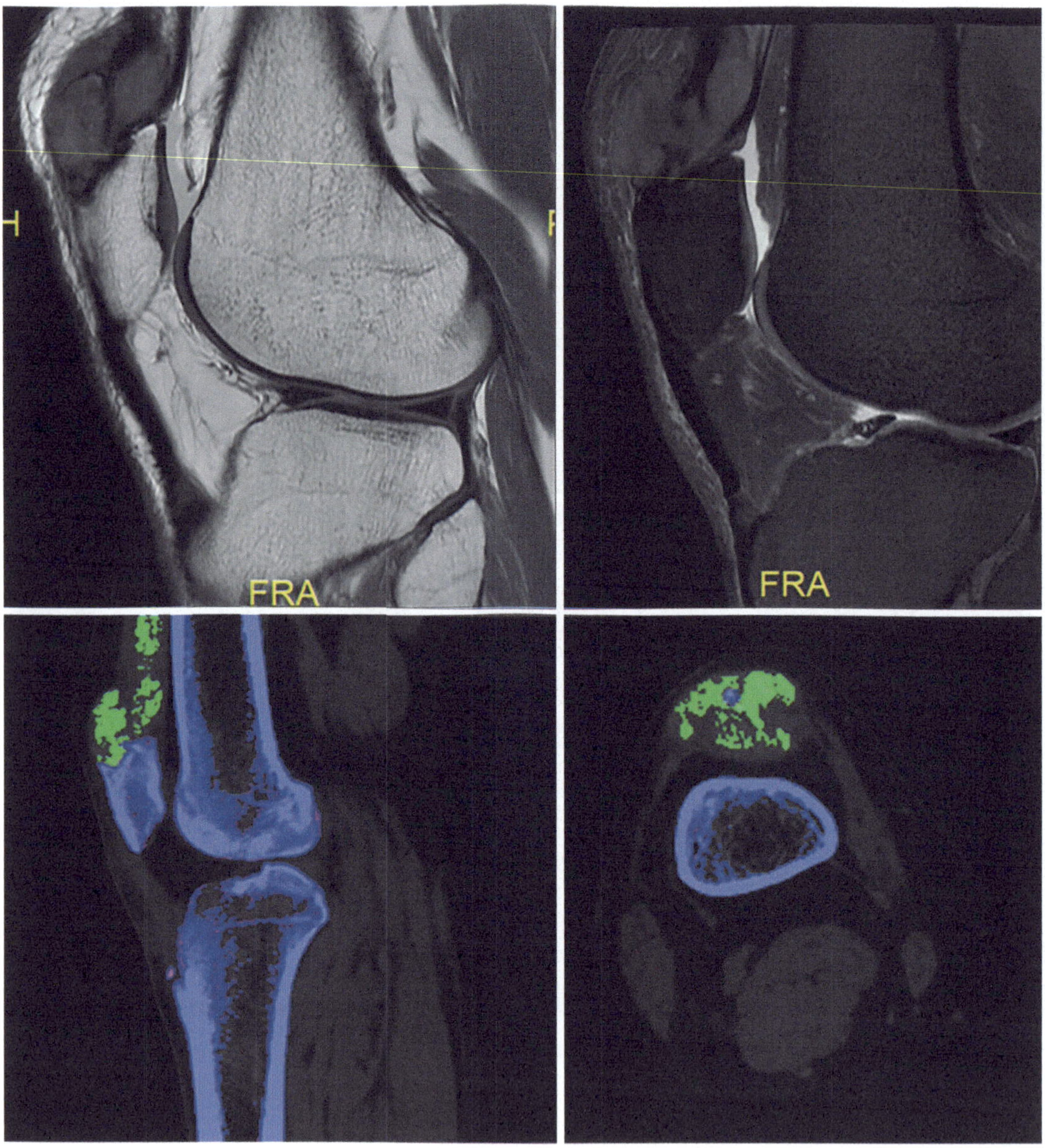

▪ Companion case: Another case of gout involving the extensor mechanism with dual-energy CT highlighting the monosodium urate crystals

Tophaceous Gout of the Extensor Mechanism of the Knee

Definition & Pathophysiology

- Tophaceous gout is the chronic, advanced stage of gout characterised by the deposition of monosodium urate (MSU) crystals in soft tissues, bones, and joints, forming destructive, inflammatory masses known as tophi.
- Mechanism: Chronic hyperuricemia leads to the supersaturation of body fluids with uric acid, resulting in the crystallisation of MSU. These crystals are deposited in soft tissues, bones, and joints, forming destructive, inflammatory masses known as tophi.
- In the knee, these tophi are most commonly deposited in the extensor mechanism.

Clinical Presentation

- Typically, middle-aged to elderly males with a long history of poorly controlled gout.
- Pain: chronic, often dull ache over the anterior knee. It can be acutely painful during a "gout flare".
- Palpable mass: firm, sometimes chalky, subcutaneous nodules or diffuse thickening of the tendon.
- Stiffness & limited motion: difficulty with full knee flexion or extension.
- Skin changes: tophi can erode through the skin, leading to draining sinuses and a white, pasty discharge (urate crystals).

Complications

- Tendon weakness or rupture: due to infiltration and destruction of collagen fibres.
- Patellar bone destruction: intraosseous tophi can cause significant osteolysis.
- Secondary infection.

Imaging Findings

Imaging is crucial for diagnosis, as the presentation can mimic a tumour or infection.

- Radiography
  - "Punched-out" erosions: well-defined, sclerotic-marginated lytic lesions in the patella or adjacent bones.
  - "Overhanging edge" sign: a classic sign where a rim of bone projects over the erosion.
  - Preserved joint space: unlike inflammatory arthritis, the joint space is often preserved until very late stages.
  - Soft tissue swelling & calcification: amorphous cloud-like soft tissue densities due to calcified tophi.
- Ultrasound
  - "Double-contour" sign: a hyperechoic line of MSU crystals on the surface of the articular cartilage.
  - Tophus appearance: hyperechoic, heterogeneous masses with an anechoic halo. May show posterior acoustic shadowing.
  - Tendon involvement: shows hyperechoic foci within the quadriceps or patellar tendon, disrupting the normal fibrillar architecture.
- MRI
  - T1-weighted: low to intermediate signal intensity.
  - T2-weighted/PDFS: heterogeneously low to intermediate signal intensity. This is a key feature—most masses (tumours, infections) are hyperintense on T2, but tophi are low-signal due to their crystalline structure and fibrosis.
  - T1-weighted post-contrast: solid, heterogeneous enhancement of the tophus and surrounding synovium due to the intense inflammatory reaction.
- Dual-energy computed tomography (DECT) is a relatively recent development in the imaging of gouty arthritis. DECT is a non-invasive method for the visualisation, characterisation and quantification of monosodium urate crystal deposits, which aids the clinician in the early diagnosis, treatment and follow-up of this condition.

Differential Diagnosis

- Pigmented villonodular synovitis (PVNS): Also shows low T2 signal due to hemosiderin.
- Amyloid deposition: can be identical on MRI; requires clinical history (renal failure) or biopsy.
- Synovial sarcoma: A malignant tumour that may contain calcifications and show triple sign on MRI.
- Xanthoma: Associated with hyperlipidemia, but MRI signal is often brighter on T2.

- Infection (e.g., tuberculosis): Can cause erosions and soft tissue masses, but typically has more surrounding marrow oedema, collection and lymphadenopathy.

Management

- Medical management
  - Goal: Reduce serum uric acid to <6 mg/dL (or < 5 mg/dL for severe tophaceous gout).
  - Allopurinol or Febuxostat (XOI inhibitors).
  - Probenecid (Uricosuric).
  - Acute flare management: Colchicine, NSAIDs, or corticosteroids.
- Surgical management: Surgery is adjunctive to medical therapy, not a replacement. Indications:
  - Tendon rupture or impending rupture.
  - Large, painful, or disabling tophi limiting function.
  - Recurrent infection or sinuses.
  - Neurovascular compression.

Suggested Reading

Kester C, Wallace MT, Jelinek J, Aboulafia A. Gouty involvement of the patella and extensor mechanism of the knee mimicking aggressive neoplasm. A case series. Skeletal Radiol. 2018;47(6):865–9.

Vansevenant M, Vanhoenacker FM, Catry F. Tophaceous gout of the extensor mechanism of the knee. J Belg Soc Radiol. 2015;99(1):93–4.

Case 99

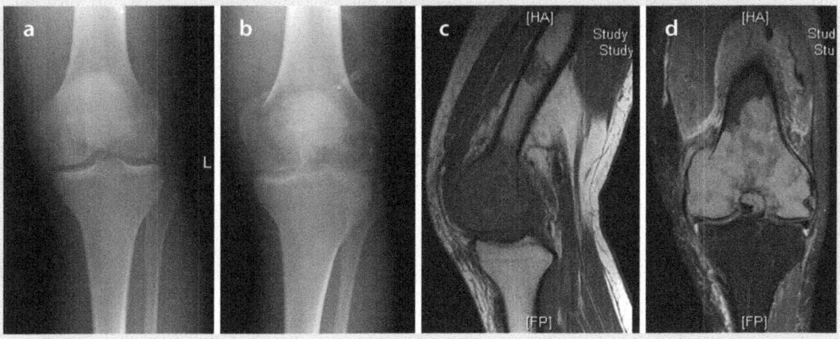

■ A 55-year-old male presented with pain in the knee joint. The second radiograph is obtained 1 month after the first radiograph

S. Saran et al., *101 Knee Imaging Case Series*, 101 MSK Imaging 1,
https://doi.org/10.1007/978-3-032-21567-3_99

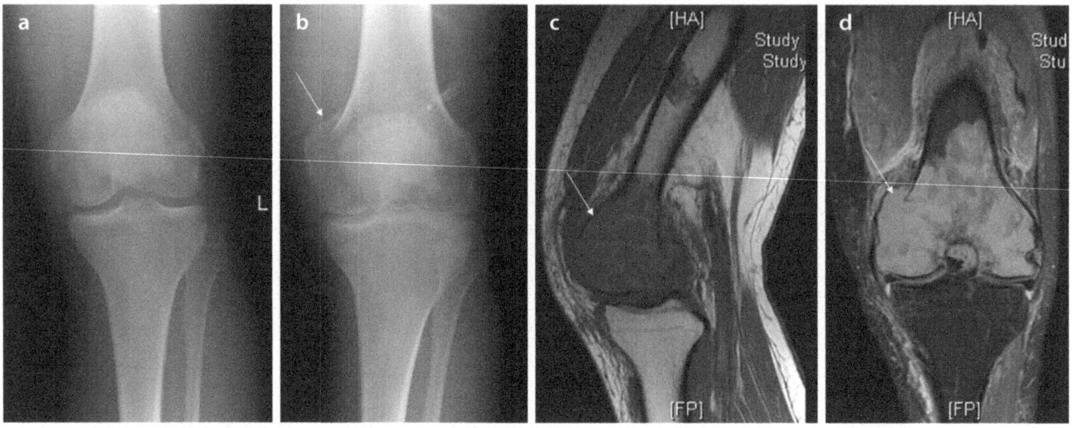

Anteroposterior radiographs **a**, **b** show a rapidly progressing osteolytic lesion in the distal femur with a wide zone of transition and a pathological fracture (arrow). MRI Knee **c**, **d** shows the presence of a diffusely infiltrative lesion (arrows) involving the distal femur metaphyseal and epiphyseal region, showing hypointense signals on T1-weighted sagittal **c** and hyperintense signals on T2FS coronal sequences **d**. Imaging findings represent the possibility of a rapidly progressing neoplastic aetiology. Histopathology turned out to be lymphoma

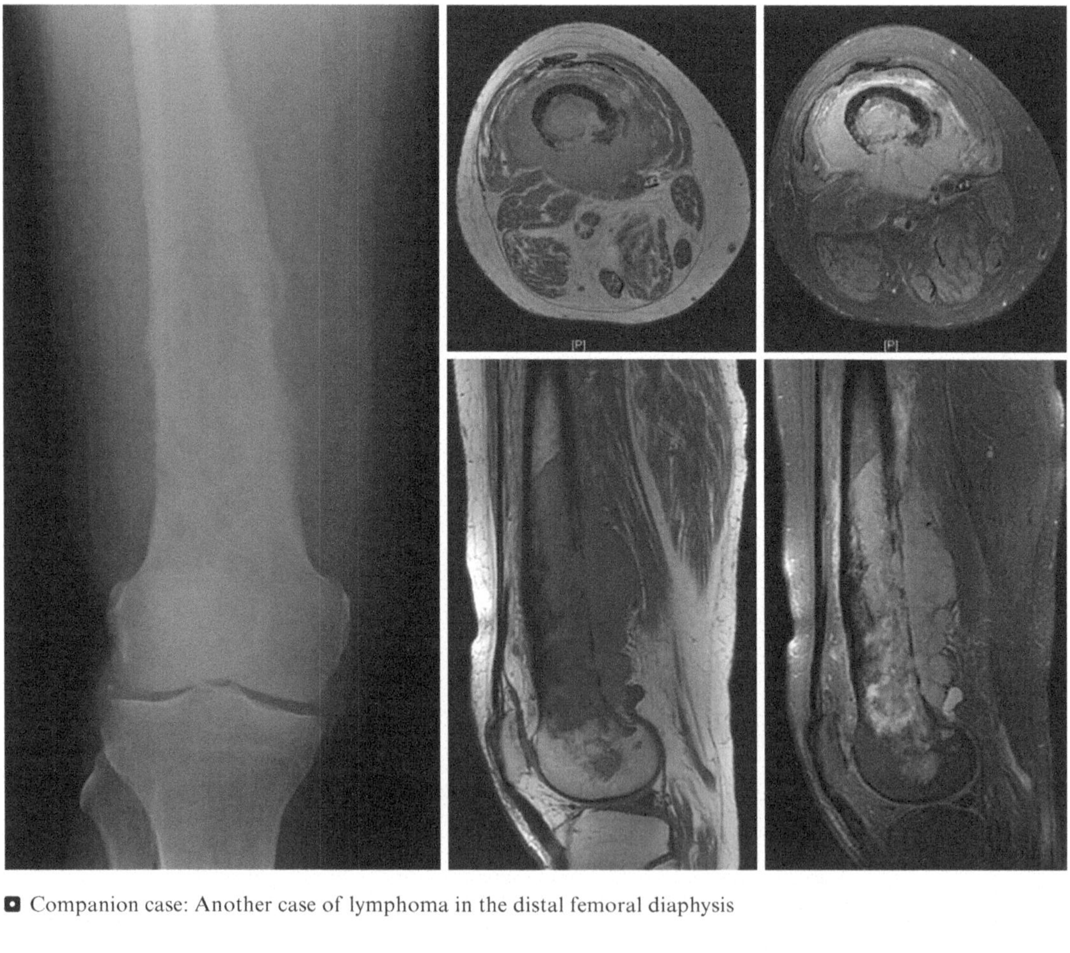

Companion case: Another case of lymphoma in the distal femoral diaphysis

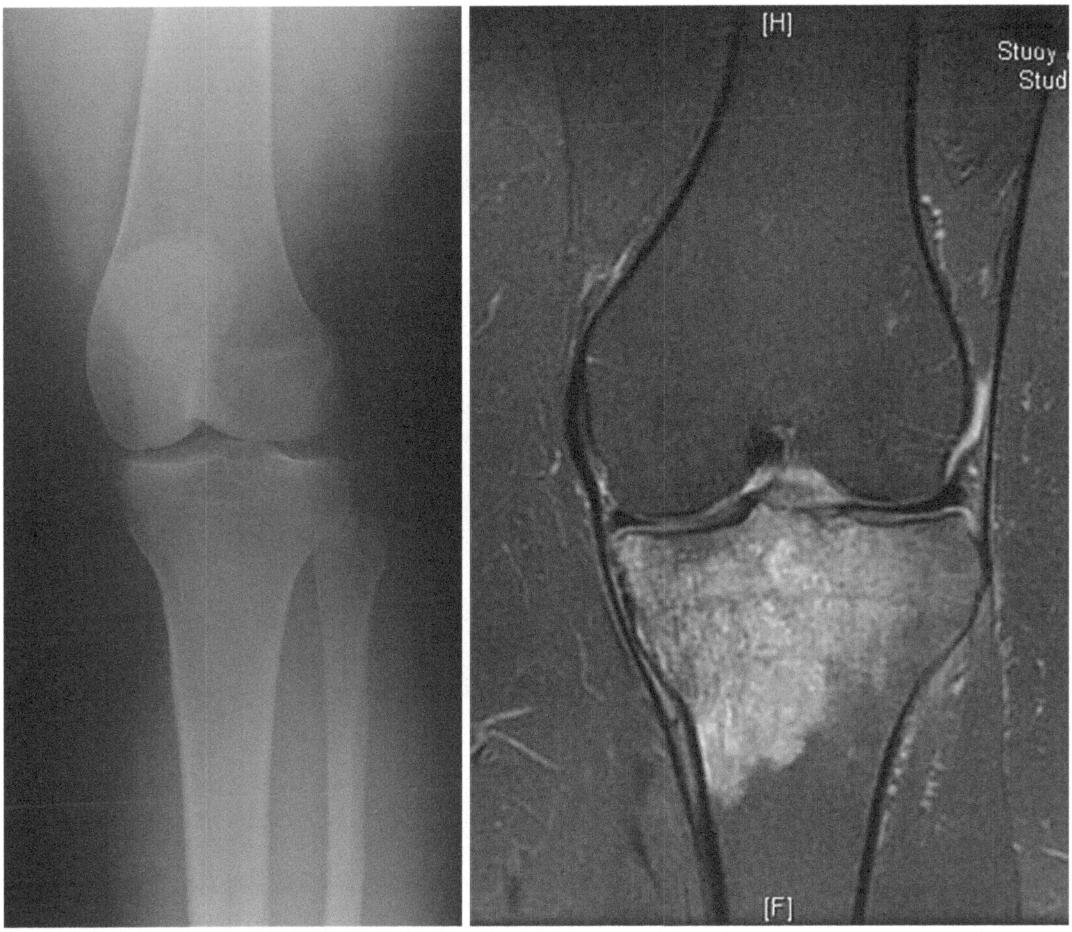

Companion case: Another case of lymphoma in the proximal tibial epi-metaphysis

Primary Bone Lymphoma

Definition & Pathophysiology

- Primary bone lymphoma (PBL) is a rare malignant tumour consisting of lymphomatous cells that arises within the bone marrow, with no evidence of systemic nodal or extranodal involvement at the time of diagnosis. Over 90% of cases are Diffuse Large B-Cell Lymphoma (DLBCL).
- The soft tissue component is often disproportionately large compared to the degree of bone destruction.

Clinical Presentation

- Demographics: Most common in adults aged 40–60, with a slight male predominance.
- Location: The femur (especially the metaphysis/diaphysis) is the most common site, followed by the pelvis and spine.

Symptoms

- Persistent, dull, aching pain at the site, often worse at night. This is the most common symptom.
- Palpable mass or swelling.
- Pathologic fracture occurs in ~20% of cases.
- "B" Symptoms (fever, night sweats, weight loss) are uncommon in true PBL, as its definition requires the absence of systemic disease.

Imaging Findings

- Radiography
  - A permeative or "moth-eaten" pattern of bone destruction with a wide zone of transition. A large soft tissue mass may be visible.
  - The degree of bone destruction is often less dramatic than the large associated soft tissue mass.
- MRI
  - MRI is crucial for defining the full extent.
  - T1-weighted: The tumour is homogeneously hypointense to muscle, completely replacing the normal bright fatty marrow.
  - T2-weighted/STIR (fat-saturated): The tumour is heterogeneously hyperintense. The extensive bone marrow involvement and large soft tissue mass are clearly visible.
  - T1-weighted post-contrast: Shows intense, homogeneous enhancement of the tumour and soft tissue mass.
  - Diffusion-weighted imaging (DWI): Shows markedly restricted diffusion, a characteristic feature of highly cellular tumours like lymphoma.
  - Classic MRI triad for PBL:
    - Permeative bone lesion.
    - Large, surrounding soft tissue mass.
    - Relative preservation of the bony architecture despite the massive soft tissue component.

- FDG-PET/CT (crucial for systemic staging)
  - The primary bone lesion shows intense FDG avidity.
  - It is the best modality to confirm the "primary" nature of the disease by ruling out other skeletal or nodal involvement.

Differential Diagnosis

- Fibrosarcoma: can be indistinguishable from lymphoma on imaging. However, a large soft tissue mass as compared to the osseous component favours lymphoma.
- Metastatic carcinoma: More common in older patients. Often multiple, but a solitary metastasis can be indistinguishable. A known primary cancer is the key.
- Ewing sarcoma: The main differential in younger patients (<30). It can appear identical, but Ewing's is rare in patients over 30.
- Osteosarcoma: Typically shows tumour bone (osteoid) formation ("cloud-like" mineralisation), which is absent in lymphoma.
- Multiple myeloma: Also a "punched-out" lytic lesion in an older adult, but it is typically more purely lytic and less likely to have a large soft tissue mass.

Diagnosis

- Core needle biopsy: mandatory for diagnosis. The tissue must be sent for histology, immunohistochemistry (e.g., CD20, CD3, CD45), and flow cytometry to confirm the subtype (usually DLBCL).

Management

- PBL is highly sensitive to both chemotherapy and radiation. Treatment is primarily non-surgical and requires a multidisciplinary team (Oncology, Radiation Oncology).
- Regimen: R-CHOP (Rituximab, Cyclophosphamide, Doxorubicin, Vincristine, Prednisone) is the standard for DLBCL.
- Surgical intervention: for pathologic fracture.

Sugeested Reading

Duffy P, Ecklund K. MR features of primary bone lymphoma in children. Pediatr Radiol. 2023;53(12):2400–10.

Winn J, Stock H. Primary lymphoma of bone. Conn Med. 2015;79(3):173–5. PMID: 26244226.

Case 100

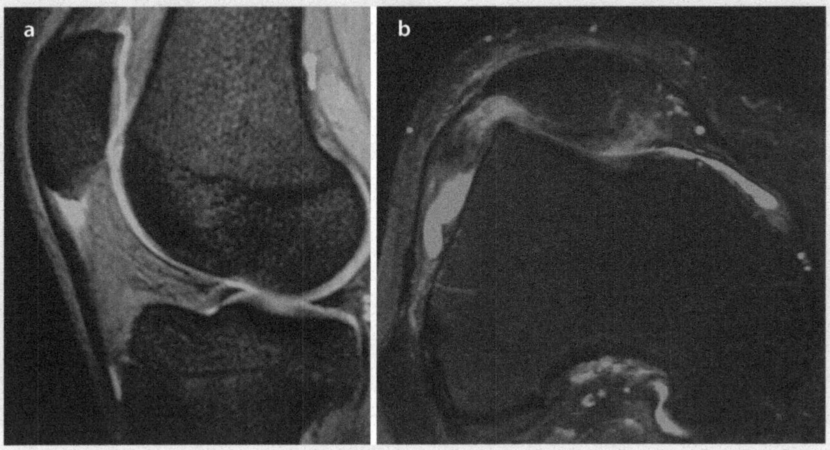

A 27-year-old male presented with anterior knee pain exacerbated by hyperextension and point tenderness at the inferior pole of the patella

S. Saran et al., *101 Knee Imaging Case Series*, 101 MSK Imaging 1,
https://doi.org/10.1007/978-3-032-21567-3_100

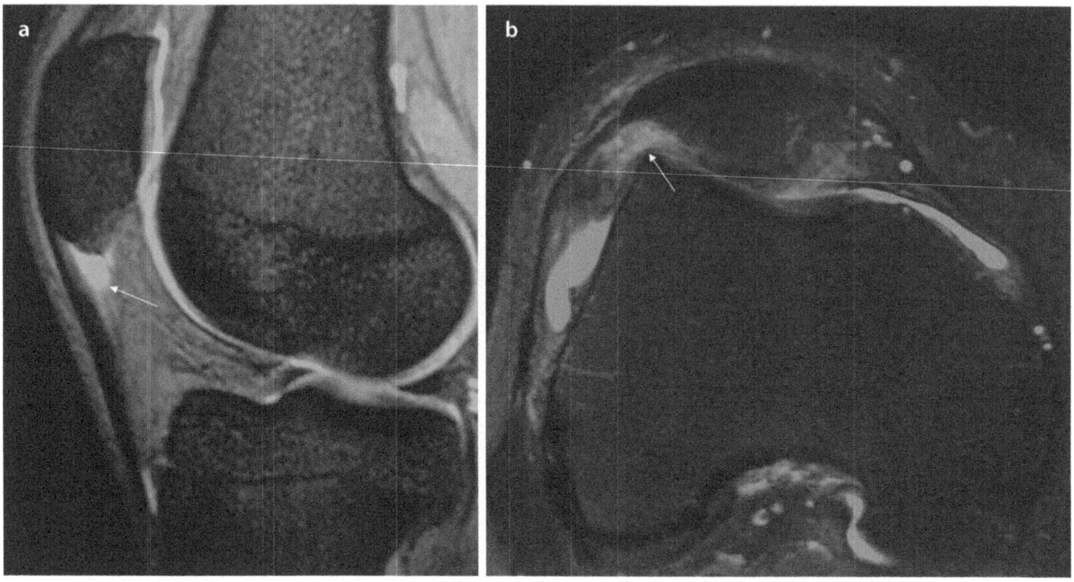

MRI knee sagittal T2 gradient echo **a**, and PDFS axial **b** show the presence of a focal area of high signal intensities (arrows) at the superolateral aspect of the Hoffa's fat pad between the inferior pole of the patella and lateral femoral condyle, appearances are of Patellar tendon-lateral femoral condyle friction syndrome or Hoffa's fat pad impingement syndrome or Hoffa's disease

Patellar Tendon-Lateral Femoral Condyle Friction Syndrome, or Hoffa's Fat Pad Impingement Syndrome, or Hoffa's Disease

Definition & Pathophysiology

- It is thought to be due to patellar maltracking or imbalance of the forces between the medial and lateral vastus muscles, causing impingement of the superolateral aspect of the Hoffa's fat pad between the inferior patella and the lateral femoral condyle.
- This repetitive microtrauma leads to inflammation, swelling, and oedema within the fat pad, leading to progressive fibrosis and scarring.

Clinical Presentation

- Pain location: anterior knee pain, deep to the patellar tendon. Pain is often localised to the inferior and/or lateral aspects of the patella.
- Aggravating factors: full knee extension, hyperextension, prolonged standing, and descending stairs.

- Hoffa's test (hyperextension test): pain is reproduced when the clinician presses on the fat pad just adjacent to the patellar tendon and then passively hyperextends the patient's knee.

MRI Findings

- The diagnosis is confirmed on MRI by the presence of oedema within the superolateral aspect of the Hoffa's fat pad between the inferior pole of the patella and the lateral femoral condyle.

Management

- Conservative: activity modification and physical therapy.
- Ultrasound-guided corticosteroid injection: into the fat pad to break the cycle of inflammation.
- Surgical (refractory cases): arthroscopic debridement.

Suggested Reading

Dragoo JL, Johnson C, McConnell J. Evaluation and treatment of disorders of the infrapatellar fat pad. Sports Med. 2012;42(1):51–67.

Saddik D, McNally EG, Richardson M. MRI of Hoffa's fat pad. Skeletal Radiol. 2004;33(8):433–44.

Case 101

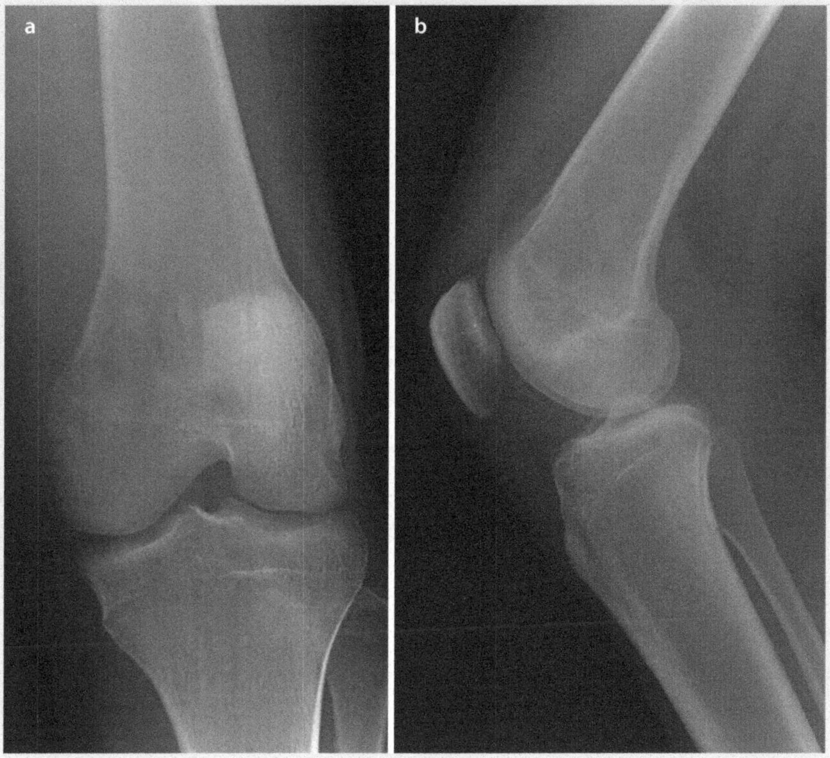

■ A 24-year-old male presented with a 6-week history of progressive, deep-seated pain with swelling in his left knee

S. Saran et al., *101 Knee Imaging Case Series*, 101 MSK Imaging 1,
https://doi.org/10.1007/978-3-032-21567-3_101

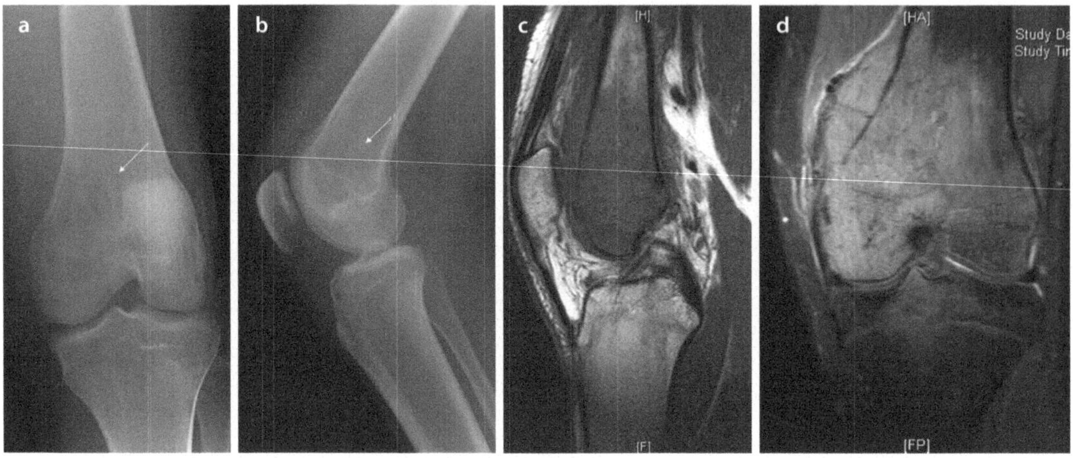

Radiographs anteroposterior **a**, and lateral **b** show a permeative, purely lytic lesion (arrows) in the metaphysis of the distal femur, extending to the subchondral bone with a wide "zone of transition" between the lesion and normal bone and no evidence of any matrix mineralisation within the lesion. The differentials on the radiograph will be: (1) Osteosarcoma (lytic variant) (2) Giant cell tumour of bone (3) Ewing's sarcoma (4) Osteomyelitis (5) Metastatic disease (less likely at this age). MRI shows an ill-defined lesion appearing hypointense on the T1-weighted sagittal sequence **c**, replacing marrow and hyperintense on the T2 FS coronal sequence **d**, with breach in the cortex and extra-osseous extension. Considering the age and imaging findings, the possibility of Osteosarcoma and Ewing's sarcoma appears most likely. The histopathology revealed osteosarcoma

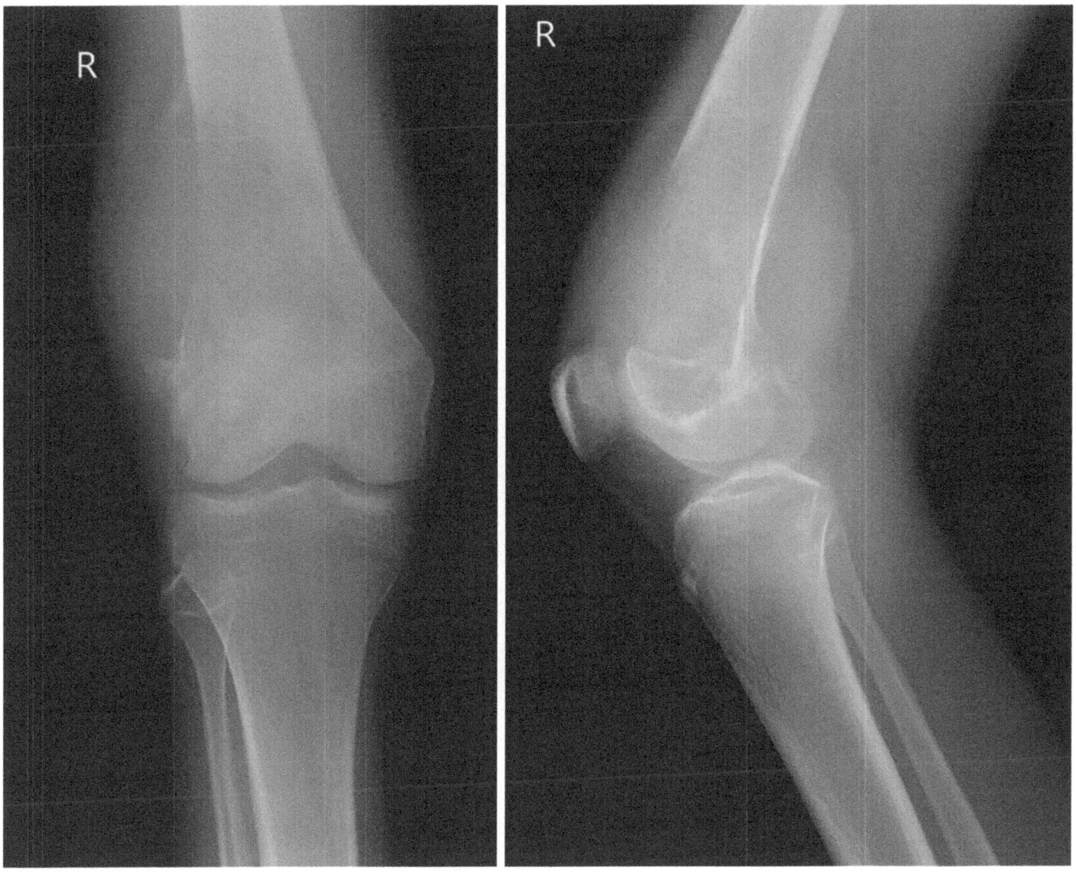

Companion case: An adolescent male with a mass in the distal thigh. Radiograph shows a lytic lesion with a wide zone of transition in the distal femoral metaphysis with osseous matrix and Codman angle type of aggressive periosteal reaction, along with soft tissue extension, appearance are of conventional osteosarcoma

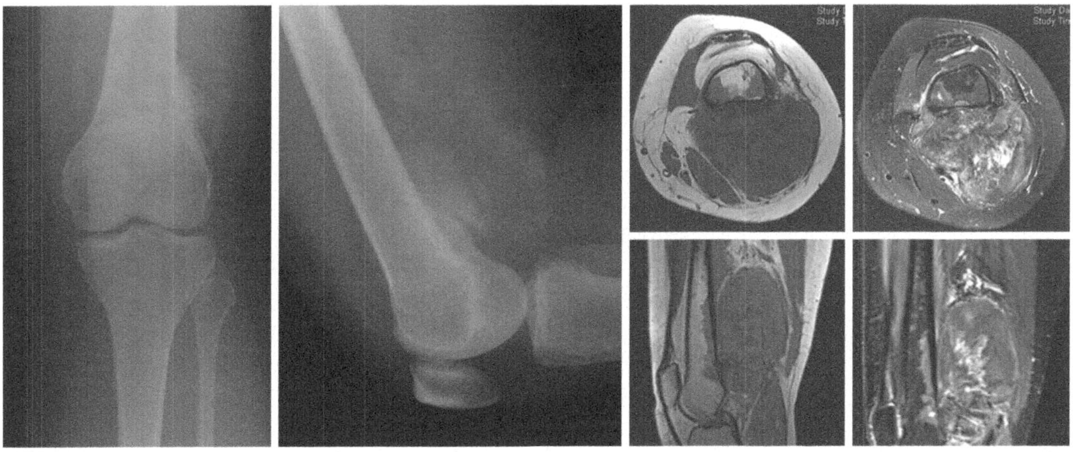

Companion case: Another case of conventional osteosarcoma of the distal femur with "sunburst" type of periosteal reaction and osseous matrix

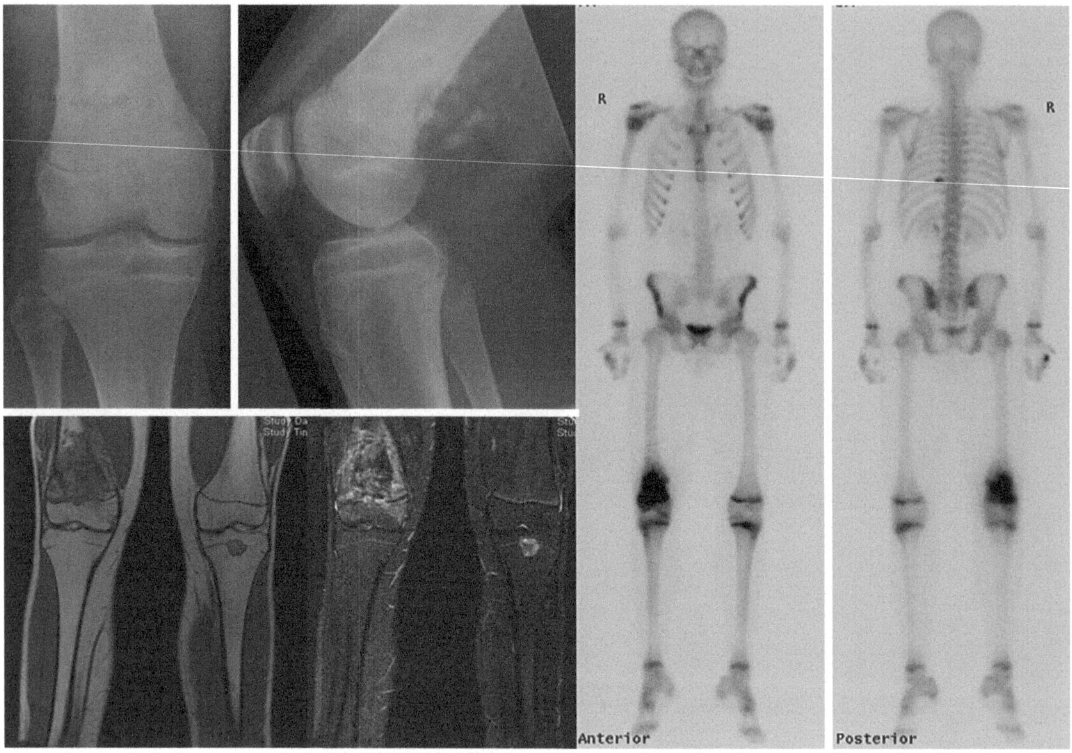

▪ Companion case: Osteoarcoma right distal femur with contralateral tibial metastasis

Lytic Variant of Osteosarcoma

Definition & Pathophysiology

- The lytic variant of osteosarcoma is a highly aggressive malignant bone tumour characterised by predominant bone destruction with little to no visible osteoid formation on imaging. It represents a histologic subtype where the malignant cells produce minimal matrix, leading to its purely destructive appearance.
- The classic "cloud-like" or "fluffy" opacities of tumour bone seen in conventional osteosarcoma are absent or minimal. This makes it one of the most challenging bone tumours to diagnose radiographically, as it mimics other purely lytic lesions.
- Despite the lack of radiographically visible matrix, histology confirms the diagnosis by revealing sarcomatous (spindle-shaped) stroma and the production of malignant osteoid (even in small quantities), which is the definitive diagnostic feature.

Clinical Presentation

- Age & location: similar to conventional osteosarcoma, it most commonly affects adolescents and young adults in the metaphysis of long bones (especially distal femur, proximal tibia, proximal humerus).
- Symptoms:
  - Pain: progressive, deep, aching pain, often worse at night and not relieved by rest.
  - Swelling: a palpable, often tender mass.
  - Pathologic fracture: a common presenting symptom due to the extensive bone destruction.
  - Systemic symptoms: weight loss and fever can occur in advanced stages.

Imaging Findings

- Radiography
  - Purely lytic (moth-eaten/permeative pattern) area with a wide zone of transition.
  - Cortical destruction: aggressive erosion, breakthrough, and often a large soft tissue mass.
  - Lack of sclerosis: the absence of the typical "cloud-like" osteoid matrix is the key differentiator from conventional osteosarcoma.
  - Periosteal reaction: may show aggressive patterns like a "sunburst" or, more classically, a Codman's triangle.
- CT
  - Confirms the extensive bone lysis and cortical destruction.
  - May reveal subtle matrix mineralisation not visible on X-ray.
  - Excellent for staging the chest to look for pulmonary metastases.
- MRI: MRI is essential to define the true intramedullary extent and the soft tissue component with neurovascular involvement, skip lesions and joint involvement.
  - T1-weighted: The tumour is heterogeneously low to intermediate signal intensity, replacing the normal bright fatty marrow.
  - T2-weighted/PDFS: The lesion is heterogeneously hyperintense. Areas of haemorrhage or necrosis can create fluid-fluid levels.
  - Post-contrast (T1 + C): Shows marked, heterogeneous enhancement of the viable tumour tissue.
  - Soft tissue mass: a large, enhancing soft tissue mass is almost always present, a critical feature that helps distinguish it from benign lytic lesions.

Differential Diagnosis

The purely lytic appearance leads to a broad differential diagnosis, which is why biopsy is mandatory.

- Giant cell tumour of bone (GCT): A purely lytic lesion that is subchondral and occurs in skeletally mature patients (20–40 years). It has a narrow zone of transition, unlike the permeative pattern of a lytic osteosarcoma.
- Telangiectatic Osteosarcoma: A specific subtype that is also purely lytic and cystic, often with prominent fluid-fluid levels on MRI.
- Metastasis (e.g., from renal or thyroid cancer): Especially in older patients. A known primary cancer is the key.
- Lymphoma of bone: can be purely lytic and permeative, often with a large soft tissue mass disproportionate to the bone destruction.
- Ewing sarcoma: also occurs in children/young adults, and is characterised by lytic and permeative lesions. It is a "small round blue cell tumour" and lacks malignant osteoid.
- Malignant fibrous histiocytoma of bone: a purely lytic sarcoma that is histologically identical to osteosarcoma except for the absence of malignant osteoid.
- Osteomyelitis: can be aggressive and lytic, but usually has more systemic signs of infection.

Management

Management is identical to conventional osteosarcoma and requires a multidisciplinary team at a specialist sarcoma centre.

- Neoadjuvant chemotherapy:
  - The standard first step. Uses multi-agent regimens (often including Doxorubicin, Cisplatin, and Methotrexate).
  - Goals: Treat micrometastases, shrink the primary tumour to facilitate surgery.
- Surgical resection:
  - Wide surgical excision: The tumour is removed with a margin of normal tissue to ensure complete removal.
  - Limb-salvage surgery is the goal in more than 90% of cases, using a metal endoprosthesis (a custom-made implant) or an allograft to reconstruct the defect.
  - Amputation: Required if the tumour involves critical neurovascular structures.
- Adjuvant chemotherapy:
  - Continues after surgery based on the tumour's response to neoadjuvant chemo (as seen on histologic analysis of the resected specimen).

Prognosis

- The prognosis for lytic osteosarcoma is generally similar to conventional osteosarcoma.
- The most important prognostic factor is the response to neoadjuvant chemotherapy. A good response (>90% tumour necrosis) correlates with better long-term survival.
- The presence of detectable metastases at diagnosis significantly worsens the prognosis.

Suggested Reading

Cè M, Cellina M, Ueanukul T, Carrafiello G, Manatrakul R, Tangkittithaworn P, Jaovisidha S, Fuangfa P, Resnick D. Multimodal imaging of osteosarcoma: from first diagnosis to radiomics. Cancers (Basel). 2025;17(4):599.

Crombé A, Simonetti M, Longhi A, Hauger O, Fadli D, Spinnato P. Imaging of osteosarcoma: presenting findings, metastatic patterns, and features related to prognosis. J Clin Med. 2024;13(19):5710.

The manufacturer's authorised representative in the EU is Springer
Nature Customer Service Centre GmbH, Europaplatz 3, 69115 Heidelberg,
Germany. If you have any concerns regarding our products, please
contact ProductSafety@springernature.com

Printed and bound by CPI Group (UK) Ltd, Croydon, CR0 4YY
16/10/2026
02234448-0001